The Nurses'
Handbook of

Intravenous
Medications

The Nurses'
Handbook of

J.B. LIPPINCOTT COMPANY
Philadelphia

New York   St. Louis
London   Sydney   Tokyo

Intravenous Medications

Sharon M. Weinstein

RN, CRNI, MS

Executive Director, Alternative Care Today

Vice Chairperson, Intravenous Nurses' Society, Certification
Corporation Executive Board

Formerly, Administrative Director, University Clinics, Chicago Medical
School, North Chicago, Illinois

Director of Nursing, VNA of Texas, Dallas, Texas

IV Therapy Coordinator, Southwest Texas Methodist Hospital,
San Antonio, Texas

Acquisitions Editor: Ellen Campbell
Project Editor: Grace R. Caputo
Indexer: Alexandra Weir Nickerson
Designer: Doug Smock
Production Manager: Helen Ewan
Production Coordinator: Kathryn Rule
Compositor: Circle Graphics
Printer/Binder: R.R. Donnelley & Sons Company

6   5   4   3   2   1

Library of Congress Cataloging-in-Publication Data

Weinstein, Sharon.
    The nurses' handbook of intravenous medications / Sharon M. Weinstein.
      p.   cm.
    Includes bibliographical references.
    ISBN 0-397-54765-X
    1. Intravenous therapy—Handbooks, manuals, etc.   2. Nursing—Handbooks, manuals, etc.   I. Title.
    [DNLM: 1. Infusions, Intravenous—handbooks.   2. Infusions, Intravenous—nurses' instruction.   3. Pharmacology—handbooks.   4. Pharmacology—nurses' instruction.   WB 39 W424n]
    RM170.W433   1991
615.8'55—dc20
DNLM/DLC
for Library of Congress   90-6684
                                                CIP

Any procedure or practice described in this book should be applied by the health-care practitioner under appropriate supervision in accordance with professional standards of care used with regard to the unique circumstances that apply in each practice situation. Care has been taken to confirm the accuracy of information presented and to describe generally accepted practices. However, the author, editors, and publisher cannot accept any responsibility for errors or omissions or for any consequences from application of the information in this book and make no warranty, express or implied, with respect to the contents of the book.

Every effort has been made to ensure drug selections and dosages are in accordance with current recommendations and practice. Because of ongoing research, changes in government regulations and the constant flow of information on drug therapy, reactions and interactions, the reader is cautioned to check the package insert for each drug for indications, dosages, warnings and precautions, particularly if the drug is new or infrequently used.

Reviewers

ANNE MARIE FREY, RN, CRNI, BSN
IV Nurse Clinician, St. Christopher's Hospital for Children, Philadelphia, Pennsylvania

CHRISTINE C. HEILIG, RPH
Pharmacist Consultant, O'Fallon, Illinois

SUSAN Y. PAULEY, RN, CRNI
Supervisor, IV Therapy, Massachusetts General Hospital, Boston, Massachusetts

BETH PERDUE, RN, MSN
Instructor, El Centro College, Brookhaven Campus, Dallas, Texas

Preface

The practice of infusion therapy has changed dramatically over the past few years; nowhere has this been more evident than in the clinical environment in which intravenous care is delivered. As nursing practice moves from the inpatient, acute care setting to the confines of a patient's home, it becomes increasingly important for all nurses, as clinical practitioners, to have a sound knowledge of intravenous drugs and solutions.

Because of the overwhelming number of new drugs on the market and advances in medical science and practice, nurses responsible for the delivery of intravenous therapy require more than ever before an accurate, complete, concise, and readily available reference tool as an adjunct to practice. *The Nurses' Handbook of Intravenous Medications* is that resource. This text provides both new and experienced clinicians with a reference based on the latest information available.

Each drug monograph is written in the following easy-to-use format:

Generic Name: in large type.
Trade Names: those most frequently used, divided into US and Canadian. A cross-reference of Canadian trade names can be found in Appendix 17.
Drug Classification: in smaller type.
pH: where available; listed in the lower righthand corner of the monograph; represents the pH of the undiluted drug after addition of manufacturer-supplied diluents or after initial reconstitution.
Action: a concise statement describing the drug's actions within the human body and the method of drug excretion.

Indications/Uses: the manufacturer's recommendations concerning use of each drug; investigational uses are indicated if known.

Usual Dose: the usual range for adult patients unless otherwise indicated. Specific dosing requirements relevant to disease entities are presented in detailed format. Where available, pediatric dosing information is provided.

Preparation/Reconstitution: specific, detailed information about dilution, preparation, and admixture. This is a significant responsibility of the nurse administering intravenous therapy, particularly in alternative care environments and critical care units.

Incompatibilities: listed by generic drug name. They are provided to alert the intravenous nursing clinician to the dangers inherent in a specific admixture. Order and method of mixing often influence a drug's compatibility and stability. In addition, product literature should be reviewed before administration of a specific drug or solution.

Rate/Mode of Administration: listed in easily read outline format: IV push, intermittent, continuous, filter. Definitions of these terms are listed on the inside of the back cover. It is thought that such a concise format enables the reader to determine quickly and accurately the appropriateness of a physician's written order. Filtration information ensures delivery of a particulate-free solution to the patient.

Nursing Considerations: broad category further broken down into the following subsections:

- Nursing Diagnoses: potential drug-related nursing diagnoses are provided to assist the clinician in developing a nursing care plan in any clinical setting. Nursing diagnoses provided are those most commonly used; others are possible.

- Acute Care: specific information relevant to clinical practice in the acute care setting.

- Precautions: drug-specific; provide all essential considerations before drug administration.

- Contraindications: those specifically provided by the drug's manufacturer; other contraindications may be patient specific, as determined by the physician.

- Side Effects: listed according to bodily systems; easily understood and recognized.
- Patient/Caregiver Teaching: consistent with the intended use of this book by nurses in all clinical environments, patient/caregiver teaching parameters are provided to simplify the teaching process.
- Home Care: the growth of the home infusion business necessitates attention to the relative safety of intravenous drug administration in the home setting.
- Administration in Other Clinical Settings: further information for the needs of the nurse with intravenous nursing responsibilities in the ambulatory or long-term care setting.
- Nursing Interventions: specific nursing actions to reverse undesirable side effects, along with emergency resuscitative information.

Appendices: comprehensive appendices address a wealth of subjects and provide specific information concerning such issues as drug monitoring, handling of cytotoxic waste, and extravasation of vesicant and irritant drugs.

The Nurses' Handbook of Intravenous Medications is designed for use by the nursing student, new practitioner, established nurse in a diversity of clinical environments from community health to acute care, and the intravenous team nursing clinical specialist. Complete and concise, the *Handbook* can facilitate the delivery of intravenous therapy in the clinical setting and can enhance the quality of care.

Sharon M. Weinstein, RN, CRNI, MS

Acknowledgments

The Nurses' Handbook of Intravenous Medications is the result of a great deal of work and the ongoing support and encouragement on the part of my husband, Steve, and my children, Heidi, Jason, and Marla. To each I extend my gratitude.

I also would like to acknowledge the excellent reviewers: Anne Marie Frey, Susan Pauley, Beth Perdue, and Chris Heilig.

Finally, a special thank you to Ellen Campbell and Nancy Mullins of J.B. Lippincott Company, whose assistance made the initial manuscript a publication of this quality; to Mary Larkin, Executive Director of The Intravenous Nurse's Society, Inc., for her guidance; and to Alick Torchinsky, Director of the Pharmacy Department, The Sir Mortimer B. Davis–Jewish General Hospital, for his assistance in the use of Canadian trade names.

Contents

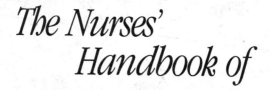

The Nurses'
Handbook of
Intravenous Medications

Acetazolamide sodium

US: Diamox
CAN: Acetazolam (ICN),
Apo-Acetazolamide (Apotex)

Sulfonamide   pH 9.2

ACTION

Depresses tubular reabsorption of sodium, potassium, and bicarbonate. Excreted unchanged in the urine, producing diuresis, alkalinization of urine, mild degree of metabolic acidosis.

INDICATIONS/USES

Used in the treatment of glaucoma, congestive heart failure, epilepsy, elevated intracranial pressure, drug-induced edema, drug overdosage (aspirin and phenobarbital). Used investigationally in the treatment of hypokalemia- or hyperkalemia-induced paralysis.

USUAL DOSE

5 mg/kg body wt over 24 h, or 250 mg to 1 g over 24 h. Give in
  divided doses over 250 mg.
Epilepsy. Dosage may range from 8–30 mg/kg body wt over 24-h
  period in divided doses.

PREPARATION/RECONSTITUTION

Reconstitute each 500 mg in 5 ml sterile water for injection for a concentration of 100 mg/ml.

INCOMPATIBILITIES

Specific information is not available.

RATE/MODE OF ADMINISTRATION

IV push: 500 mg or fraction thereof over 1–5 min (preferred).
Intermittent: Add dose to IV fluid to be given over 4–8 h.
Continuous: As above.
Filter: Applicable; use according to institutional guidelines.

1

NURSING CONSIDERATIONS
Nursing Diagnoses
1. Impaired sensorium, related to effect of medication.
2. Impaired electrolyte balance, related to diuresis.

Acute Care
Use with caution in respiratory acidosis. Hypokalemia may result from concurrent administration of steroids. Toxicity may occur with digitalis.

Precautions
Potentiates absorption of amphetamines, ephedrine, procainamide, quinidine. Inhibits absorption of primidone, salicylates, urinary antiinfectives, lithium, methotrexate, phenobarbital.

Contraindications
Not indicated for the patient with hypokalemia or hyponatremia; do not give to patients with sensitivity to sulfonamides or adrenocortical insufficiency. Do not give in first trimester of pregnancy.

Side Effects
Neurologic: Confusion, drowsiness, paresthesias.
Hematologic: Bone marrow depression, thrombocytopenic purpura, hemolytic anemia.
Other: Fever, rash, renal calculus.

Patient/Caregiver Teaching
Instruct patient (1) to report all side effects immediately and (2) to discontinue drug if necessary.

Home Care
May be safely administered in the home with careful blood level monitoring.

Administration in Other Clinical Settings
Appropriate in the outpatient environment.

Nursing Interventions

The physician should be notified of all side effects. Drug should be discontinued if necessary. Allergic reactions should be treated as indicated.

Acyclovir

US: Zovirax
CAN: Zovirax (B.W., Inc.)

Antiviral agent   pH 11

ACTION

Displays inhibitory action against the following viruses: herpes simplex, varicella zoster, Epstein-Barr, cytomegalovirus. Onset of action is prompt and therapeutic level is maintained for 8 h. Excreted in the urine.

INDICATIONS/USES

Used in the treatment of initial and recurrent mucosal and cutaneous herpes simplex infections in immunosuppressed adults and children.

USUAL DOSE

Adults: 5 mg/kg body wt every 8 h for 7 days. Reduce length of treatment to 5 days in presence of severe initial clinical episodes of herpes genitalis.
Children: 250 mg/m² every 8 h for 7 days.

PREPARATION/RECONSTITUTION

Reconstitute 500-mg vial with 10 ml sterile water for injection, producing 50 mg/ml. Use of bacteriostatic water containing parabens causes precipitation. Shake well to dissolve completely. Withdraw appropriate dose and further dilute in amount of solution to provide concentration less than 7 mg/ml (70-kg adult at 5 mg/kg equals 350 mg dissolved in 100 ml of solution, or 3.5 mg/ml).

INCOMPATIBILITIES
Compatible with most IV solutions.

RATE/MODE OF ADMINISTRATION
IV push: No.
Intermittent: Yes, a single dose must be administered at constant rate over 1 h; infusion pump recommended.
Continuous: No.
Filter: Applicable; use according to institutional guidelines.

NURSING CONSIDERATIONS
Nursing Diagnoses
1. Decreased urine output, related to too rapid infusion.
2. Impaired sensorium, related to effect of medication.
3. Decreased appetite, related to side effects of medication.

Acute Care
Rotate IV site and confirm patency of vein.

Precautions
Confirm diagnosis by culture. Use with caution in impaired renal function. Use with caution in patients with underlying neurologic abnormalities, in patients receiving intrathecal methotrexate or interferon, or those with previous neurologic reactions to anti-neoplastic drug agents.

Contraindications
Hypersensitivity to acyclovir.

Side Effects
Neurologic: Coma, agitation, confusion, hallucinations, headache, lethargy, seizures, tremors.
Circulatory: Hypotension, acute renal failure, phlebitis.
Gastrointestinal: Nausea, obtundation.

Patient/Caregiver Teaching
Instruct patient (1) to report all side effects immediately and (2) to maintain adequate hydration.

Home Care
Appropriate in home IV programs.

Administration in Other Clinical Settings
Not recommended.

Nursing Interventions
The physician should be notified of all side effects. Discontinue acyclovir therapy with onset of CNS side effects.

Alteplase, recombinant
US: Activase

Enzyme (Tissue Plasminogen Activator [tPA])   pH 7.3

ACTION
Binds to fibrin in a thrombus and converts plasminogen to plasmin. Cleared from plasma by liver within 5–10 min after infusion is complete. Some side effects may linger.

INDICATIONS/USES
Used in management of acute myocardial infarction to lyse thrombi obstructing coronary arteries.

USUAL DOSE
Adults: 100 mg over 3 h; give 6–10-mg bolus followed by 50–54 mg (total 60-mg dose) over the first hour. Follow with 20 mg/h for 2 h. Follow with 30 ml of normal saline or 5% dextrose in water by sideport to ensure administration of total dose.

Children: Calculate total dose using 1.25 mg/kg body wt for those under 65 kg. Give three fifths of this total calculated dose divided into a bolus and first-hour dose. Administer one fifth of this dose per hour for 2 h.

Geriatrics: Same as above.

PREPARATION/RECONSTITUTION

May be diluted with sterile water for injection without preservatives 1-mg/ml concentration. Use large-bore needle and direct stream of diluent into lyophilized cake. Do not use if vacuum is not present. Slight foaming is expected. Allow to stand for several minutes to dissolve large bubbles. May be further diluted to 0.5 mg/ml immediately prior to administration with equal volume of normal saline or 5% dextrose for injection. Avoid agitation of container during reconstitution.

INCOMPATIBILITIES

Manufacturer warns against adding to any other drugs or solutions.

RATE/MODE OF ADMINISTRATION

IV push: Initial bolus over 2 min.
Intermittent: No.
Continuous: Balance of initial dose over 1 h; succeeding doses over 1 h followed by final flush over 30 min. May be administered with microdrip set or electronic flow control device.
Filter: No.

NURSING CONSIDERATIONS

Nursing Diagnoses

1. Potential disturbance in bleeding mechanisms, related to drug side effects.
2. Potential impairment of skin integrity, related to drug side effects.

Acute Care

This drug is to be administered in the acute care setting only. Administer under direction of a licensed physician knowledgeable in the use of alteplase; have appropriate diagnostic and laboratory facilities readily available. Attain baseline parameters including ECG, CPK, PT, PTT, CBC, fibrinogen level, platelet count, and baseline physical assessment. Monitor ECG continuously and record strips with greatest ST segment elevation initially and every 15 min for 4 h.

Precautions

Reperfusion dysrhythmias occur frequently. Exercise bleeding precautions. Simultaneous therapy with continuous infusion of heparin (without a loading dose) is frequently ordered to reduce risk of rethrombosis. Use extreme caution in major surgery, trauma, GU or GI bleeding, puncture of noncompressible vessels within previous 10 days, cerebrovascular disease, hypertension, subacute bacterial endocarditis, coagulation disorders, liver dysfunction, pregnancy and first 20 days postpartum, septic thrombophlebitis, patients over age 75.

Contraindications

Active internal bleeding, bleeding diathesis, cerebral vascular accident within 2 mo, intracranial neoplasm, uncontrolled hypertension, arteriovenous malformation, or aneurysm.

Side Effects

Hematologic: Bleeding.
Gastrointestinal: Nausea, vomiting.
Circulatory: Hypotension, fever.
Dermatologic: Urticaria.

Patient/Caregiver Teaching

Instruct patient (1) to avoid use of sharp instruments, including razors and other devices; (2) to report all episodes of bleeding; (3) to control minor bleeding by local pressure; and (4) to expect oozing at IV sites.

Home Care

Not recommended.

Administration in Other Clinical Settings

Not recommended.

Nursing Interventions

The physician should be notified of all side effects. For severe bleeding in a critical site, discontinue alteplase and heparin therapy immediately. Prepare to administer whole blood, packed RBC, cryoprecipitate, fresh frozen plasma, or aminocaproic acid. Resuscitate as necessary.

Amikacin sulfate

US: Amikin
CAN: Amikin (Bristol)

Aminoglycoside antibiotic   pH 4.5

ACTION

Amikacin sulfate has neuromuscular blocking action and is bactericidal against many gram-negative organisms resistant to other antibiotics, including aminoglycosides such as gentamicin, kanamycin, tobramycin. Well distributed through all body fluids, its usual half-life is 2–3 h. Crosses the placental barrier. Excreted in the kidneys.

INDICATIONS/USES

Used in short-term treatment of serious infections caused by susceptible organisms resistant to alternative drugs IV with less potential toxicity.

USUAL DOSE

Adults: Up to 15 mg/kg body wt over 24 h in 2–3 equal divided doses. Dosage is based on ideal weight of lean body mass. Not to exceed total adult dose of 15 mg/kg/24 h in average-weight patient or 1.5 g in heavier patients by all routes in 24 h.

Neonates: 10 mg/kg body wt as loading dose; then 7.5 mg/kg every 24 h. Lower doses may be appropriate in immature kidney function.

PREPARATION/RECONSTITUTION

Reconstitute each 500 mg or fraction thereof with 100–200 ml IV 5% dextrose in water, 5% dextrose in normal saline, or 0.9% normal saline solution. Decrease diluent proportionately with children and infants.

INCOMPATIBILITIES

Follow manufacturer's recommendations for separate administration. Inactivated by carbenicillin, ticarcillin, other penicillins. Do not administer with amphotericin B, cephalothin, chlorothiazide, heparin sodium, phenytoin, thiopental, vitamin B complex with C.

RATE/MODE OF ADMINISTRATION

Single dose over 30–60 min; administer to infants as a 1–2-h infusion.

NURSING CONSIDERATIONS

Nursing Diagnoses

1. Possible impaired renal function, related to drug side effects.
2. Impaired sensory-perceptual alteration: olfactory, related to drug toxicity.
3. Alteration in patterns of urinary elimination, related to drug side effects.

Acute Care

Monitor serum peak and trough levels to avoid peak serum concentrations above 35 μg/ml and trough concentrations above 10 μg/ml. Therapeutic level is 8–15 μg/ml. All aminoglycosides are potentiated by anticholinesterases, antineoplastics, barbiturates, muscle relaxants, phenothiazines.

Precautions

Use with extreme caution if therapy is indicated over 7–10 days. Reduce daily dose commensurate with degree of renal impairment. Maintain adequate hydration. Do not administer concurrently with any ototoxic or nephrotoxic agents. Superinfection may occur from overgrowth of nonsusceptible organisms.

Contraindications

Known amikacin or aminoglycoside sensitivity.

Side Effects

Circulatory: Fever, headache, hypotension, respiratory arrest.
Neurologic: Paresthesias, tremors, ototoxicity, arthralgia, neuromuscular blockade.
Dermatologic: Skin rash.
Hematologic: Anemia.

Patient/Caregiver Teaching

Instruct patient (1) to report any known side effects; (2) to discontinue drug and notify physician if side effects persist; and (3) to report other medications and therapies to physician.

Home Care

Appropriate for short-term use in home IV programs.

Administration in Other Clinical Settings

Appropriate as indicated.

Antidote

Exchange transfusion in the newborn. Calcium salts or neostigmine may reverse neuromuscular blockade. Resuscitate as necessary.

Aminocaproic acid

US: Amicar
CAN: Amicar (Lederle)

Plasma activation inhibitor   pH 6.0–7.6

ACTION

A monoaminocarboxylic acid that inhibits plasminogen activator substances. Increases fibrinogen activity in clot formation by inhibiting the enzyme required for destruction of formed fibrin. Readily excreted in the urine. Prompt onset of action that lasts up to 3 h.

INDICATIONS/USES

Used in hemorrhage caused by overactivity of the fibrinolytic system; systemic hyperfibrinolysis, which may result from heart surgery, hepatic cirrhosis, aplastic anemia, or carcinoma of the prostate, lung, stomach, and cervix; urinary fibrinolysis resulting from severe trauma, anoxia, shock, surgery on the genitourinary system, or carcinoma of the genitourinary system. Used investigationally to prevent recurrence of subarachnoid hemorrhage and to reduce need for platelet transfusion in management of amegakaryocytic thrombocytopenia.

USUAL DOSE

Adults: Initial dose 4–5 g. Follow with 1–1.25 g/h or at hourly intervals for 6–8 h. To achieve and maintain plasma levels at 0.13 mg/ml, maximum dose is 30 g/24 h.

- Prevention of recurrent subarachnoid hemorrhage: 36 g/24 h in 6 divided doses.
- Reduction of need for platelet transfusion in amegakaryocytic thrombocytopenia: 8–24 g/24 h for 3 days–13 mo.

Children: Initial doses of 100 mg/kg or 3 g/m² during first hour, followed by continuous infusion of 33.3 mg/kg/h or 1 g/m² h. Total dosage should not exceed 18 g/m² in 24 h.

Geriatrics: Same as for adults.

PREPARATION/RECONSTITUTION

1 g equals 4 ml of prepared solution. Further dilute with 0.9% saline solution, 5% dextrose in 0.9% saline solution, Ringer's solution, or distilled water: 50 ml of diluent to 1 g.

INCOMPATIBILITIES

Sodium lactate.

RATE/MODE OF ADMINISTRATION

IV push: No.

Intermittent: 5 g or fraction thereof over first hour in 250 ml of solution, then each succeeding 1 g over 1 h in 50–100 ml of solution.

Continuous: Yes, as above for 6–8 h or until bleeding is controlled.

Filter: Applicable; use according to institutional guidelines.

NURSING CONSIDERATIONS

Nursing Diagnoses

1. Possible alteration in bowel elimination: diarrhea, related to drug side effects.
2. Possible sensory-perceptual alteration: visual and olfactory, related to drug side effects.
3. Possible alteration in tissue perfusion, related to too rapid administration of drug.

Acute Care

Rapid administration may cause hypotension, bradycardia, or dysrhythmia. Monitor the patient carefully.

Precautions

Should be used in conjunction with general and specific tests to determine the degree of fibrinolysis present. Whole blood transfusions may be needed. Avoid large doses in the presence of anticoagulants to prevent induction of coagulability.

Contraindications

Disseminated intravascular coagulation, evidence of thrombosis, first and second trimester of pregnancy.

Side Effects

Gastrointestinal: Cramps, diarrhea, nausea.
Neurologic: Tinnitus, dizziness, headache, grand mal seizure.
Circulatory: Malaise, thrombophlebitis, tearing.
Dermatologic: Skin rash.

Patient/Caregiver Teaching

Instruct patient to report all side effects immediately.

Home Care

Not recommended.

Administration in Other Clinical Settings

Not recommended.

Nursing Interventions

The physician should be advised immediately of all side effects. Treat symptomatically. Discontinue use of drug if thrombophlebitis is suspected.

Ammonium chloride

Acidifying agent   pH 4.5–6.0

ACTION
Ammonium chloride is an acidifying agent.

INDICATIONS/USES
Used in treatment of metabolic alkalosis due to chloride loss from vomiting, gastric fistula drainage, gastric suction, or excessive alkalinizing medication to prevent tetany.

USUAL DOSE
In absence of edema or hyponatremia, estimated total dose in mEq of chloride ion is equal to 20% of body weight in kilograms times serum chloride deficit in mEq/L. Administer with caution; give half the calculated dose and redetermine pH. Maximum effect of a dose is not complete for several days. A 26.75% solution contains 5 mEq/ml ammonium and 5 mEq/ml chloride.

PREPARATION/RECONSTITUTION
Dilute 26.75% solution in 500–1000 ml 0.9% sodium chloride for infusion at a ratio of 10 ml for each ml of ammonium chloride. Potassium chloride, 20–40 mEq/L, may be added to the ammonium infusion.

INCOMPATIBILITIES
Chlortetracycline, codeine, dimenhydrinate, levorphanol, methadone hydrochloride, warfarin, all alkalis.

RATE/MODE OF ADMINISTRATION
IV push: No.
Intermittent: No.
Continuous: Infuse at a rate not exceeding 5 ml/min for adults; reduce rate for infants.
Filter: Applicable; use according to institutional guidelines.

NURSING CONSIDERATIONS

Nursing Diagnoses

1. Possible impaired gas exchange, related to side effects.
2. Alteration in cardiac output: decreased, related to drug side effects.

Acute Care

Obtain blood chemistry baseline prior to administration and after therapy to avoid serious metabolic acidosis and other electrolyte disturbances. Sodium and potassium replacement may be needed. Slow infusion rate for pain along the venipuncture site. If crystals form, warm in warm water to room temperature prior to administration.

Precautions

Observe respirations closely for evidence of acidosis. Record intake and output. Use caution in impaired renal function, pulmonary insufficiency, or cardiac edema.

Contraindications

Sodium loss resulting in excretion of sodium bicarbonate in the urine of a patient with renal dysfunction; primary respiratory acidosis with high total carbon dioxide and buffer base; marked hepatic impairment.

Side Effects

Circulatory: Bradycardia, hypokalemia, hyperglycemia, metabolic acidosis, pallor.
Neurologic: EEG abnormalities, excitability, headache, stupor, twitching, weakness, depression, disorientation, calcium-deficient tetany.
Gastrointestinal: Vomiting, nausea.
Respiratory: Irregular Kussmaul respirations.

Patient/Caregiver Teaching

Instruct patient (1) to report all side effects and (2) to discontinue drug and notify the physician.

Home Care

Generally not administered in the home environment.

Administration in Other Clinical Settings
Not recommended.

Nursing Interventions
Reduce rate of administration or discontinue drug and notify physician of all side effects. Treat hypokalemia with potassium and tetany with calcium. Acidosis may be treated with sodium lactate, $^{1}/_{6}$ molar sodium lactate, or sodium bicarbonate IV.

Amobarbital sodium
US: Amytal Sodium

Hypnotic barbiturate   pH 9.6–10.4

ACTION
Amobarbital is a CNS depressant, sedative, and hypnotic barbiturate with anticonvulsant effects. Onset of action is rapid and duration is 4–6 h. Rapidly absorbed by all body tissues and excreted quickly in changed form in the urine. Crosses placental barrier and is secreted in breast milk.

INDICATIONS/USES
Used to control convulsive seizures due to eclampsia, psychiatric abnormality, and drug poisoning. Used as a sedative hypnotic, for narcoanalysis and narcotherapy.

USUAL DOSE
Adults: 65–500 mg (1–7.5 gr); 1 g (15 gr) is maximum single dose.
Children over 6 yr: 65–250 mg (1–3.75 gr); 500 mg (7.5 gr) is maximum dose.

PREPARATION/RECONSTITUTION
Reconstitute each 125 mg (2 gr) in 1.25 ml of sterile water for injection to create a 10% solution for a final concentration of 100 mg/ml. Inject diluent slowly and rotate dial to dissolve. Do not shake.

INCOMPATIBILITIES

Cefazolin, cephalothin, chlorpromazine, cimetidine, clindamycin, codeine, dimenhydrinate, diphenhydramine, hydrocortisone sodium succinate, hydroxyzine, levarterenol, levorphanol, meperidine, methadone, morphine, oxytetracycline, penicillin G, pentazocine, penicilling potassium, phytonadione, procaine, prochlorperazine, streptomycin, tetracycline, thiamine, trifluoperazine, vancomycin.

RATE/MODE OF ADMINISTRATION

IV push: Administer each 100 mg or fraction thereof over 1 min for adults and 60 mg/min for children. Titrate slowly to desired effect. Not to exceed 1 ml/min of a 10% solution.
Intermittent: No.
Continuous: No.
Filter: Inappropriate for doses less than 0.5 ml.

NURSING CONSIDERATIONS

Nursing Diagnoses

1. Possible impaired tissue perfusion, related to drug side effects.
2. Possible ineffective thermoregulation, related to drug side effects.
3. Possible ineffective breathing pattern, related to drug side effects.

Acute Care

IV route is for emergency use only. Use large veins to avoid thrombosis. Intraarterial injection results in gangrene. Use only adequate medication to achieve desired results. Keep emergency resuscitative equipment available. Inhibits corticosteroids, doxycycline, oral anticoagulants, theophylline and β-adrenergic blockers.

Precautions

Hydrolyzes in dry or solution form when exposed to air. Use only clear solutions. Record blood pressure, pulse, and respiration every 3–5 min. Patient must be constantly observed. Maintain a patent airway. Use with caution in asthma, cardiovascular diseases, hypertension or hypotension, pulmonary diseases, depressive states after convulsions, shock, trauma, and in the elderly. May cause birth defects. May interact with many drugs.

Contraindications

Impaired liver function, known hypersensitivity, severe respiratory depression, history of porphyria.

Side Effects

Respiratory: Asthma, bronchospasm, neonatal apnea, respiratory depression.
Circulatory: Facial edema, fever, hypotension.
Neurologic: Depression.
Dermatologic: Dermatitis.
Overdose: Apnea, coma, cough reflex depression, flat EEG, pulmonary edema, renal shutdown, respiratory depression.

Patient/Caregiver Teaching

Instruct patient to report all side effects immediately, no matter how slight.

Home Care

Not recommended.

Administration in Other Clinical Settings

Not recommended.

Antidote

The physician must be immediately notified of any side effects. Maintain adequate airway with artificial ventilation if indicated. IV volume expanders and other fluids may be administered. Osmotic diuretics or hemodialysis promotes elimination of drug. Vasopressors maintain blood pressure.

Amphotericin B

US: Fungizone
CAN: Fungizone (Squibb)

Antifungal antibiotic   pH 5.7

ACTION

Injures membrane of the fungi. Remains in the body at a therapeutic level up to 20 h after infusion and is excreted slowly in the urine.

INDICATIONS/USES

Used in treatment of systemic fungal infections that are progressive in nature and may be fatal, such as cryptococcosis, blastomycosis, moniliasis, coccidioidomycosis, histoplasmosis, mucomycosis, sporotrichosis, aspergillosis. Establish diagnosis by culture of histologic study.

USUAL DOSE

Test: 1 mg in 20 ml 5% dextrose given over 10–30 min.
Usual: 0.25 mg/kg body wt/24 h, gradually increased to 1 mg/kg/24 h as tolerated. Up to 1.5 mg/kg/24 h may be given on alternate-day therapy. Dosage must be adjusted for each patient.

PREPARATION/RECONSTITUTION

Reconstitute a 50-mg vial with 10 ml of distilled water for injection without bacteriostatic agent for a final concentration of 5 mg/ml. Shake well until clear. Further dilute each 1 mg in 10 ml of 5% dextrose in water for injection with a pH above 4.2. Do not use any other diluent. Do not wipe vials with alcohol sponges. Use a 20-gauge or larger sterile needle, maintaining asepsis.

INCOMPATIBILITIES

Do not mix with any other drug unless absolutely necessary. Incompatibilities include amikacin, benzyl alcohol preservatives, calcium chloride, calcium gluconate, carbenicillin, chlorpromazine, chlortetracycline, cimetidine, diphenhydramine, dopamine, electrolyte solutions, gentamicin, heparin sodium, kanamycin, penicillin G potassium or sodium, potassium chloride, saline solutions, tetracycline.

RATE/MODE OF ADMINISTRATION

IV push: No.
Intermittent: Yes, as indicated.
Continuous: Yes, by slow infusion over 6 h at concentration of 0.1 mg/ml.
Filter: To 1-μ range.

NURSING CONSIDERATIONS

Nursing Diagnoses

1. Possible ineffective thermoregulation, related to drug side effects.
2. Possible alteration in tissue perfusion, related to drug toxicities.

Acute Care

Use only fresh solutions without evidence of foreign matter. Light sensitive; should be protected from light if solution will be exposed more than 8 h. Monitor vital signs and intake and output. A small amount of heparin sodium added to the infusion may minimize incidence of thrombophlebitis. May potentiate digitalis and skeletal muscle relaxants.

Precautions

Potentiates antifungal effects of other antibiotics. Monitor renal and liver function tests, blood counts, and electrolyte panels during therapy. If not given for a period of 7 days, restart treatment at lowest dosage level. Hydrocortisone 0.7 mg/kg body wt added to the infusate may prevent chills.

Contraindications

Known sensitivity; pregnancy.

Side Effects

Neurologic: Convulsions, headache.
Circulatory: Fever, cardiac disturbances, hypo- or hypertension, hypokalemia, phlebitis.
Gastrointestinal: Anorexia, diarrhea, vomiting.
Hematologic: Anemia, coagulation defects.

Patient/Caregiver Teaching

Instruct patient (1) to report any evidence of side effects and (2) to be aware that some symptoms may reverse after treatment ends.

Home Care

Although administration generally is limited to the acute care setting, many companies providing IV care at home offer this type of treatment.

Administration in Other Clinical Settings

May be administered in a closely monitored outpatient setting.

Nursing Interventions

Notify physician of all side effects. Urinary alkalizers may minimize renal tubular acidosis. Reduce dose if BUN exceeds 40 mg/200 ml or serum creatinine level exceeds 3 mg/100 ml.

Ampicillin sodium

US: Omnipen-N, Polycillin N, Totacillin-N
CAN: Ampicin (Bristol), Ampilean (Organon)

Semisynthetic penicillin   pH 8.5–10.0

ACTION

Ampicillin sodium is bactericidal against many gram-positive and some gram-negative organisms. Crosses the placental barrier and is excreted in the urine and secreted in breast milk.

INDICATIONS/USES

A highly effective agent against severe infections caused by gram-positive and gram-negative organisms, except penicillinase-producing staphylococci.

USUAL DOSE

Adults: 1–12 g/24 h in equally divided doses every 6 h.
- Severe renal impairment: Increase interval to 12 h.

Children: 50–200 mg/kg body wt/24 h in equally divided doses at 6–8-h intervals.

Neonates
- Over 2 kg and up to 7 days: 75 mg/kg body wt in divided doses every 8 h; 150 mg/kg/24 h for meningitis.
- Over 2 kg and over 7 days: 100 mg/kg/24 h in divided doses every 6 h; 200 mg/kg/24 h for meningitis.
- Under 2 kg and up to 7 days: 50 mg/kg/24 h in divided doses every 12 h; 100 mg/kg/24 h for meningitis.
- Under 2 kg and under 7 days: 75 mg/kg/24 h in divided doses every 8 h; 150 mg/kg/24 h for meningitis.

PREPARATION/RECONSTITUTION

Reconstitute every 500 mg or fraction thereof with 5 ml of sterile water for injection. May further dilute in 50 ml or more of one of the following and administer intermittently over not more than 4 h: 5% dextrose in water, 5% dextrose in 0.45% sodium chloride solution, 10% invert sugar in water, or ⅙ molar sodium lactate solution. *Note: When admixed in isotonic sodium chloride, stability is maintained over 8 h. May be added to the final 100 ml of a compatible IV solution after initial preparation/reconstitution.*

INCOMPATIBILITIES

Incompatible with all other drugs and solutions other than those listed.

RATE/MODE OF ADMINISTRATION

IV push: As a single dose over 10–15 min.
Intermittent: In 100 ml or more of solution per schedule described.
Continuous: Not to exceed 4 h as described.
Filter: Applicable; use according to institutional guidelines.

NURSING CONSIDERATIONS

Nursing Diagnoses

1. Potential sensory-perceptual alteration, related to drug side effects.

2. Potential for infection, related to potential for overgrowth of susceptible organisms.

Acute Care

Watch for early signs of allergic reaction. Use within 1 h of reconstitution unless diluted in solutions indicated. Monitor SGOT for possible increase. Monitor renal, hepatic, and hematopoietic functions during prolonged treatment. If used concurrently with aminoglycosides, administer in separate infusions to avoid aminoglycoside inactivation. May create false-positive glucose reaction with Clinitest and Benedict's or Fehling's solution.

Precautions

Inactivated by chloramphenicol, erythromycin, and tetracyclines. May potentiate action of heparin sodium. Neuromuscular excitability or convulsions may be caused by excessive dosing. Drug elimination rate is reduced in neonates. Sensitivity studies are indicated prior to use of this drug. Rapid administration may cause seizures.

Contraindications

Known penicillin or cephalothin sensitivity.

Side Effects

Dermatologic: Dermatitis, rashes, urticaria.
Hematologic: Anemia, leukopenia, thrombocytopenia.
Circulatory: Anaphylaxis.

Patient/Caregiver Teaching

Instruct patient to report any side effects immediately.

Home Care

Appropriate if consideration is given to stability guidelines.

Administration in Other Clinical Settings

Appopriate if consideration is given to stability guidelines.

Nursing Interventions

The physician should be notified of all side effects. Severe symptoms require discontinuing the drug; allergy manifestations and resuscitation are treated as necessary. Overdose may be effectively treated with hemodialysis or peritoneal dialysis.

Ampicillin sodium and sulbactam sodium

US: Unasyn

Antibacterial antibiotic   pH 7

ACTION

A broad-spectrum, semisynthetic penicillin that improves ampicillin's bactericidal activity against β-lactamase–producing strains resistant to penicillins and cephalosporins. Crosses the placental barrier and is excreted in the urine and secreted in breast milk.

INDICATIONS/USES

Used in the treatment of skin and skin structure, intraabdominal, and gynecologic infections due to susceptible strains of indicated organisms.

USUAL DOSE

Adults: 1.5 g (1 g ampicillin plus 0.5 g sulbactam) to 3 g (2 g ampicillin plus 1 g sulbactam) every 6 h not to exceed 4 g sulbactam/24 h.

Children: Safety for use in infants and children has not been established.

PREPARATION/RECONSTITUTION

Reconstitute each initial 1.5 g with 4 ml of sterile water for injection (375 mg/ml). Further dilute in 50 ml or more of one of the following solutions: 5% dextrose in water, 5% dextrose in 0.45 sodium chloride solution, 10% invert sugar in water, lactated Ringer's injection,

$1/6$ molar sodium lactate, or isotonic sodium chloride to a concentration of 3–45 mg/ml.

INCOMPATIBILITIES

Do not mix with any other drug or solution; may be administered sideport through an ongoing infusion if solution is compatible.

RATE/MODE OF ADMINISTRATION

IV push: Slow, single dose over 10–15 min.
Intermittent: In 50–100 ml of diluent, over 15–30 min.
Continuous: No.
Filter: Applicable; refer to institutional guidelines.

NURSING CONSIDERATIONS

Nursing Diagnoses

1. Potential for vascular injury, related to burning, discomfort, and pain at injection site.
2. Potential alteration in bowel elimination: diarrhea, related to side effects of medication.

Acute Care

Obtain patient history of drug sensitivity to penicillins. Monitor patient for signs of untoward reaction. Do not exceed stability parameters for drug to ensure safety and efficacy of solution. Monitor for development of thrombophlebitis at infusion site; rotate sites per institutional guidelines and national standards. Monitor SGOT levels.

Precautions

Avoid prolonged use of ampicillin sodium and sulbactam sodium to prevent superinfection caused by overgrowth of nonsusceptible organisms. Concurrent use of β-adrenergic blockers may increase risk of anaphylaxis. May potentiate action of heparin sodium. False-positive glucose reaction with Clinitest or Benedict's or Fehling's solution may occur. Too rapid administration may result in development of seizures.

Contraindications

Known sensitivity to penicillin or cephalothin.

Side Effects

Dermatologic: Rash, itching, mucosal bleeding.

Hematologic: Decreased hemoglobin, hematocrit, RBC, WBC, neutrophils, platelets, serum albumin, total protein; increased alkaline phosphatase, BUN, creatinine, LDH, SGOT, SGPT, basophils, eosinophils, monocytes. *Caution: Lymphocyte and platelet counts may either increase or decrease significantly.*

Gastrointestinal: Nausea, vomiting, glossitis, diarrhea, abdominal distention, flatulence.

Urologic: RBC and hyaline casts in urine.

EENT: Facial swelling, epistaxis.

Circulatory: Thrombophlebitis at injection site with pain, discomfort, and burning.

Neurologic: Headache, fatigue.

Patient/Caregiver Teaching

Instruct patient (1) to report any side effects immediately; (2) to report incidence of pain or burning at injection site immediately; and (3) to ensure adequate fluid intake.

Home Care

Not recommended, unless patient/caregiver can be taught to mix fresh solution; check manufacturer's recommendation.

Administration in Other Clinical Settings

Appropriate if parameters can be monitored.

Nursing Interventions

The physician should be notified of any side effects immediately. Severe symptoms may require discontinuing the drug and initiating appropriate treatment with antihistamines, epinephrine, and corticosteroids. Resuscitate as necessary. Overdose may be treated with hemodialysis or peritoneal dialysis.

Amrinone lactate

US: Inocor

Inotropic agent   pH 3.2—4.0

___

ACTION

An inotropic and vasodilator that reduces afterload and preload by direct relaxation of vascular smooth muscle. Increases cardiac output without measurable increase in myocardial oxygen consumption or changes in arteriovenous oxygen difference. Decreases pulmonary capillary wedge pressure, total peripheral resistance, diastolic blood pressure and mean arterial pressure. Amrinone lactate is metabolized by conjugated pathways and excreted in the urine.

INDICATIONS/USES

Used in the short-term management of congestive heart failure in those who have been unresponsive to conventional therapies including digitalis, diuretics, or vasodilators.

USUAL DOSE

Initial: 0.75 mg/kg body wt (52.5 mg [10.5 ml] for a 70-kg adult); may repeat in 30 min.

Maintenance: 5–10 µg/kg/min (350–700 µg/min for a 70-kg adult); not to exceed total dose of 10 mg/kg/24 h, including boluses.

PREPARATION/RECONSTITUTION

May be administered undiluted, or each 5 mg (1 ml) may be diluted to a concentration of 1–3 mg/ml in 1 ml 0.9% saline solution or 0.45% saline for injection. To infuse, dilute 250 mg (50 ml) in 50 ml 0.95% saline solution or 0.45% saline solution (2.5 mg/ml); 1 ml is equal to 2500 µg/min.

INCOMPATIBILITIES

Solutions containing dextrose in direct preparation/reconstitution and furosemide.

RATE/MODE OF ADMINISTRATION

IV push: Yes, over 2–3 min.

Intermittent: Microdrip administration set recommended.

Continuous: Follow manufacturer's recommendations for use by electronic infusion device titrated to patient's condition.

Filter: Applicable; use according to institutional guidelines.

NURSING CONSIDERATIONS

Nursing Diagnoses

1. Potential alteration in cardiac output, related to drug toxicities.
2. Potential fluid volume deficit, related to insufficient cardiac filling pressure.

Acute Care

Monitor ECG, cardiac index, pulmonary capillary wedge pressure, and central venous pressure continuously. Monitor plasma concentration, blood pressure, urine output, and body weight. Observe patient for development of orthopnea, dyspnea, fatigue.

Precautions

Use with caution in renal or hepatic dysfunction. May increase ventricular response in atrial flutter/fibrillation and required pretreatment with digitalis. Additional fluids and electrolytes may be required. Not recommended for use in acute phase of myocardial infarction due to lack of clinical trials at this time. Safety for use during pregnancy and lactation and in children not yet established. May be used in pregnancy only if potential benefit justifies potential risk.

Contraindications

Hypersensitivity to amrinone or bisulfites; severe aortic or pulmonic valvular disease in lieu of surgical correction of the obstruction.

Side Effects

Gastrointestinal: Abdominal pain, anorexia, nausea, vomiting.

Circulatory/respiratory: Chest pain, dysrhythmias, hypotension, pericarditis, vasculitis with nodular pulmonary densities, hypoxemia, jaundice.

Other: Pain and burning at injection site.

Patient/Caregiver Teaching
Instruct patient to report all side effects immediately.

Home Care
Not recommended.

Administration in Other Clinical Settings
Not recommended.

Nursing Interventions
The physician should be notified of all side effects. Dose may remain constant, be decreased, or be discontinued consistent with intensity of side effects. At first sign of marked hypotension, reduce rate or discontinue drug and notify physician. Vasopressors may be required; resuscitate as necessary.

Antihemophilic factor (human)

US: Hemofil T, HT Factorate, HT Factorate Generation II, Kryobulin VH (Immuno)

Coagulation factor VIII

ACTION
A lyophilized or dried concentrate of coagulation factor VIII (antihemophilic factor or AHF) obtained from fresh human plasma (less than 3 h old) and prepared, irradiated, and dried.

INDICATIONS/USES
Used in the treatment of congenital deficiency of factor VIII or to control unexpected hemorrhagic episodes during emergency or elective surgery; used prophylactically to maintain status of known hemophilic patients.

USUAL DOSE

Prophylaxis of spontaneous hemorrhage: 10 AHF IU/kg body wt to increase by 20%; minimum of 30% of normal is indicated.

Moderate hemorrhage/minor surgery: 15–25 AHF IU/kg to increase by 30%–50% of normal. Maintain with 10–15 AHF IU/kg every 8–12 h.

Severe hemorrhage: 40–50 AHF IU/kg to increase to 80%–100% of normal. Maintain with 20–25 AHF IU/kg every 8–12 h.

Major surgery: Adequate dose to increase to 80%–100% of normal administered 1 h before surgery. Confirm with AHF level assays just before surgery. Administer a second dose of half the first dose in 5 h and maintain at 30% of normal for 10–14 days.

PREPARATION/RECONSTITUTION

Follow manufacturer's recommendations on package insert, using only the provided diluent.

INCOMPATIBILITIES

Do not mix with other drugs; sufficient information is unavailable.

RATE/MODE OF ADMINISTRATION

IV push: 10–20 ml over 3 min if less than 34 AHF IU/ml; greater concentrations require administration at rate of 2 ml/min.
Intermittent: No.
Continuous: No.
Filter: No.

NURSING CONSIDERATIONS

Nursing Diagnoses

1. Potential for infection, related to transmission of blood-borne diseases.
2. Potential alteration in tissue perfusion, related to side effects of drug.

Acute Care

Maintain strict aseptic technique in preparation of this agent; use of a plastic syringe prevents binding of drug to glass surfaces. Reduce rate of infusion if a significant increase in pulse rate is evident. Identify baseline deficiency with level assays before administration and during treatment. Must be refrigerated and given within 3 h of reconstitution. Monitor patient for development of signs of dissemi-nated intravascular coagulation (DIC) including blood pressure and pulse rate changes, respiratory discomfort, chest pain, prolonged clotting tests, sudden cough.

Precautions

May transmit AIDS and hepatitis. Intravascular hemolysis may occur when large volumes are administered to individuals with blood groups A, B, and AB. Type-specific cryoprecipitate may be used to maintain adequate factor VIII levels.

Contraindications

None when used as listed. Ineffective in bleeding episodes caused by von Willebrand's disease.

Side Effects

Dermatologic: Hives, erythema.
Hematologic/immunologic: Acute hemolytic anemia, increased bleed-ing tendencies, and hyperfibrinogenemia may follow massive dose; AIDS; hepatitis.
Other: Backache, fever.

Patient/Caregiver Teaching

Instruct patient of the risks and benefits associated with administra-tion of factor VIII and of the likelihood of transmission of blood-borne diseases.

Home Care

Appropriate.

Administration in Other Clinical Settings

Appropriate.

Nursing Interventions

The physician should be notified of all side effects. Discontinue drug; may be resumed later at a decreased rate or replaced with an alternative product. Treat anaphylaxis accordingly.

Antivenin (*Crotalidae*) polyvalent

US: North and South American Anti–Snake-Bite Serum

Snake bite neutralizer

ACTION
Neutralizes the venom of rattlesnakes, copperheads, and cottonmouth moccasins; refer to package insert for additional information.

INDICATIONS/USES
Used in the emergency treatment of patients with symptoms of envenomation sustained as a result of a bite of a rattlesnake, copperhead, cottonmouth moccasin, or pit viper species of snake.

USUAL DOSE
Usual: Consistent with degree of envenomation:
- None: No dose needed.
- Minimal: 2–4 vials.
- Moderate: 5–9 vials.
- Severe: 10–15 vials.

Additional: Further antivenin use is based on patient's clinical response and progression of symptoms. A maximum of 1–5 additional vials may be administered. Most effective within 4 h of the bite; less effective after 8 h. In presence of envenomation, should be given even after 24 h.

Children: Not weight based; see above.

PREPARATION/RECONSTITUTION
Reconstitute each vial with diluent provided (10 ml sterile water for injection). Must be further diluted with 0.9% sodium chloride or 5% dextrose in water to a 1:1–1:10 solution. Gentle swirling of solution will prevent foaming.

INCOMPATIBILITIES

Do not mix with any other drug or solution; sufficient information is not yet available.

RATE/MODE OF ADMINISTRATION

IV push: 5–10 ml over 3–5 min; remaining initial dose at maximum rate of administration.
Continuous: No.
Filter: No.

NURSING CONSIDERATIONS

Nursing Diagnoses

1. Potential alteration in cardiac output, related to drug side effects.
2. Potential impairment of skin integrity, related to skin testing technique.

Acute Care

Evaluate status of each patient individually; determine history of previous allergic-type reactions. Sensitivity testing is mandatory prior to administration, beginning with conjunctival test and proceeding to scratch test and skin test; refer to manufacturer's recommendations for use and administration of testing. Monitor all vital signs frequently. Baseline CBC, hematocrit, platelet count, PT, clot retraction, bleeding and coagulation times, BUN, electrolytes, and bilirubin should be established.

Precautions

Familiarize yourself with manufacturer's product literature prior to use of antivenin. Obtain blood type and crossmatch prior to administration. Patient requires two IV lines, one for supportive therapy and the other for antivenin and electrolyte therapy. Emergency resuscitative equipment should be readily available.

Contraindications

Hypersensitivity to horse serum unless it is the only treatment available.

Side Effects

Dermatologic: Urticaria, local pain, local erythema.
Circulatory/respiratory: Respiratory distress, vascular collapse, anaphylaxis.

Patient/Caregiver Teaching
Instruct patient to report all side effects immediately.

Home Care
Not recommended.

Administration in Other Clinical Settings
Not recommended.

Nursing Interventions
The physician should be notified of all side effects. Discontinue drug and treat anaphylaxis immediately. Resuscitate as necessary.

Antivenin (*Latrodectus mactans*)

US: Black Widow Spider Antivenin

Snake bite neutralizer

ACTION
Neutralizes one lethal (for average-size mouse) dose of black widow spider venom.

INDICATIONS/USES
Used in the treatment of patients with black widow spider bites.

USUAL DOSE
Entire contents of 1 vial (2.5 ml) of antivenin; a second vial may be needed. Symptoms usually subside in 1–3 h.

PREPARATION/RECONSTITUTION
Reconstitute single dose with 2.5 ml sterile water for injection (supplied). Maintain needle in rubber stopper of antivenin vial and shake to completely dissolve contents. Further dilute in 10–50 ml of normal saline for IV use.

INCOMPATIBILITIES
Do not mix with any other drug; sufficient information is not yet available.

RATE/MODE OF ADMINISTRATION
IV push: Preferred route of administration in severe cases as a single dose over 15-min minimum.
Intermittent: No.
Continuous: No.
Filter: Not applicable.

NURSING CONSIDERATIONS
Nursing Diagnoses
1. Potential for impairment of skin integrity, related to skin testing technique.
2. Potential alteration in cardiac output: decreased due to drug side effects.

Acute Care
Familiarize yourself with manufacturer's recommendations for use. Evaluate symptoms and status of each patient individually. Determine previous sensitivity reactions with clinical history and conjunctival/skin testing. Observe patient carefully for development of respiratory depression.

Precautions
Treatment with 10 ml 10% calcium gluconate may control muscle pain; morphine sulfate may be needed. Safety for use in pregnancy and lactation has not been established.

Contraindications
Hypersensitivity to horse serum unless other treatment is not available.

Side Effects
Dermatologic: Urticaria, local pain, local erythema.
Circulatory/respiratory: Respiratory distress, vascular collapse, anaphylaxis.

Patient/Caregiver Teaching
Instruct patient to report all side effects immediately.

Home Care
Not recommended.

Administration in Other Clinical Settings
Not recommended.

Nursing Interventions
The physician should be notified of all side effects. Discontinue drug and treat anaphylaxis immediately. Resuscitate as needed.

Antivenin (*Micrurus fulvius*)

US: North American Coral Snake Antivenin

Snake bite neutralizer   pH 6.5–7.5

ACTION
Neutralizing agent for venom of eastern and Texas coral snakes.

INDICATIONS/USES
Used in the treatment of snake bite caused by eastern and Texas coral snakes.

USUAL DOSE
3–5 vials is recommended; up to 10 vials may be required.

PREPARATION/RECONSTITUTION
Reconstitute each vial with 10 ml sterile water for injection.

INCOMPATIBILITIES
Do not mix with any other drug or solution; sufficient information is not available.

RATE/MODE OF ADMINISTRATION
IV push: Initial 2-ml dose; if no reaction, begin intermittent administration.

Intermittent: Remaining dose by sideport through an ongoing infusion of 250–500 ml 0.9% saline solution.

Continuous: No.

Filter: Not applicable.

NURSING CONSIDERATIONS
Nursing Diagnoses
1. Potential for alteration in cardiac output: decreased, related to drug side effects.
2. Potential impairment of skin integrity, related to skin testing technique.

Acute Care
Familiarize yourself with manufacturer's recommendations for use. Evaluate patient on an individual basis for possible sensitivities using conjunctival/scratch testing. Observe patient constantly; symptoms may develop in 1–18 h.

Precautions
Resuscitative equipment should be readily available. Patient's extremity should be immobilized. Supportive therapy may be indicated. Respiratory depressants should be used with great caution.

Contraindications
Hypersensitivity to horse serum unless no other treatment is available.

Side Effects
Dermatologic: Urticaria, local pain, local erythema.

Circulatory/respiratory: Respiratory distress, vascular collapse, anaphylaxis.

Patient/Caregiver Teaching
Instruct patient to report all side effects immediately.

Home Care
Not recommended.

Administration in Other Clinical Settings
Not recommended.

Nursing Interventions
The physician should be notified of all side effects. Discontinue drug and treat anaphylaxis immediately. Resuscitate as needed.

Arginine hydrochloride
US: R-Gene 10

Diagnostic aid   pH 5.0–6.5

ACTION
An IV stimulant to the pituitary gland given to induce an increase in plasma level of human growth hormone in normal patients.

INDICATIONS/USES
Used as an IV stimulant to the pituitary gland as a diagnostic tool for patients with panhypopituitarism, pituitary dwarfism, hypophysectomy, acromegaly, gigantism, and other growth disorders. Investigationally used to reverse ammonium intoxication.

USUAL DOSE
Adult: 300 ml as a test dose.
Children: 5 ml/kg body wt.

PREPARATION/RECONSTITUTION
10% solution in 500-ml bottles is available.

INCOMPATIBILITIES

Do not mix with any other drug or solution; specific information not available.

RATE/MODE OF ADMINISTRATION

IV push: No.
Intermittent: Single dose over 30 min.
Continuous: No.
Filter: Not applicable.

NURSING CONSIDERATIONS

Nursing Diagnoses

1. Potential for alteration in cardiac output: decreased, related to drug side effects.
2. Potential for alteration in bowel elimination: diarrhea, related to drug side effects.

Acute Care

Patient must be fasting overnight prior to use. Draw venous samples from opposite extremity 30 min before, at time infusion is initiated, and every 30 min times five. Baseline serum electrolyte balance should be obtained.

Precautions

May cause bicarbonate deficit or hyperkalemia. Use with caution in renal dysfunction. False-positive results may be obtained during pregnancy or with oral contraceptives. Do not use cloudy solution or container without vacuum.

Contraindications

Known allergic tendency.

Side Effects

Circulatory: Flushing.
Gastrointestinal: Nausea, vomiting.
Neurologic: Numbness, headache.
Dermatologic: Rash.
Other: Local venous irritation.

Patient/Caregiver Teaching
Instruct patient to report all side effects immediately.

Home Care
Not recommended.

Administration in Other Clinical Settings
Appropriate in the outpatient environment.

Nursing Interventions
The physician should be notified of all side effects. Reduction in rate of administration may be needed to reduce side effects; continue infusion within 30 min to ensure accuracy of test results. Treat allergic reaction by discontinuing infusion and administering diphenhydramine or epinephrine. Resuscitate as needed.

Ascorbic acid

US: Cenolate, sodium ascorbate, vitamin C

Water-soluble vitamin   pH 5.5–7.0

ACTION
Necessary to the formation of collagen in all fibrous tissue, carbohydrate metabolism, connective tissue repair, and other body processes.

INDICATIONS/USES
Used in pre- and postoperative management, prolonged IV therapy, and to meet vitamin needs in severe burns, extensive injuries, and extreme infections. Used to meet clinical needs in prematurity, wasting disorders, decreased wound healing, and scurvy.

USUAL DOSE
Adults: 200 mg–2 g/24 h; up to 6 g/24 h without toxicity.

Infants: 100–300 mg/24 h.
Premature infants: 75–100 mg/24 h.

PREPARATION/RECONSTITUTION
May be administered undiluted; soluble in most IV solutions.

INCOMPATIBILITIES
Bleomycin, chloramphenicol, dextran, erythromycin, hydrocortisone, nafcillin, sodium bicarbonate.

RATE/MODE OF ADMINISTRATION
IV push: 100 mg or fraction thereof over 1 min.
Intermittent: No.
Continuous: No.
Filter: Not applicable in less than 1-ml dose.

NURSING CONSIDERATIONS
Nursing Diagnosis
1. Potential for impaired physical mobility, related to drug side effects.

Acute Care
Slight discoloration does not affect the potency of this medication. Protect from temperature extremes and light.

Precautions
May potentiate barbiturates, salicylates, and sulfonamides and antagonize anticoagulants. Use with caution in pregnancy, cardiac patients, diabetics, and those prone to development of recurrent renal calculi. Inhibits amphetamines and tricyclic depressants and is inhibited by smoking.

Contraindications
None known.

Side Effects
Neurologic: Faintness and dizziness following too rapid injection.
Gastrointestinal: Diarrhea following large doses.
Urologic: Renal calculi following large doses.

Patient/Caregiver Teaching
Instruct patient to report all side effects immediately.

Home Care
Appropriate.

Administration in Other Clinical Settings
Appropriate.

Nursing Interventions
Temporarily discontinue dose and resume administration at a decreased rate of flow. For persistent side effects, notify physician and discontinue drug.

Asparaginase
US: Elspar

Enzyme   pH 7.4

ACTION
Derived from *Escherichia coli,* aspariginase is an enzyme that depletes asparaginine from cells.

INDICATIONS/USES
Used to induce remission in acute lymphocytic leukemia.

USUAL DOSE
Skin Testing: Required prior to initial dose or when 7 days or more elapse between doses. 0.1 ml (2 IU) is administered intradermally; patient must be observed for 1 h.

Other: Per patient-specific dosing regimen; 1000 IU/kg/day for 10 days beginning on day 22 of prednisone/vincristine regimen.

As a single agent: 200 IU/kg/day for 28 days.

PREPARATION/RECONSTITUTION

Reconstitute each 10-ml vial with 5 ml of sterile water for injection or sodium chloride to yield solution of 2000 IU/ml.

Skin test: Further dilute 0.1 ml with 9.9 ml sodium chloride; 0.1 ml of this solution equals 2 IU.

Direct IV: Use 2000 IU/ml solution.

INCOMPATIBILITIES

Considered incompatible in syringe or solution; specific information not available.

RATE/MODE OF ADMINISTRATION

IV push: Through sideport of free-flowing infusion of 5% dextrose in water or 0.9% sodium chloride solution over 30 min.

Intermittent: No.

Continuous: No.

Filter: To 0.5-μm range per institutional policies.

NURSING CONSIDERATIONS

Nursing Diagnoses

1. Possible hyperthermia, related to anaphylactic drug reaction.
2. Potential for impaired physical mobility, related to drug side effects.

Acute Care

Follow guidelines for handling cytotoxic agents; refer to Appendix. Have resuscitative equipment readily available prior to administering this highly toxic drug. Rarely used as single-agent therapy. Monitor blood counts, bone marrow, serum amylase, blood sugar, and liver/kidney function frequently. Monitor for elevated uric acid level; may require allopurinol therapy, increase in fluid intake, and alkalization of urine. Use only clear solutions and follow manufacturer's recommendations for use and storage.

Precautions

May increase toxicities of other drugs. Increases toxicity associated with vincristine and prednisone if given before or as concurrent treatment. Inhibits action of methotrexate. A mutagenic drug, asparaginase will produce teratogenic effects on the fetus; it is excreted in breast milk. Prophylactic administration of antiemetics may decrease incidence of nausea and vomiting.

Contraindications

Known hypersensitivity to this drug; history of pancreatitis.

Side Effects

Gastrointestinal: Nausea, vomiting.

Hematologic: Bleeding, bone marrow depression, hypofibrinogenemia, depression of other clotting factors, hyperglycemia.

Neurologic: Depression, fatigue, hallucinations, agitation.

Other: Allergic reactions, anaphylaxis, fatal hyperthermia, fatal fulminating pancreatitis.

Patient/Caregiver Teaching

Instruct patient to report all side effects immediately.

Home Care

Not recommended.

Administration in Other Clinical Settings

Generally not recommended in the absence of resuscitative equipment.

Nursing Interventions

None specific. The physician should be notified of all side effects. Resuscitative equipment should be available. Anaphylaxis may be treated with epinephrine, corticosteroids, oxygen, antihistamines.

Atropine sulfate

Anticholinergic drug   pH 3.5–6.5

ACTION

An anticholinergic drug and belladonna alkaloid that affects smooth muscle, cardiac muscle, and gland cells. Excreted through all body fluids; crosses the placental barrier and is secreted in breast milk.

INDICATIONS/USES

Used in the treatment of sinus bradycardia, syncope occurring as a result of Stokes-Adams syndrome, and atrioventricular block with bradycardia. Also used to treat cardiac asystole and to suppress salivary, gastric, pancreatic, and respiratory secretions.

USUAL DOSE

Adults

- Acute poisoning: Maximum of 3 mg as a single dose.
- Bradyarrhythmias: 0.5–1 mg bolus every 5 min not to exceed 2 mg; subsequent doses of 0.3–1 mg at 4–6-h intervals may be administered.
- Cardiac asystole: 1-mg bolus; may be repeated in 5 min.
- Smooth muscle relaxant/control of secretions: 0.4–0.6 mg every 3–4 h.
- Surgery: Same as bradyarrhythmias with exception of concurrent administration of cyclopropane anesthesia; reduce dose to 0.4 mg or less and administer slowly to avoid incidence of ventricular dysrhythmias.

Children

- Bradyarrhythmias: 0.02 mg/kg body wt in a distressed infant under 6 mo to achieve pulse rate of 80; may repeat in 5 min. *Note: Maximum dose not to exceed 1 mg for a child and 2 mg for an adolescent.*
- Smooth muscle relaxant/control of secretions: Administered subcutaneously.

PREPARATION/RECONSTITUTION

May be administered undiluted; may also be diluted in 10 ml of sterile water for injection; do not add to IV solutions.

INCOMPATIBILITIES

Amobarbital, ampicillin, chloramphenicol, cimetidine, epinephrine, heparin sodium, isoproterenol, levarterenol, metaraminol, methicillin, pentobarbital, promazine, sodium bicarbonate, thiopental.

RATE/MODE OF ADMINISTRATION

IV push: 1 mg or fraction thereof over 1 min.
Intermittent: No.
Continuous: No.
Filter: Not applicable.

NURSING CONSIDERATIONS

Nursing Diagnoses

1. Potential for sensory-perceptual alteration: visual, related to drug side effects.
2. Potential for urinary retention and alteration in patterns of urinary elimination, related to drug side effects.
3. Potential for impaired swallowing, related to gastroesophageal reflux.

Acute Care

Atropine is potentiated by many other drugs; check manufacturer's product literature carefully to avoid potentiation with antidepressants, antihistamines, MAO inhibitors, and adverse effects associated with other drugs. Antagonistic to many drug classifications and antagonized by many others.

Precautions

Use with caution in chronic lung disease, prostatic hypertrophy, and in the very young and elderly patient. Safety for use in pregnancy and lactation and in children has not been established. Capable of producing excitation, drowsiness, agitation in the elderly patient.

Contraindications

Known hypersensitivity to atropine, glaucoma, acute hemorrhage and unstable cardiovascular status, asthma, hepatic/renal dysfunction, myocardial ischemia, paralytic ileus, pyloric stenosis, tachycardia, and ulcerative colitis.

Side Effects

Neurologic: Blurred vision, dilation of pupils, postural hypotension.
Gastrointestinal: Vomiting, gastroesophageal reflux.
Urologic: Urinary retention, urinary hesitation.

Circulatory: Bradycardia (reversible), anhidrosis, dryness of mouth, flushing, heat prostration.

Patient/Caregiver Teaching

Instruct patient to report all side effects immediately.

Home Care

Not recommended.

Administration in Other Clinical Settings

Not generally recommended.

Nursing Interventions

Emergency resuscitation as indicated. Physostigmine salicylate reverses many cardiovascular and CNS effects, but it may cause asystole, bradycardia, or seizures.

Azathioprine sodium

US: Imuran

Immunosuppressive agent   pH 9.6

ACTION

A derivative of mercaptopurine, azathioprine sodium is an immunosuppressant. Readily metabolized and excreted in small amounts in the urine.

INDICATIONS/USES

Used as an adjunct to prevent rejection in renal homotransplantation.

USUAL DOSE

Adults: 3–5 mg/kg body wt/24 h. Treatment should begin within 24 h of renal transplantation.
- Pretransplantation: 1–5 mg/kg for several days.
- Maintenance: 1–3 mg/kg/24 h adjusted on an individual basis.

PREPARATION/RECONSTITUTION

Reconstitute each 100 mg with 10 ml of sterile water for injection; ensure complete dissolution. If desired, may dilute further with minimum of 50 ml of 0.9% sodium chloride or 5% dextrose in water for infusion purposes.

INCOMPATIBILITIES

Administer separately; insufficient information available at this time.

RATE/MODE OF ADMINISTRATION

IV push: As single dose for not less than 5 min.
Intermittent: Yes.
Continuous: Administered in appropriate diluent and run over 30–60 min; may administer over as long as 8 h.
Filter: Not applicable.

NURSING CONSIDERATIONS

Nursing Diagnoses

1. Potential for infection, related to immunosuppression.
2. Potential alteration in patterns of urinary elimination, related to drug side effects.
3. Potential for injury, related to bleeding tendencies.

Acute Care

Oral dosage is preferred; IV solution must be used within 24 h. Monitor bone marrow function, RBC and WBC counts, BUN, and platelet count. Administer with caution when other myelosuppressive drugs or radiation therapy is being used

Precautions

Reduce dosage if patient is receiving allopurinol. Reduce dosage in renal dysfunction and in persistent negative nitrogen balance. Azathioprine sodium has mutogenic and teratogenic potential, and safety for use in pregnancy and lactation and in those capable of conception has not been established. May increase possibility of malignant tumor growth.

Contraindications

Known hypersensitivity, anuria, severe case of organ rejection.

Side Effects

Hematologic: Anemia, bleeding, leukopenia, thrombocytopenia.
Gastrointestinal: Vomiting, anorexia, diarrhea, pancreatitis, nausea.
Neurologic: Arthralgia.
Dermatologic: Skin rash, alopecia.

Patient/Caregiver Teaching

Instruct patient (1) to report all side effects immediately and (2) that alopecia may be reversible.

Home Care

Appropriate.

Administration in Other Clinical Settings

Appropriate.

Nursing Interventions

The physician should be notified of all side effects. Symptomatic treatment is preferred; however, hematologic side effects may require withholding of treatment on a permanent or temporary basis.

Azlocillin sodium

US: Azlin

Broad-spectrum penicillin   pH 6–8

ACTION

Azlocillin sodium is bactericidal against a diversity of gram-negative and gram-positive organisms, including aerobic and anaerobic strains. Crosses the placental barrier and is excreted in urine and is secreted in breast milk. Prompt onset of action.

INDICATIONS/USES

Most effective against *Pseudomonas*. Used in the treatment of severe infections of lower respiratory tract, urinary tract, skin, bone and joints, and bacterial septicemia. Also effective in acute pulmonary exacerbation of cystic fibrosis in children; refer to package insert for dosing information.

USUAL DOSE

100–300 mg/kg body wt daily in 4–6 equally divided doses; not to exceed 24 g/day.

PREPARATION/RECONSTITUTION

Reconstitute each gram or fraction thereof in 10 ml sterile water, 5% dextrose in water, or 0.9% sodium chloride solution. Shake vigorously and further dilute to desired volume (50–100 ml) with compatible infusion solution according to package insert.

INCOMPATIBILITIES

Amikacin, gentamicin, kanamycin, streptomycin, tobramycin, amphotericin B, chloramphenicol, lincomycin, promethazine, tetracycline, vitamin B with C.

RATE/MODE OF ADMINISTRATION

IV push: Only as a 10% solution over 5 min or longer.
Intermittent: Preferred method of administration by IV piggyback infused over 30 min in 50–100 ml of compatible diluent, or sideport infusion.
Continuous: No.
Filter: Applicable consistent with institutional guidelines.

NURSING CONSIDERATIONS

Nursing Diagnoses

1. Potential for injury, related to bleeding tendencies.
2. Potential for impaired physical mobility, related to neuromuscular excitability and convulsions.
3. Potential for alteration in bowel elimination: diarrhea, related to drug side effects.

Acute Care

Slightly darkened color does not affect potency of drug. May be used concomitantly with aminoglycosides, but must be given in separate containers due to incompatibilities. Pretreatment sensiuvity studies are indicated. Monitor patient for signs of allergic reaction or sensitivities to drug. Avoid extravasation; azlocillin is an irritant (refer to Appendix 16).

Precautions

Superinfection may occur with prolonged use. Monitor patient's renal, hepatic, and hematopoietic functions regularly. Azlocillin should be continued for 2 days following cessation of symptoms. Risk of bleeding increases with heparin sodium therapy. Potentiates the action of cefotaxime. Higher than usual doses may cause neuromuscular excitability; monitor patient carefully for development of these symptoms.

Contraindications

Known sensitivity to penicillin or other drugs.

Side Effects

Hematologic: Bleeding; decreased hemoglobin/hematocrit levels; elevated SGOT, SGPT, BUN; thrombocytopenia; neutropenia; leukopenia.
Dermatologic: Urticaria, skin rash, pruritus.
Urinary: Pseudoproteinuria, interstitial nephritis.
Neurologic: Neuromuscular excitability, abnormal taste sensation, convulsions.
Gastrointestinal: Vomiting, nausea, diarrhea.
Other: Anaphylaxis, thrombophlebitis.

Patient/Caregiver Teaching

Instruct patient (1) to report all side effects immediately and (2) in methodology for home administration of this drug.

Home Care

Appropriate.

Administration in Other Clinical Settings

Appropriate.

Nursing Interventions

The physician should be notified of all side effects. Discontinue drug in event of severe symptoms and treat allergic reactions as indicated. Resuscitative equipment should be available for initial dosing in inpatient environment. Hemodialysis or peritoneal dialysis may be effective to counteract overdosage.

Aztreonam

US: Azactam

Monobactam antibiotic   pH 4.5–7.5

ACTION

The bactericidal action causes inhibition of bacterial cell wall synthesis due to high attraction for penicillin-binding protein.

INDICATIONS/USES

Aztreonam may inhibit most species of *Enterobacteriaceae*, especially those resistant to gentamicin, tobramycin, and amikacin. Also inhibits strains of *Escherichia coli* and *Klebsiella* organisms resistant to the third-generation cephalosporin, cefoperazone; therefore, effective in the treatment of serious lower respiratory tract, urinary tract, skin, and intraabdominal infections.

USUAL DOSE

Pseudomonas aeruginosa: 2 g every 6–8 h; maximum dose is 8 g. *Other:* 500 mg–2 g every 6, 8, or 12 h in divided doses.

PREPARATION/RECONSTITUTION

Available in 15-ml vials containing either 0.5, 1, or 2 g of drug. Reconstitute each vial with at least 3 ml of sterile water for injection; further dilute to a concentration of no greater than 2% solution. Also available in 100-ml premixed containers.

INCOMPATIBILITIES

Cephradine, metronidazole, nafcillin sodium.

RATE/MODE OF ADMINISTRATION

IV push: Reconstitute with at least 6–10 ml of sterile water for injection and administer over 3–5 min.

Intermittent: Preferred method of administration; dilute each dose with 3 ml sterile water for injection; may further dilute in 50–100 ml of 5% dextrose in water, 0.9% sodium chloride solution, or other compatible infusate to run over 20–60 min.
Continuous: No.
Filter: Applicable consistent with institutional guidelines.

NURSING CONSIDERATIONS

Nursing Diagnoses

1. Potential for alteration in bowel elimination: diarrhea, related to drug side effects.
2. Potential for alteration in comfort, related to development of thrombophlebitis.
3. Potential for alteration in tissue integrity, related to development of mouth ulcers.
4. Potential for alteration in cardiac output: decreased, related to drug toxicity.

Acute Care

Monitor patient's ECG, hematology, and chemistry studies frequently. Symptomatic treatment of side effects. Prevent falls; remove safety hazards. Rotate IV site carefully to avoid development of thrombophlebitis. Monitor peak and trough levels.

Precautions

Observe patient for hypotension, dizziness, dyspnea, bleeding, and ECG changes and treat accordingly. Aztreonam excreted mainly in the urine; serum half-life in healthy individuals averages 1.7 h. For renal uremic patients, reduce dose but maintain similar schedule *or* administer usual dose with longer dose interval.

Contraindications

Known sensitivity to aztreonam.

Side Effects

Gastrointestinal: Nausea, vomiting, diarrhea, abdominal cramping, colitis.
Dermatologic: Skin rash, jaundice, mouth ulcer, petechiae, pruritus, purpura, urticaria.

Neurologic: Vertigo, tinnitus, seizures, insomnia, dizziness, diplopia, paresthesias.
Circulatory/respiratory: ECG changes, hypotension.
Other: Local pain at injection site.

Patient/Caregiver Teaching

Instruct patient (1) to report all side effects immediately and (2) in the principles of home self-administration and related monitoring.

Home Care

Appropriate.

Administration in Other Clinical Settings

Appropriate.

Nursing Interventions

The physician should be notified immediately of all side effects. Allergic reactions are treated symptomatically; emergency drugs should be available for home use. Initial dose should be given in inpatient environment.

Benzquinamide hydrochloride

US: Emete-Con

Antiemetic sedative   pH 3–4

ACTION

Displays antiemetic, antihistaminic, mild anticholinergic, and sedative effects; the mechanism of action is unknown.

INDICATIONS/USES

Used in the prevention and treatment of nausea and vomiting during anesthesia and surgery.

USUAL DOSE

0.2–0.4 mg/kg body wt, or 25 mg as initial dose; additional doses may be given IM.

PREPARATION/RECONSTITUTION

Reconstitute each 50 mg with 2.2 ml of sterile water for injection for a concentration of 25 mg/ml.

INCOMPATIBILITIES

Chlordiazepoxide, diazepam, pentobarbital, phenobarbital, sodium chloride, thiopental.

RATE/MODE OF ADMINISTRATION

IV push: Yes, sideport through an ongoing infusion.
Intermittent: No.
Continuous: No.
Filter: Not applicable in less than 1-ml dose.

NURSING CONSIDERATIONS

Nursing Diagnoses

1. Potential for alteration in cardiac output: decreased, related to drug side effects.
2. Potential for injury, related to neurologic manifestations of drug therapy.

Acute Care

Use under the direction of an anesthesiologist and monitor patient's blood pressure carefully. Discard unused solution after 14 days at room temperature.

Precautions

Dosage should be reduced substantially in patients receiving pressor agents. Sudden hypertension, PVCs, and transient PACs may develop with IV injection. Safety for use in pregnancy and children has not been established.

Contraindications

Patients with cardiovascular disease, hypersensitivity to this drug and other phenothiazide preparations.

Side Effects

EENT: Blurred vision, dry mouth, salivation.
Neurologic: Tremors, weakness, excitation, dizziness, nervousness.
Cardiovascular/respiratory: PVCs, PACs, atrial fibrillation, diaphoresis, hypo- or hypertension.

Patient/Caregiver Teaching

Instruct patient (1) to report all side effects immediately and (2) to keep siderails up to avoid falls.

Home Care

Inappropriate.

Administration In Other Clinical Settings

Not recommended.

Nursing Interventions

The physician should be notified of all side effects and may choose to discontinue therapy. Resuscitative equipment should be readily available.

Benztropine mesylate
US: Cogentin

Anticholinergic/antihistaminic   pH 5–8

ACTION

Relieves tremor, rigidity, drooling, dysphagia, gait disturbances, and other symptoms of parkinsonism. Excreted in the urine, onset of action is prompt.

INDICATIONS/USES

Used as a treatment to relieve drug-induced, postencephalitic, idiopathic, or arteriosclerotic symptoms of parkinsonism.

USUAL DOSE

1–2 mg; may be gradually increased to 4–6 mg/24 h as needed.

PREPARATION/RECONSTITUTION

1 ml of solution equals 1 mg of benztropine mesylate; administer undiluted.

INCOMPATIBILITIES

None known at this time.

RATE/MODE OF ADMINISTRATION

IV push: Yes; used only in acute drug reactions or for psychotic patients.
Intermittent: No.
Continuous: No.
Filter: Not applicable in this dose range.

NURSING CONSIDERATIONS

Nursing Diagnoses

1. Potential for sensory-perceptual alteration, related to side effects of drug.
2. Potential for injury, related to development of weakness, dizziness, nervousness.
3. Potential alteration in cardiac output: decreased, related to overdose.

Acute Care

Monitor patient carefully for development of untoward reactions to drug. Due to potential for potent cumulative action, the patient must be observed closely. Do not discontinue other antiparkinsonian drugs abruptly; decrease dosage gradually to wean patient and allow system to adjust appropriately.

Precautions

Drug action may be potentiated by alcohol, antihistamines, barbiturates, narcotic analgesics, phenothiazines, and tricyclic antidepressants. Patient must be observed closely for any and all side effects. May inhibit lactation.

Contraindications

Known hypersensitivity, pregnancy, children under age 3.

Side Effects

Dermatologic: Skin rash.
Neurologic: Depression, dry mouth, listlessness, nervousness, numbness of fingers.
Gastrointestinal: Vomiting, nausea.
Overdose: Anhidrosis, circulatory collapse, coma, respiratory depression, tachycardia, urinary retention.

Patient/Caregiver Teaching

Instruct patient (1) to report all side effects immediately and (2) to prevent falls and keep siderails elevated.

Home Care

Inappropriate.

Administration in Other Clinical Settings

Inappropriate.

Nursing Interventions

The physician should be notified of all side effects immediately. Physostigmine salicylate reverses symptoms of anticholinergic intoxication. Patient should be observed for possible relapse for a minimum of 12 h. CNS excitation may be alleviated by administration of diazepam. Resuscitative equipment should be readily available.

Biperiden lactate

US: Akineton, Akineton

Anticholinergic   pH 4.8–5.8

ACTION

Inhibits the parasympathetic nervous system.

INDICATIONS/USES
Used to control drug-induced extrapyramidal disorders and for postencephalitic, arteriosclerotic, and idiopathic parkinsonism.

USUAL DOSE
2 mg; may be repeated every 30 min until symptoms have been relieved. Not to exceed 4 doses in 24 h.

PREPARATION/RECONSTITUTION
Administer undiluted.

INCOMPATIBILITIES
None known.

RATE/MODE OF ADMINISTRATION
IV push: 2 mg or fraction thereof over 1 min.
Intermittent: No.
Continuous: No.
Filter: Not applicable in less than 1-ml dose form.

NURSING CONSIDERATIONS
Nursing Diagnoses
1. Potential disturbance of self-concept, related to side effects of drug.
2. Potential for sensory-perceptual alteration, related to development of blurred vision.
3. Potential for alteration in cardiac output: depression, related to toxic effects of drug.

Acute Care
IV route used in acute drug reactions and psychotic patients; not recommended for use in children. Monitor patient carefully for potential development of symptoms related to cumulative effect of drug. Side effects may be potentiated by alcohol, antihistamines, barbiturates, narcotic analgesics, phenothiazines, tricyclic antidepressants. Maintain accurate drug profile.

Precautions
Use caution in presence of hypo- or hypertension, tachycardia, and cardiac, liver, and renal disorders. May potentiate oral digoxin and may inhibit lactation.

Contraindications
Known hypersensitivity.

Side Effects
Dermatologic: Skin rash.
Gastrointestinal: Vomiting, nausea, constipation.
Neurologic: Depression, dizziness, listlessness, numbness of fingers, nervousness.
EENT: Blurred vision.
Overdose: Anhidrosis, circulatory collapse, coma, paralytic ileus, respiratory depression, tachycardia, urinary retention.

Patient/Caregiver Teaching
Instruct patient (1) to report all side effects immediately and (2) to keep siderails elevated at all times.

Home Care
Inappropriate.

Administration in Other Clinical Settings
Inappropriate.

Nursing Interventions
The physician should be notified of all side effects. Resuscitative equipment should be readily available. Treat overdose symptomatically, including provision of adequate respiratory support. Observe patient for possible relapse for a minimum of 12 h.

Bleomycin sulfate
US: Blenoxane
CAN: Blenoxane (Bristol)

Antibiotic antineoplastic   pH 4.5–6.0

ACTION
A cell-cycle-specific antibiotic antineoplastic agent, which acts by

splitting and fragmenting double-stranded DNA, causing chromosomal damage. 40% is excreted in the urine.

INDICATIONS/USES

Used in the treatment of testicular carcinoma or as palliative treatment in patients unresponsive to other protocols used to treat squamous cell carcinoma of the skin, head, esophagus, neck, GU tract, and other lymphomas.

USUAL DOSE

0.25–0.5 U/kg body wt/24 h or 10–20 U/m², once or twice weekly. *Note: Test dose is required prior to administration.*
Hodgkin's disease: As above; following a 50% response, administer maintenance dose of 1 U/24 h or 5 U weekly.

PREPARATION/RECONSTITUTION

See precautions relevant to technique on package insert. Reconstitute each 15 U or fraction thereof with 5 ml or more of sterile water for injection, 5% dextrose in water, or 0.9% sodium chloride solution resulting in a solution of not more than 3 U/ml. Further dilute with 50–100 ml of identical solution.

INCOMPATIBILITIES

Amino acids, ascorbic acid, diazepam, furosemide, theophylline.

RATE/MODE OF ADMINISTRATION

IV push: No.
Intermittent: Administer each 15 U or fraction thereof through side-port of freely flowing infusion over 10 min.
Continuous: Yes, by electronic infusion device. Continuous infusion is thought to minimize pulmonary toxicities.
Filter: Applicable consistent with institutional guidelines.

NURSING CONSIDERATIONS

Nursing Diagnoses

1. Potential alteration in cardiac output: decreased, related to toxic effect up to 6 h after test dose.
2. Potential alteration in self-concept, related to alopecia and weight loss.

3. Potential alteration in body temperature, related to drug side effects.

Acute Care

Follow guidelines for recommended handling of cytotoxic agents; see Appendix 14. Determine patency of vein to avoid extravasation; see Appendix 15 for treatment of vesicant extravasation. Obtain baseline chest radiograph and monitor every 1 or 2 wk to determine evidence of pulmonary changes. Dosage is based on patient's average weight in presence of edema or ascites. Maintain adequate hydration. Observe patient for signs of infection.

Precautions

Administration requires test dosing; may cause severe anaphylactic reaction. Pulmonary toxicity is increased with larger dosages. Most toxic when total cumulative dose exceeds 350–450 U. Diluted solution is stable at room temperature for 24 h. Crosses placental barrier.

Contraindications

Known hypersensitivity to this drug; elderly patients with pulmonary disease.

Side Effects

Dermatologic: Alopecia and skin tenderness, toxicity, and hyperpigmentation are the major side effects.
Neurologic: Pain at tumor site.
Gastrointestinal: Anorexia, nausea, vomiting, weight loss.
Circulatory/respiratory: Dyspnea, chills, hypotension, rales, pulmonary fibrosis, pneumonitis.

Patient/Caregiver Teaching

Instruct patient (1) to report all side effects immediately; (2) to avoid chills caused by drafts; and (3) that hair loss is reversible.

Home Care

Not generally administered in the home care setting.

Administration in Other Clinical Settings

Appropriate if nursing personnel have been adequately trained to monitor the patient.

Nursing Interventions

The physician must be notified of all side effects immediately. Provide symptomatic treatment for minor side effects. If major side effects occur, discontinue drug immediately and notify physician at once. Treat anaphylaxis with epinephrine or diphenhydramine hydrochloride.

Bretylium tosylate

US: Bretylol, Bretylate
CAN: Bretylate (B.W., Inc.)

Group III antiarrhythmic   pH 5–7

ACTION

Exerts transient adrenergic stimulation through release of norepinephrine; suppresses aberrant impulses and increases refractory period without increasing heart rate. Effect occurs within minutes; requires constant plasma levels. Half-life ranges from 4–17 h. Excreted in the urine.

INDICATIONS/USES

Used in the prophylaxis and treatment of ventricular fibrillation and treatment of life-threatening ventricular dysrhythmias that have failed to respond to adequate doses of lidocaine or procainamide.

USUAL DOSE

Adults
- Ventricular fibrillation: 5 mg/kg body wt; increase to 10 mg/kg and repeat at 15–30-min intervals if dysrhythmia persists. Not to exceed total dose of 30 mg/kg/24 h.
- Other ventricular dysrhythmias: 5–10 mg/kg by infusion; may be repeated in 1–2 h if dysrhythmia persists.
- Maintenance: By infusion at 1–2 mg/min.

Children: Not recommended.
Geriatrics: Same as for adults.

PREPARATION/RECONSTITUTION

May be given undiluted (50 mg/ml) in ventricular fibrillation. For other use, reconstitute 500 mg of drug in 50 ml of 5% dextrose in water or 0.9% sodium chloride solution for a concentration of 10 mg/ml and infuse over minimum of 8 min or reconstitute greater amount of drug in comparable amount of solution (1 g in 1000 ml equals 1 mg/ml).

INCOMPATIBILITIES

Effect may be increased or decreased when used with quinidine, procainamide, propranolol. May increase effects of drug when used with antihypertensives or digitalis preparations.

RATE/MODE OF ADMINISTRATION

IV push: Single dose over 15–30 sec.
Intermittent: Single dose over 20–30 min.
Continuous: 1–2 mg/min by electronic infusion device titrated to patient's clinical condition.
Filter: Applicable; use according to institutional guidelines.

NURSING CONSIDERATIONS

Nursing Diagnoses

1. Potential for sensory-perceptual alteration, related to effect of medication.
2. Potential for alteration in cardiac output: decreased, related to dysrhythmias.
3. Potential for fluid volume deficit, related to medication administration.

Acute Care

Monitor the patient's ECG and blood pressure continuously; bretylium causes hypotension. Monitor for signs of dehydration or hypovolemia. May aggravate digitalis toxicity. Use dilute solution. Reduce dose of drug after 3–5 days of monitored therapy, then discontinue.

Precautions

Observe patient for postural hypotension; maintain supine position. Use with caution if patient is receiving digitalis. Use during pregnancy or in children only in life-threatening situations. Use with caution in patients with renal failure or impaired renal function.

Contraindications
None when used as indicated.

Side Effects
Neurologic: Dizziness, light-headedness, syncope, vertigo.
Circulatory: Anginal attacks, bradycardia, hypotension, increased frequency of PVCs, transitory hypertension.
Gastrointestinal: Nausea, vomiting.

Patient/Caregiver Teaching
Instruct patient (1) to report all side effects immediately (including nausea and vomiting); (2) to remain in a supine position; and (3) to exercise caution when change of position is necessary.

Home Care
Not recommended.

Administration in Other Clinical Settings
Not recommended.

Nursing Interventions
The physician should be notified of all side effects. Reduction in rate of administration may be needed to relieve nausea and vomiting. Dopamine is indicated to correct hypotension. Resuscitative equipment should be available. Overdose may be reversed by dialysis.

Brompheniramine maleate
US: Codimal-A, Dehist, Dimetane-Ten, Histaject

Antihistaminic/anticholinergic   pH 6.8—7.0

ACTION
Acts by blocking effects of histamine at receptor sites.

INDICATIONS/USES

Used in prevention or reduction of allergic reactions to whole blood and plasma; in treatment of anaphylactic reactions and other allergic conditions.

USUAL DOSE

Initial: 10 mg; 5–20 mg may be administered.
Maintenance: Every 3–12 h as indicated, not to exceed 40 mg/24 h.

PREPARATION/RECONSTITUTION

May be given undiluted (10 mg/ml); side effects are minimized with further preparation/reconstitution in 0.9% sodium chloride solution or 5% dextrose in water.

INCOMPATIBILITIES

Insulin, pentobarbital, theophylline.

RATE/MODE OF ADMINISTRATION

IV push: As a single dose over 1 min.
Intermittent: Diluted as above.
Continuous: No.
Filter: Not applicable when administered IV push in less than 1 ml.
Note: Although some manufacturers state that brompheniramine maleate injection may be added to whole blood prior to transfusion, most authorities believe that antihistamines should not be added to blood.

NURSING CONSIDERATIONS

Nursing Diagnoses

1. Potential for alteration in cardiac output: decreased, related to drug side effects.
2. Potential for injury, related to transient effects of drug.

Acute Care

Note the label carefully: only 10 mg/ml form may be administered by IV. Administer with patient in recumbent position. Solution is light sensitive.

Precautions

Use with caution in patients with history of bronchial asthma, cardiovascular or renal disease, diabetes, hypertension, hyperthyroidism, or increased intravascular pressure and in the elderly.

Contraindications

Hypersensitivity to antihistamines; pregnancy; lactation; newborn or premature infants; patients with lower respiratory disease.

Side Effects

Neurologic: Confusion, convulsions, dizziness, hallucinations, hysteria, paresthesias, sedation.
Urinary: Urinary retention.
Gastrointestinal: Nausea, vomiting.
Cardiovascular/respiratory: Tachycardia, wheezing, hypo- or hypertension.
Other: Respiratory or cardiac arrest, leading to death.

Patient/Caregiver Teaching

Instruct patient to report all side effects immediately.

Home Care

Not recommended in IV form.

Administration in Other Clinical Settings

Not recommended in IV form.

Nursing Interventions

Inform physician of all side effects. Resuscitative equipment should be readily available. Most side effects are reversible when drug is discontinued.

Bumetanide

US: Bumex

Sulfonamide diuretic   pH 7

ACTION

A loop diuretic agent related to the thiazides.

INDICATIONS/USES
Used in the treatment of congestive heart failure, acute pulmonary edema, cirrhosis of the liver, edema unresponsive to other diuretic agents, and as an alternative to furosemide in sensitive patients.

USUAL DOSE
0.5 to 1 mg; may be repeated at 2–3-h intervals not to exceed a maximum of 10 mg/24 h.

PREPARATION/RECONSTITUTION
May be administered undiluted (0.25 mg/ml).

INCOMPATIBILITIES
Dobutamine.

RATE/MODE OF ADMINISTRATION
IV push: As a single dose over 1–2 min, or sideport through an ongoing infusion of 5% dextrose in water, 0.9% sodium chloride solution, or lactated Ringer's infusion.
Intermittent: No.
Continuous: No.
Filter: Not applicable in dose less than 1 ml.

NURSING CONSIDERATIONS
Nursing Diagnoses
1. Potential for alteration in cardiac output: decreased, related to drug side effects.
2. Potential for sensory-perceptual alteration, related to drug side effects.
3. Potential for impairment of skin integrity, related to drug side effects.

Acute Care
Can be administered to patients who are sensitive to furosemide therapy; ratio for calculation of dose is 1 mg bumetanide to 40 mg furosemide. Use only freshly prepared solutions for infusion; discard after 24 h. Monitor urine output carefully to avoid excessive diuresis and subsequent water/electrolyte depletion. Baseline and routine electrolyte parameters are required.

Precautions

May increase blood glucose and precipitate diabetes mellitus. May potentiate antihypertensive drugs. May cause transient deafness if used concomitantly with ototoxic drugs.

Contraindications

Known sensitivity to bumetanide; anuria; hepatic coma; advanced cirrhosis.

Side Effects

Gastrointestinal: Abdominal pain, nausea.
Neurologic: Dizziness, headache, encephalopathy, impaired hearing.
Dermatologic: Pruritus, rash.
Major: Anaphylaxis, blood volume reduction, circulatory collapse, vascular thrombosis, embolism.

Patient/Caregiver Teaching

Instruct patient (1) to report all side effects immediately and (2) that hearing loss may be reversible.

Home Care

Not recommended.

Administration in Other Clinical Settings

Not recommended.

Nursing Interventions

The physician should be notified of all side effects. Discontinue drug and advise physician for evidence of minor side effects; therapy may be continued and symptomatic treatment provided. Fluid and electrolyte therapy is needed for treatment of major side effects. Resuscitative equipment should be readily available.

Buprenorphine hydrochloride

US: Buprenex

Narcotic agonist-antagonist   pH 3.5–5.5

ACTION
A synthetic narcotic agonist-antagonist analgesic product.

INDICATIONS/USES
Used in the relief of moderate to severe pain.

USUAL DOSE
0.3 mg/1 ml; may repeat in 30–60 min if required. Repeat every 6 h as needed.
Geriatrics/Debilitated: Reduce dose accordingly.

PREPARATION/RECONSTITUTION
May be given undiluted.

INCOMPATIBILITIES
Diazepam, lorazepam.

RATE/MODE OF ADMINISTRATION
IV push: As a single dose over 3–5 min.
Intermittent: No.
Continuous: No.
Filter: Not applicable in dose less than 1 ml.

NURSING CONSIDERATIONS
Nursing Diagnoses
1. Potential for alteration in cardiac output: decreased, related to toxic effects of drug.
2. Potential for alteration in bowel elimination: constipation, related to drug side effects.

69

Acute Care

May precipitate withdrawal symptoms if abruptly discontinued after prolonged administration of opiate drugs. Oxygen and emergency drugs must be available. Monitor vital signs and observe patient frequently.

Precautions

Potentiated by phenothiazines and other CNS depressants. Use with caution in asthma, respiratory depression, impaired renal/hepatic function, CNS depression or coma, acute alcoholism. Crosses placental barrier; safety for use in pregnancy not established. *Caution: Use this drug only when clearly indicated.*

Contraindications

Children under age 12; hypersensitivity to buprenorphine.

Side Effects

Neurologic: Hypersedation, dizziness, headache, vertigo.
EENT: Visual disturbances.
Circulatory/respiratory: Hyper- or hypotension, dyspnea, respiratory depression, tachycardia, bradycardia, cyanosis.
Gastrointestinal: Vomiting, constipation.
Other: Anaphylaxis.

Patient/Caregiver Teaching

Instruct patient (1) to report all side effects immediately (including dizziness) and (2) to keep siderails raised.

Home Care

Not recommended.

Administration in Other Clinical Settings

Not recommended.

Nursing Interventions

Discontinue drug and notify physician immediately of any side effects. Administration of naloxone hydrochloride helps to reverse respiratory depression. Maintain patent airway and resuscitate as needed.

Butorphanol tartrate
US: Stadol

Narcotic analgesic   pH 4.5

ACTION
Exhibits narcotic agonist-antagonist effects; action is similar to that of morphine sulfate. Pain relief is immediate and peaks at 30 min, lasting 3 h. Metabolized in the liver and excreted in the urine.

INDICATIONS/USES
Used to provide relief of moderate to severe pain and as a preoperative sedative.

USUAL DOSE
0.5–2 mg IV; usually 1 mg. May repeat every 3–4 h as needed.

PREPARATION/RECONSTITUTION
May be given undiluted. Available in concentrations of 1 and 2 mg/ml.

INCOMPATIBILITIES
Pentobarbital.

RATE/MODE OF ADMINISTRATION
IV push: Administer 2 mg over 3–5 min; may titrate consistent with patient's clinical condition.
Intermittent: No.
Continuous: No.
Filter: Not applicable in dose less than 1 ml.

NURSING CONSIDERATIONS
Nursing Diagnoses
1. Potential for ineffective breathing pattern, related to respiratory depression.
2. Potential for alteration in cardiac output: decreased, related to side effects of drug.

Acute Care

Monitor patient carefully to ensure adequate respiratory function. Oxygen and respiratory equipment should be readily available.

Precautions

Do not use for narcotic-dependent patients; can produce further dependent states. Use with caution in obstructive respiratory conditions, head injury, or hepatic/renal dysfunction. Potentiated by secobarbital, cimetidine, and other tranquilizers.

Contraindications

Known hypersensitivity, biliary surgery, pregnancy, lactation, and in children under age 18.

Side Effects

Dermatologic: Clammy skin, flushing, sensitivity to cold, sweating, warmth.
Neurologic: Confusion, diplopia, dizziness, hallucinations, headache, lethargy, sedation.
Gastrointestinal: Vomiting, nausea.
Respiratory: Respiratory depression.

Patient/Caregiver Teaching

Instruct patient to report all side effects immediately.

Home Care

Not applicable.

Administration in Other Clinical Settings

Not applicable.

Nursing Interventions

Notify physician of all side effects. Administration of naloxone hydrochloride reverses symptoms of respiratory depression. Resuscitative equipment must be readily available.

Caffeine and sodium benzoate injection

CNS stimulant   pH 6.5–8.5

ACTION
Constricts intracranial blood vessels to lower intracranial pressure; a CNS stimulant and xanthine derivative that is excreted in the urine. Caffeine–sodium benzoate crosses the placental barrier and is secreted in breast milk.

INDICATIONS/USES
Given IV in emergency situations only as a narcotic poisoning antidote if naloxone is unavailable.

USUAL DOSE
Adults: 500 mg to 1 g not to exceed 2.5 g/24 h.
Children: 8 mg/kg body wt up to 500 mg every 4 h.
Neonates: For neonatal apnea, 10 mg/kg of caffeine followed with maintenance dose of 2.5 mg/kg/day. Monitor plasma drug concentrations. *Caution: Do not use sodium benzoate in neonates.*

PREPARATION/RECONSTITUTION
May be given undiluted.

INCOMPATIBILITIES
Chlorpromazine.

RATE/MODE OF ADMINISTRATION
IV push: 250 mg or fraction thereof over 1 min.
Intermittent: No.
Continuous: No.
Filter· Not applicable in less than 1-ml dose.

NURSING CONSIDERATIONS
Nursing Diagnoses
1. Potential for altered cardiac output: decreased, related to drug side effects.

2. Potential for anxiety, related to drug side effects.

Acute Care
History of smoking promotes elimination of caffeine and may inhibit efficacy of this drug. Monitor patient for all side effects.

Precautions
Death has been reported following IV administration.

Contraindications
Myocardial infarction.

Side Effects
Neurologic: Excessive irritability, insomnia, twitching.
Cardiovascular: Tachycardia, palpitations, dysrhythmias.
Other: Bradycardia and tremors, hypotension, and acidosis may occur in neonates.

Patient/Caregiver Teaching
Instruct patient (1) to report all side effects immediately; (2) to report history of caffeine intake; and (3) to report drug history.

Home Care
Not recommended.

Administration in Other Clinical Settings
Not recommended.

Nursing Interventions
The physician should be notified of all side effects immediately. Administration of short-acting sedatives may relieve anxiety and CNS stimulation. Resuscitative equipment should be readily available.

Calcium chloride

Replacement element   pH 6.0–8.2

ACTION

A replacement element essential to bones, muscles, blood coagulation, and glands and cardiovascular tone. Excreted in the urine and feces.

INDICATIONS/USES

Used in the treatment of tetany associated with hypocalcemia, as an antidote for magnesium sulfate, and in cardiac resuscitation to treat hypocalcemia, hyperkalemia, or calcium channel block toxicity related to overdose of verapamil.

USUAL DOSE

Adults

- Cardiac resuscitation: 2 ml repeated in 20 min; follow product literature recommendations for whole blood replacement.
- Hyperkalemic disturbances of cardiac function: 1–10 ml titrated to ECG changes.
- Hypocalcemia: 5–10 ml every 1–3 days.
- Magnesium intoxication: 5 ml.

Infants: 0.2 ml of 10% solution/kg (20 mg/kg).

PREPARATION/RECONSTITUTION

May be given undiluted as a 10% solution, or with an equal amount of distilled water or 0.9% sodium chloride to create a 5% solution.

INCOMPATIBILITIES

Amphotericin B, cephalothin, epinephrine, oxytetracycline, sodium bicarbonate, tetracycline, calcium salts not mixed with carbonates, phosphates, sulfates, tartrates.

RATE/MODE OF ADMINISTRATION

IV push: 100 mg of 10% solution over 1 min.
Intermittent: No.

Continuous: Only as an additive to nutritional support solution.
Filter: Applicable with nutritional support solution only.

NURSING CONSIDERATIONS

Nursing Diagnoses

1. Potential for anxiety, related to side effects of drug and subsequent depression.
2. Potential for alteration in cardiac output: decreased, related to drug side effects.

Acute Care

Monitor patient carefully; calcium chloride is three times as potent as calcium gluconate. Always confirm patency of vessel prior to administration and avoid extravasation with this irritant drug. (Incompatible with sodium bicarbonate; flush IV administration set with normal saline solution after bicarbonate administration and prior to calcium administration.) Keep patient recumbent following injection to avoid danger of postural hypotension.

Contraindications

Ventricular fibrillation.

Side Effects

Cardiovascular: Bradycardia, cardiac arrest, cardiac contractions.
Neurologic: Tingling.

Patient/Caregiver Teaching

Instruct patient (1) to report all side effects immediately and (2) to report accurate history of medication administration.

Home Care

Not recommended unless a component of nutritional support formula.

Administration in Other Clinical Settings

Not recommended unless a component of nutritional support formula.

Nursing Interventions

The physician should be notified of all side effects immediately. Resuscitative equipment should be readily available. Critical overdosage may be treated with calcium disodium edetate. Treat extravasation with 1% procaine hydrochloride and hyaluronidase.

Calcium disodium edetate
US: Calcium EDTA, Edetate Calcium Disodium
CAN: Calcium Disodium Versenate (Riker/3M)

Chelating agent   pH 6.5—7.5

ACTION
An iron chelation agent used to remove metals from the bloodstream.

INDICATIONS/USES
Used to treat acute and chronic lead poisoning and lead encephalopathy.

USUAL DOSE
Adults: 1 g followed by second dose in 6 h; give 2 times in 24 h for 3–5 days. Not to exceed 50 mg/kg body wt/24 h.
Children: Do not exceed 70 mg/kg/24 h in 2 or 3 equal doses.

PREPARATION/RECONSTITUTION
Reconstitute 5 ml in 250–500 ml of 5% dextrose in water or 0.9% sodium chloride solution.

INCOMPATIBILITIES
Do not mix with other diluents or other medications.

RATE/MODE OF ADMINISTRATION
IV push: No.
Intermittent: Administer over 1 h by electronic infusion device if available.

Continuous: Administer over 1 h by electronic infusion device if available.

Filter: Applicable consistent with institutional guidelines.

NURSING CONSIDERATIONS

Nursing Diagnosis

1. Potential for alteration in patterns of urinary elimination, related to side effects of drug and renal toxicities.

Acute Care

Monitor patient's urinary output carefully; essential to establish kidney function prior to administration of this drug. Monitor vital signs and cardiac function. Too rapid injection may cause hypocalcemia tetany.

Precautions

May produce toxic and fatal side effects. Resuscitative equipment must be readily available. Read drug label carefully to avoid confusing this with other calcium preparations.

Contraindications

Renal dysfunction, anuria.

Side Effects

Urinary: Hematuria, proteinuria, renal acute tubular necrosis.
Neurologic: Cramping, malaise, tetany.

Patient/Caregiver Teaching

Instruct patient (1) to report all side effects immediately and (2) to provide accurate clinical history.

Home Care

Not recommended.

Administration in Other Clinical Settings

Not recommended.

Nursing Interventions

The physician must be notified of all side effects immediately. Prepare to resuscitate as needed. Discontinuation of this drug may be necessary to deter further renal damage.

Calcium gluceptate

CAN: Calcium salt

Replacement element   pH 6–7

ACTION
Replacement for the basic element, as an additive to nutritional support formula, and for normal coagulation of the blood.

INDICATIONS/USES
Used in the treatment of hypocalcemia caused by neonatal tetany or alkalosis; used to prevent hypocalcemia during exchange transfusion treatment; and used in cardiac resuscitation to treat hypocalcemia and hyperkalemia.

USUAL DOSE
Adults: 5–20 ml.
- Cardiac resuscitation: 5–7 ml; repeat in 10 min if indicated.

Newborn exchange transfusion: 0.45 mEq after each 100 ml of exchanged blood.

PREPARATION/RECONSTITUTION
May be given undiluted (220 mg/ml).

INCOMPATIBILITIES
Cefamandole, cefazolin, cephalothin, magnesium sulfate, prochlorperazine, tetracycline, carbonates, phosphates, sulfates, tartrates.

RATE/MODE OF ADMINISTRATION
IV push: 1 ml or fraction thereof over 1 min.
Intermittent: Only as an additive to nutritional support solution.
Continuous: Only as an additive to nutritional support solution.
Filter: Not applicable in dose less than 1 ml.

NURSING CONSIDERATIONS
Nursing Diagnoses
1. Potential for impairment of skin integrity, related to sloughing

and necrosis with IM or subcutaneous injection or IV extravasation.

2. Potential for injury, related to development of hypotension.

Acute Care

Maintain patient in supine position following administration to avoid postural hypotension. Avoid extravasation and determine patency of vein. Warm solution to body temperature prior to administration.

Precautions

May increase digitalis toxicity; use with extreme caution. Do not administer calcium salts through scalp vein needles in children.

Contraindications

Existing digitalis toxicity; refer to manufacturer's recommendations prior to administration to infants and children.

Side Effects

Neurologic: Tingling, heat waves.
Overdose: Coma, lethargy, weakness, marked nausea and vomiting, death.

Patient/Caregiver Teaching

Instruct patient (1) to report all side effects immediately and (2) to provide accurate medication history.

Home Care

Not recommended unless a component of nutritional support formula.

Administration in Other Clinical Settings

Not recommended unless a component of nutritional support formula.

Nursing Interventions

The physician should be notified of all side effects. Resuscitative equipment should be readily available. Treat extravasation with 1% procaine hydrochloride and hyaluronidase to reduce venospasm.

Calcium gluconate

US: Kalcinate
CAN: H-F Antidote Gel
(Pharmascience)

Replacement element   pH 6.0–8.2

ACTION

A basic element affecting bone, nerves, glands, and normal blood coagulation.

INDICATIONS/USES

Calcium gluconate is used to treat calcium deficiency caused by hypoparathyroidism, osteomalacia, vitamin D deficiency, and uremia; as an antidote for magnesium sulfate toxicity; and following blood transfusion to maintain calcium-potassium ratio.

USUAL DOSE

Adults: 0.5–2.0 g; repeat as needed up to 30 g or up to 60 ml by continuous IV.
- Cardiac resuscitation: Refer to product literature, 5–8 ml; repeat in 10 min if indicated.

Children: 2–5 ml/24 h every 2–3 days to a maximum of 500 mg/kg body wt/24 h in divided doses.

PREPARATION/RECONSTITUTION

May be given undiluted as a 10% solution.

INCOMPATIBILITIES

Amphotericin B, cefamandole, cefazolin, cephalothin, dobutamine, epinephrine, kanamycin, magnesium sulfate, potassium phosphate, promethazine, sodium bicarbonate, tetracycline. Do not mix with carbonates, phosphates, sulfates, or tartrates.

RATE/MODE OF ADMINISTRATION

IV push: 0.5 ml over 1 min.
Intermittent: Not applicable.

Continuous: Further diluted in 1000 ml of normal saline over 12–24 h.
Filter: Applicable; use according to institutional guidelines.

NURSING CONSIDERATIONS

Nursing Diagnoses

1. Potential impairment of skin integrity, related to extravasation of drug.
2. Potential alteration in cardiac output: decreased, related to drug side effects.

Acute Care

IV use is preferred in adult patients and is mandatory for infants and children. Avoid extravasation: may cause necrosis and sloughing of tissue. Confirm patency of vein.

Precautions

Use with caution in patients receiving digitalis (may increase toxicity). Vasodilation may cause mild hypotension. Respiratory and cardiac arrest may occur.

Contraindications

Digitalis toxicity.

Side Effects

Cardiovascular: Bradycardia, cardiac arrest, flushing, heat waves, prolonged cardiac contraction.
Neurologic: Tingling sensations, depressed neuromuscular function.

Patient/Caregiver Teaching

Instruct patient to report all side effects immediately.

Home Care

Not recommended.

Administration in Other Clinical Settings

Not recommended.

Nursing Interventions

The physician must be notified of all side effects immediately. Discontinue drug; resuscitate as needed. Emergency equipment should be available.

Carbenicillin disodium
US: Geopen, Pyopen

Bactericidal penicillin   pH 5.9—8.0

ACTION

An extended spectrum penicillin; bactericidal against many gram-positive, gram-negative, and anaerobic organisms.

INDICATIONS/USES

Used in the treatment of urinary tract infections, severe systemic infections, and septicemia caused by susceptible organisms; used to treat severe respiratory infections and soft tissue infections.

USUAL DOSE

Adults: 1–10 g every 4–6 h; not to exceed 40 g/24 h.
Children: 50–500 mg/kg body wt 24 h in divided doses; not to exceed the lesser of 500 mg/kg/24 h or 40 g/24 h.

PREPARATION/RECONSTITUTION

Reconstitute 1 g in 2–2.6 ml sterile water for injection; further dilute with at least 5 ml sterile water for injection prior to IV push administration.

INCOMPATIBILITIES

Aminoglycosides, amphotericin B, bleomycin, chloramphenicol, lincomycin, promethazine, tetracycline, vitamin B with C.

RATE/MODE OF ADMINISTRATION

IV push: Following dilution requirements over 3–5 min.
Intermittent: Appropriate in 50–100 ml fluid over 30–120 min.
Continuous: Not recommended.
Filter: Applicable; use according to institutional guidelines.

NURSING CONSIDERATIONS

Nursing Diagnoses

1. Potential for injury or trauma, related to neurologic effects of drug.
2. Potential for alteration in sensory-perceptual function, related to drug side effects.

Acute Care

Assess patient for history of penicillin sensitivities. Sensitivity studies are indicated prior to administration of this drug. Administer within 24 h of preparation to avoid deactivation. Avoid extravasation and confirm patency of vein prior to administration. Avoid prolonged use to avoid superinfection caused by overgrowth. Baseline and periodic evaluations of renal, hepatic, and hematopoietic systems are recommended.

Precautions

Watch for early symptoms of allergic reaction/sensitivity to this drug. Inactivated by chloramphenicol, erythromycin, and tetracyclines. Risk of bleeding in the patient receiving anticoagulant therapy is increased. Drug elimination is reduced in neonates.

Contraindications

History of sensitivity to penicillins; pregnancy.

Side Effects

Hematologic: Increased clotting or PT, anemia, eosinophilia.
Dermatologic: Urticaria, itching.
Neurologic: Irritability, convulsions.
Other: Change in taste in mouth, elevated temperature, anaphylaxis.

Patient/Caregiver Teaching
Instruct patient (1) to report all side effects immediately, and (2) to report known penicillin sensitivities.

Home Care
Appropriate.

Administration in Other Clinical Settings
Appropriate.

Nursing Interventions
The physician should be notified of all side effects immediately. Resuscitative equipment should be readily available. Test dose should be given in the presence of a licensed physician prior to home administration of this drug.

Carmustine (BCNU)
US: BiCNU
CAN: BiCNU (Bristol)

Alkylating agent   pH 5.6–6.0

ACTION
An alkylating agent with antitumor activity, cell-cycle phase non-specific. Excreted unchanged in the urine; small amounts are excreted as respiratory carbon dioxide.

INDICATIONS/USES
Used to suppress or retard neoplastic growth of brain tumors; multiple myeloma; gastrointestinal, breast, bronchogenic, and renal carcinoma; Hodgkin's disease and some non-Hodgkin's lymphomas.

USUAL DOSE

Initial dose of 200 mg/m^2; may be given as a single dose, or half of calculated dose may be given on day 1 and half on day 2 of treatment.

PREPARATION/RECONSTITUTION

Refer to precautions listed in Appendix 14. Special techniques are required to avoid contamination with this drug agent. Reconstitute 200-mg vial with sterile diluent supplied (3 ml of absolute ethanol); further dilute with 27 ml of sterile water for injection to yield 3.3 mg/ml carmustine. Further dilute desired dose for administration as an infusion.

INCOMPATIBILITIES

Considered incompatible with all other drugs due to toxicities.

RATE/MODE OF ADMINISTRATION

IV push: No.
Intermittent: No.
Continuous: Yes, per manufacturer's recommendations in 5% dextrose or 0.9% sodium chloride solution by electronic infusion device.
Filter: Applicable; follow institutional guidelines.

NURSING CONSIDERATIONS

Nursing Diagnoses

1. Potential for alteration in skin integrity, related to possible extravasation of this nitrogen mustard preparation.
2. Potential for alteration in nutrition, related to drug side effects.

Acute Care

Obtain baseline blood laboratory studies prior to administration and adjust dose downward for platelet count below 75,000, leukocytes below 3000, and when used with other myelosuppressive agents. Allow 6 weeks between doses to avoid delayed toxicities. Avoid contact of carmustine with skin. Observe patient carefully for signs/symptoms of impending infection and maintain hydration level.

Precautions

May be potentiated by hepatotoxic or nephrotoxic medications or radiation therapy. Best administered in the inpatient environment under the direction of a licensed physician. Prophylactic administration of antiemetic agents may be needed.

Contraindications

Known hypersensitivity to carmustine; previous chemotherapy.

Side Effects

Hematologic: Bone marrow toxicity, anemia, elevated liver function tests.
Gastrointestinal: Nausea, extreme vomiting.
Renal: Abnormalities.
EENT: Retinal hemorrhage.

Patient/Caregiver Teaching

Instruct patient (1) to report all side effects immediately and (2) to provide accurate drug profile of other concurrent treatments.

Home Care

Appropriate in a controlled environment.

Administration in Other Clinical Settings

Appropriate in a controlled environment.

Nursing Interventions

The physician should be notified of all side effects immediately. Carmustine therapy may be withheld pending recovery of hematopoietic depression.

Cefamandole nafate

US: Mandol
CAN: Mandol (Lilly)

Second-generation cephalosporin   pH 6.0–8.5

ACTION

A second-generation cephalosporin antibiotic that is bactericidal to gram-positive, gram-negative, and some anaerobic organisms. Excreted in the urine and secreted in breast milk.

INDICATIONS/USES

Used in the treatment of serious respiratory, GU, bone, joint, soft tissue, and skin infections; septicemia; and peritonitis. Used to provide perioperative prophylaxis.

USUAL DOSE

Adults: 500 mg–2 g every 4–8 h according to severity of illness; not to exceed 12 g/24 h.
- Perioperative prophylaxis: 1–2 g 30–60 min before surgery followed by 1–2 g every 6 h for 24–48 h.

Children: 50 to 150 mg/kg body wt/24 h in equally divided doses every 4–8 h not to exceed 12 g/24 h.
- Perioperative prophylaxis: 50–100 mg/kg/24 h in equally divided doses for infants over 3 mo old. Administer initial dose 30–60 min preoperatively and then every 6 h for 48–72 h.

PREPARATION/RECONSTITUTION

Reconstitute each gram with 10 ml sterile water for injection, 5% dextrose in water, or 0.9% sodium chloride solution.

INCOMPATIBILITIES

All aminoglycosides, cimetidine, lidocaine, magnesium.

RATE/MODE OF ADMINISTRATION

IV push: In 10 ml of diluent as indicated.
Intermittent: Applicable in 100 ml dextrose or saline by appropriate Y-site.
Continuous: In 1000 ml compatible solution.
Filter: Applicable, consistent with institutional guidelines.

NURSING CONSIDERATIONS

Nursing Diagnoses

1. Potential for injury, related to drug side effects and tendency for bleeding disorders.
2. Potential for alteration in bowel elimination: diarrhea, related to drug side effects.
3. Potential for alteration in comfort: pain, related to thrombophlebitis.

Acute Care

Sensitivity studies are indicated to ensure susceptibility of the causative organism. Monitor patient for early signs of sensitivity reaction. Monitor renal function and calculate dosage consistent with degree of impairment. Administer within 24 h of preparation if unrefrigerated or 96 h if refrigerated, consistent with manufacturer's recommendations.

Precautions

Symptoms of acute alcohol intolerance may occur with alcohol usage. Do not mix in the same container with aminoglycosides or administer through same IV administration tubing. Avoid concurrent administration of bacteriostatic agents. Avoid storing in syringe. Monitor patient for high sodium levels due to heavy sodium content of this drug.

Contraindications

Known sensitivity.

Side Effects

Gastrointestinal: Diarrhea, nausea, vomiting, oral thrush, anorexia.
Hematologic: Anemia, bleeding episodes, leukopenia, jaundice, neutropenia.

Other: Positive direct Coombs' test, thrombophlebitis, false-positive reaction for urine glucose except with Tes-Tape or Keto-Diastix; anaphylaxis.

Patient/Caregiver Teaching

Instruct patient (1) to report all side effects immediately and (2) to provide accurate drug profile and family history.

Home Care

Appropriate.

Administration in Other Clinical Settings

Appropriate.

Nursing Interventions

The physician should be notified of all side effects. Initial dose should be administered in a monitored environment. Resuscitative equipment and emergency drugs should be readily available. Hemodialysis may be useful in event of overdose.

Cefazolin sodium

US: Ancef, Kefzol
CAN: Ancef (SK & F)

First-generation cephalosporin   pH 4.8–5.5

ACTION

A first-generation cephalosporin antibiotic that is bactericidal to some gram-positive and gram-negative organisms, including staphylococci and streptococci. Excreted in the urine and secreted in breast milk.

INDICATIONS/USES

Used in the treatment of serious infections of bone, joints, skin, soft tissue, cardiovascular system, respiratory tract, and GU tract. Used for perioperative prophylaxis.

USUAL DOSE

Adults: 250 mg–1.5 g every 6–8 h; maximum of 12 g in 24 h.
- Perioperative prophylaxis: 1 g 30–60 min before surgery; repeat 0.5–1.0 g in 2 h and every 6–8 h for 24 h for up to 5 days.

Children: 25–50 mg/kg body wt/24 h in 3–4 divided doses; may increase to 100 mg/kg/24 h for severe infections.

Neonates: Safety not established for infants less than 1 mo old; aminoglycosides preferred.

PREPARATION/RECONSTITUTION

Reconstitute each gram in 10 ml sterile water for injection. To reduce the incidence of phlebitis, further dilute in 50–100 ml of 5% dextrose in water, 0.9% sodium chloride solution, or other compatible infusate.

INCOMPATIBILITIES

Amikacin, amobarbital, ascorbic acid, bleomycin, calcium gluceptate, calcium gluconate, cimetidine, erythromycin, kanamycin, lidocaine hydrochloride, tetracycline, vitamin B with C.

RATE/MODE OF ADMINISTRATION

IV push: Yes, 500 mg or 1 g in 10 ml of diluent over 3–5 min.

Intermittent: Yes, by Y-set or additive infusion set; also available as premixed solution for piggyback administration.

Continuous: No.

Filter: Applicable; use consistent with institutional guidelines.

NURSING CONSIDERATIONS

Nursing Diagnoses

1. Potential for impaired bowel elimination: diarrhea, related to drug side effects.
2. Potential for alteration in cardiac output: decreased, related to drug side effects.

Acute Care

Sensitivity studies should be performed prior to administration of this drug. Dose is calculated according to degree of impairment in renal failure patients. Prolonged use may lead to superinfection.

Administer within 24 h of preparation, or within 96 h if refrigerated. Continuous infusion will increase the incidence of thrombophlebitis.

Precautions

Safety for use in infants has not been determined. Monitor patient for signs/symptoms of hypernatremia or other electrolyte disturbance; contains 2.1 mEq sodium per gram of medication. Avoid concurrent administration of bacteriostatic agents. Use with caution in penicillin-sensitive patients.

Contraindications

Known sensitivity to cephalosporins or penicillin antibiotics.

Side Effects

Gastrointestinal: Diarrhea, nausea, vomiting, oral thrush.
Hematologic: Elevated SGOT, SGPT, BUN, alkaline phosphatase, neutropenia, leukopenia.
Other: Phlebitis, false-positive reaction for urine glucose except with Tes-Tape or Keto-Diastix.

Patient/Caregiver Teaching

Instruct patient (1) to report all side effects immediately (including signs of allergic reaction); (2) to provide accurate drug and allergen profile; and (3) to learn principles of home self-administration and monitoring techniques.

Home Care

Appropriate.

Administration in Other Clinical Settings

Appropriate.

Nursing Interventions

The physician should be notified of all side effects immediately. Resuscitative equipment should be readily available. Initial dose should be given in inpatient environment.

Cefonicid sodium

US: Monocid

Second-generation cephalosporin   pH 3.5–6.5

ACTION
A second-generation cephalosporin antibiotic that is bactericidal to selected gram-negative, gram-positive, and anaerobic organisms. Excreted in the urine; also crosses the placental barrier and is secreted in breast milk.

INDICATIONS/USES
Used in the treatment of serious infections of the lower respiratory tract, urinary tract, skin and skin structures, and septicemia. Used for perioperative prophylaxis as indicated.

USUAL DOSE
0.5–2.0 g in 24 h.

Perioperative prophylaxis: 1 g IV 1 h before incision, except during cesarean section (given only after clamping of umbilical cord). Repeat daily dose for 2 days in patients of prosthetic arthroplasty or open heart surgery.

PREPARATION/RECONSTITUTION
Reconstitute 0.5 g in 2 ml sterile water injection for a final concentration of 220 mg/ml.

INCOMPATIBILITIES
Aminoglycosides.

RATE/MODE OF ADMINISTRATION
IV push: Yes, over 3–5 min.
Intermittent: Further dilute in 50–100 ml of 5% dextrose in water or 0.9% sodium chloride solution to be given over 20–30 min.
Continuous: No.
Filter: Applicable; use according to institutional guidelines.

NURSING CONSIDERATIONS
Nursing Diagnoses
1. Potential for alteration in bowel elimination: diarrhea, related to drug side effects.
2. Potential for alteration in cardiac output: decreased, related to sodium content of drug.

Acute Care
Sensitivity studies are indicated prior to administration of this drug. If renal function is impaired, reduce total daily dose and monitor patient carefully. Phlebitis may be avoided through strict adherence to site rotation and careful site selection. Drug is stable for 24 h at room temperature; 72 h if refrigerated. Slight yellowing does not affect potency of admixed solution.

Precautions
Do not mix with aminoglycosides in same infusion or give concurrently to avoid danger of severe nephrotoxicity. Avoid concurrent administration of bacteriostatic agents. Electrolyte imbalances may occur due to sodium content (3.7 mEq/g) of this drug.

Contraindications
Known sensitivity to cefonicid or penicillins.

Side Effects
Hematologic: Increase in platelets and eosinophils and elevated alkaline phosphatase, SGOT, SGPT, GGTP, and LDH.
Gastrointestinal: Diarrhea.
Other: Burning, discomfort at injection site.

Patient/Caregiver Teaching
Instruct patient (1) to report all side effects immediately; (2) to provide accurate history of allergic reactions and drug sensitivities; and (3) to learn principles of home self-administration.

Home Care
Appropriate.

Administration in Other Clinical Settings
Appropriate.

Nursing Interventions

The physician should be notified of all side effects. Mild cases of colitis may respond to discontinuation of drug. Resuscitative equipment should be readily available. Hemodialysis may be useful to treat overdose.

Cefoperazone sodium

US: Cefobid
CAN: Cefobid (Pfizer)

Third-generation cephalosporin   pH 4.5–6.5

ACTION

Broad-spectrum cephalosporin antibiotic effective against organisms resistant to other second- and third-generation cephalosporins; bactericidal to many gram-negative, gram-positive, and anaerobic organisms. Excreted in the bile; also crosses the placental barrier and is excreted in breast milk.

INDICATIONS/USES

Used in the treatment of infections of the respiratory tract, intraabdominal area, skin and skin structure, gynecologic system, and bacterial septicemia.

USUAL DOSE

2–4 g/24 h in divided doses every 12 h; may be increased in severe infections.

PREPARATION/RECONSTITUTION

Reconstitute each gram in 5 ml sterile water and shake vigorously; examine for clarity of solution. Further dilute each gram with 20–40 ml 5% dextrose in water, or 0.9% sodium chloride solution to maximum preparation/dilution of 50 mg/ml for intermittent infusion or 2–25 mg/ml for continuous infusate.

INCOMPATIBILITIES

Incompatible in solution or syringe with all aminoglycosides and other bacteriostatic agents.

RATE/MODE OF ADMINISTRATION

IV push: No.
Intermittent: Consistent with dilution guidelines.
Continuous: Consistent with dilution guidelines.
Filter: Applicable; use consistent with institutional guidelines.

NURSING CONSIDERATIONS

Nursing Diagnoses

1. Potential for impaired fluid volume: deficit, related to nephrotoxicity.
2. Potential for impaired bowel function: diarrhea, related to drug side effects.

Acute Care

Administer within 24 h of preparation; refer to manufacturer's recommendations concerning use of diluent to ensure stability without benefit of refrigeration. Use with extreme caution in the penicillin-sensitive patient; symptoms of acute alcohol intolerance will occur with concomitant use of alcohol. May contribute to thrombophlebitis: select site carefully and rotate sites faithfully, consistent with institutional guidelines. Monitor patient for electrolyte imbalance related to high sodium level (1.5 mEq/g) of this drug.

Precautions

Platelet dysfunction may be avoided by limiting dose to 4 g/24 h and administering vitamin K. Avoid superinfection by limiting prolonged use of drug. Do not mix with aminoglycosides in solution. Use with caution in patient with hepatic dysfunction.

Contraindications

Known sensitivity to cephalosporins or penicillins; not recommended for use in children.

Side Effects

Hematologic: Abnormal bleeding; decreased hemoglobin/hematocrit; decreased PT and platelet function; elevated SGOT, SGPT, total bilirubin, alkaline phosphatase, LDH, and BUN (transient); leukopenia; eosinophilia.

Gastrointestinal: Colitis, vomiting, diarrhea.

Respiratory: Dyspnea.

Other: Phlebitis, vaginitis, false-positive reaction for urine glucose except with Tes-Tape or Keto-Diastix.

Patient/Caregiver Teaching

Instruct patient (1) to report all side effects immediately; (2) to report accurate history of allergic reactions and drug sensitivities; and (3) to learn principles of home self-administration.

Home Care

Appropriate.

Administration in Other Clinical Settings

Appropriate.

Nursing Interventions

The physician should be notified of all side effects immediately. First dose should be administered in the inpatient environment. Vitamin K, fresh frozen plasma, packed RBC, or platelet concentrates may be indicated to treat abnormal bleeding tendencies.

Ceforanide

US: Precef

Second-generation cephalosporin   pH 5.5–8.5

ACTION

Broad-spectrum second-generation cephalosporin antibiotic; bactericidal to selected gram-negative, gram-positive, and anaerobic organisms. Excreted unchanged in the urine; also crosses the placental barrier and is secreted in breast milk.

INDICATIONS/USES

Used in the treatment of serious infections of the lower respiratory tract, urinary tract, skin and skin structure, bone, and joints and of subacute bacterial endocarditis. Used as adjunctive therapy for perioperative prophylaxis.

USUAL DOSE

Adults: 0.5 to 1.0 g/12 h.
- *Perioperative prophylaxis:* 0.5 to 1.0 g given 1 h before incision; may repeat for 2 doses in prosthetic arthroplasty or open heart surgery.

Children: 20–40 mg/kg body wt/24 h in divided doses every 12 h.

PREPARATION/RECONSTITUTION

Reconstitute each 0.5 g with 5 ml sterile water for injection or 0.9% sodium chloride solution for a concentration of 100 mg/ml.

INCOMPATIBILITIES

Incompatible in syringe or solution with any other bacteriostatic agent and all aminoglycosides.

RATE/MODE OF ADMINISTRATION

IV push: As a single dose in adequate diluent over 3–5 min.

Intermittent: Over 30 min by Y-site or piggyback administration set. Discontinuation of the primary solution while giving the drug is recommended.

Continuous: No.

Filter: Applicable in doses exceeding 1 ml; refer to institutional guidelines.

NURSING CONSIDERATIONS

Nursing Diagnoses

1. Potential for alteration in bowel elimination, related to development of colitis.
2. Potential for alteration in nutrition: less than body requirements, related to drug side effects.

Acute Care

Sensitivity studies should be performed prior to administration to ensure susceptibility of this drug to the organisms in question.

Monitor patient for early evidence of allergic reaction. Administer within 24 h of preparation; may be light yellow to amber in color depending on concentration and type of diluent used. May be administered concomitantly with aminoglycosides but never in same syringe or infusate. Potential for nephrotoxicity is increased when both drugs are used.

Precautions

Note concerns when used concomitantly with aminoglycosides. Avoid concurrent administration of bacteriostatic agents. May cause thrombophlebitis and infusion sites should be rotated carefully. Ceforanide is sodium-free.

Contraindications

Known sensitivity to cephalosporins or penicillins.

Side Effects

Gastrointestinal: Diarrhea, nausea, vomiting.
Hematologic: Elevated alkaline phosphatase, SGOT, SGPT, and BUN; transient thrombocytosis.
Other: Burning, discomfort, and pain at injection site.

Patient/Caregiver Teaching

Instruct patient (1) to report all side effects immediately and (2) to learn principles of IV home self-administration.

Home Care

Appropriate; administer initial dose in inpatient environment.

Administration in Other Clinical Settings

Appropriate; administer initial dose in inpatient environment.

Nursing Interventions

The physician should be notified of all side effects immediately. Resuscitative equipment should be readily available. Mild cases of colitis may respond to discontinuation of the drug. Hemodialysis may be useful to reverse overdose.

Cefotaxime sodium

US: Claforan
CAN: Claforan (Roussel)

Third-generation cephalosporin   pH 5–7

ACTION

Broad-spectrum third-generation cephalosporin antibiotic. Excreted in the urine; also crosses the placental barrier and is secreted in breast milk.

INDICATIONS/USES

Used in the treatment of serious infections of the respiratory tract, urinary tract, skin and skin structure, abdomen, bone and joint, and CNS; bacteremia/septicemia. Also used in perioperative prophylaxis.

USUAL DOSE

Adults: 1–2 g every 4–8 h; maximum daily dose is 12 g.
- Perioperative prophylaxis: 1 g 30–90 min before incision; then 1 g 30–120 min later.

Children
- Newborn to 1 wk: 50 mg/kg body wt every 12 h. *Note: Buildup of cephalosporins in neonates may increase half-life of drug, resulting in less frequent dosing for young infants.*
- 1–4 wk: 50 mg/kg every 8 h.
- 1 mo–12 yr: Child's weight minus 50 mg, 50–180 mg/kg/day in 4–6 divided doses.

PREPARATION/RECONSTITUTION

Reconstitute each dose with 10 ml sterile water, 5% dextrose in water, 0.9% sodium chloride solution, or other compatible infusate. Available in premixed form.

INCOMPATIBILITIES

Incompatible in syringe or solution with any other bacteriostatic agent, all aminoglycosides, all diluents with a pH of 7.5 or greater.

RATE/MODE OF ADMINISTRATION

IV push: Administer over 3–5 min.

Intermittent: Over 30 min by Y-site or piggyback administration set. Discontinue primary fluid temporarily.

Continuous: In 500–1000 ml over 6–24 h by electronic infusion device, if available.

Filter: Applicable to prevent danger of infusion phlebitis; use consistent with institutional guidelines.

NURSING CONSIDERATIONS

Nursing Diagnoses

1. Potential for alteration in bowel elimination: increase, related to development of diarrhea.
2. Potential for ineffective breathing pattern, related to dyspnea.
3. Potential for alteration in cardiac output, related to high sodium content of drug.

Acute Care

Sensitivity studies should be performed prior to administration of this drug. Avoid prolonged use which could lead to superinfection and overgrowth. Administer within 24 h of preparation, or within 5 days if refrigerated. Avoid concurrent use of bacteriostatic agents. Rotate IV sites carefully to avoid thrombophlebitis.

Precautions

Use only if absolutely necessary in pregnancy. Reduce total daily dose if patient has impaired renal function. Sodium content (2.2 mEq/g) of this drug may produce electrolyte imbalance and cardiac irregularities.

Contraindications

Known sensitivity to cephalosporins or penicillins.

Side Effects

Hematologic: Decreased hemoglobin or hematocrit; decreased PT and platelet functions; elevated SGOT, SGPT, total bilirubin, alkaline phosphatase, LDH, and BUN (transient); eosinophilia; leukopenia; transient neutropenia.

Gastrointestinal: Vomiting, diarrhea.

Respiratory: Dyspnea.
Other: Positive direct Coombs' test, pseudomembranous colitis, vaginitis, false-positive reaction for urine glucose except with Tes-Tape or Keto-Diastix, fever.

Patient/Caregiver Teaching
Instruct patient (1) to report all side effects immediately; (2) to report known sensitivity to penicillins; and (3) to learn principles of home self-administration.

Home Care
Appropriate; administer initial dose in inpatient environment.

Administration in Other Clinical Settings
Appropriate; administer initial dose in inpatient environment.

Nursing Interventions
The physician should be notified of all side effects immediately. Hemodialysis may be useful to counteract overdose. Resuscitative equipment should be readily available.

Cefotetan disodium
US: Cefotan

Third-generation cephalosporin   pH 4.5–6.5

ACTION
A third-generation cephalosporin antibiotic bactericidal to selected gram-negative, gram-positive, and anaerobic organisms. Excreted in the urine; also crosses the placental barrier and is secreted in breast milk.

INDICATIONS/USES
Used in the treatment of serious infections of the lower respiratory tract, urinary tract, skin and structure, abdomen, bone and joint infections. Also used for perioperative prophylaxis.

USUAL DOSE

1–2 g every 12 h for a period of 5–10 days; not to exceed 6 g/24 h.
Perioperative prophylaxis: 1–2 g given 30–60 min prior to incision.

PREPARATION/RECONSTITUTION

Reconstitute each gram with 10 ml sterile water for injection.

INCOMPATIBILITIES

Incompatible in syringe or solution with any other bacteriostatic agent and all aminoglycosides.

RATE/MODE OF ADMINISTRATION

IV push: As a single dose over 3–5 min.
Intermittent: Yes, over 30 min by Y-site or piggyback administration
  set; may wish to temporarily discontinue primary fluid.
Continuous: No.
Filter: Applicable; use according to institutional guidelines.

NURSING CONSIDERATIONS

Nursing Diagnoses

1. Potential for alteration in bowel elimination: increase, related to development of diarrhea.
2. Potential for alteration in fluid volume: deficit, related to side effects of drug and bleeding tendencies.

Acute Care

Perform sensitivity studies prior to use and monitor patients for evidence of allergic reaction. Avoid prolonged use to prevent superinfection caused by overgrowth. Administer within 24 h of preparation, or within 96 h if refrigerated. Drug is stable following preparation/dilution for one full week if kept frozen; thaw at room temperature prior to use and do not refreeze; slight yellowing does not affect potency of this drug.

Precautions

May be used concomitantly with aminoglycosides, but the drugs should not be mixed in same syringe or infusate. May potentiate action of oral anticoagulants; use with caution. Avoid concurrent administration of bacteriostatic agents. May cause phlebitis; avoid by rotating IV sites carefully. Contains 3.5 mEq sodium per gram and may cause electrolyte imbalance and cardiac irregularities.

Contraindications

Known sensitivity to cephalosporins or related antibiotics.

Side Effects

Hematologic: Bleeding episodes, eosinophilia, and elevated alkaline phosphatase, SGOT, SGPT, and LDH.

Gastrointestinal: Diarrhea, pseudomembranous colitis, nausea.

Other: False-positive for urine glucose with Benedict's or Fehling's solution; discomfort and pain at injection site.

Patient/Caregiver Teaching

Instruct patient (1) to report all side effects immediately; (2) to provide accurate history of allergic reactions and drug sensitivities; and (3) to learn principles of home self-administration of this drug.

Home Care

Appropriate; administer initial dose in inpatient environment.

Administration in Other Clinical Settings

Appropriate; administer initial dose in inpatient environment.

Nursing Interventions

The physician should be notified of all side effects immediately. Discontinue the drug if necessary. Resuscitative equipment should be readily available. Bleeding episodes may respond to administration of vitamin K or require discontinuation of cefotetan. Hemodialysis may reverse overdose.

Cefoxitin sodium
US: Mefoxin

Second-generation cephalosporin   pH 4.2–7.0

ACTION
A second-generation cephalosporin antibiotic; bactericidal to many gram-negative, gram-positive, and anaerobic organisms. Excreted in the urine and secreted in breast milk.

INDICATIONS/USES
Used in treatment of serious infections of the respiratory tract, GU tract, abdomen, bone and joint, skin, and skin structure and in septicemia and perioperative prophylaxis.

USUAL DOSE
Adults: 1–2 g every 6–8 h.
- Perioperative prophylaxis: 2 g given 30–60 min prior to incision followed by 2 g every 6 h for 24–72 h. Follow manufacturer's recommendations prior to use for cesarean section.

Children over 3 mo: 80–260 mg/kg body wt/24 h in equally divided doses; maximum 12 g/day.
- Perioperative prophylaxis: 30–40 mg/kg every 6 h.

Infants: 80–160 mg/kg/day in 4 to 6 equally divided doses.

PREPARATION/RECONSTITUTION
Reconstitute each gram in 10 ml sterile water, 5% dextrose in water, or 0.9% sodium chloride solution. May dilute a single dose in 50–1000 ml for continuous infusion.

INCOMPATIBILITIES
All aminoglycosides.

RATE/MODE OF ADMINISTRATION
IV push: Over 3–5 min (1–2 g/10 ml).
Intermittent: Yes, by Y-site or piggyback administration set; temporarily discontinuing other fluids at same site is recommended.

Continuous: Yes, properly dilute by electronic infusion device, if available.

Filter: Applicable; use consistent with institutional guidelines.

NURSING CONSIDERATIONS

Nursing Diagnoses

1. Potential for alteration in comfort, related to development of thrombophlebitis.

2. Potential for alteration in nutrition: less than body requirements, related to side effects of drug.

Acute Care

Obtain sensitivity studies to determine appropriateness of therapy prior to use. Avoid prolonged use of drug to prevent overgrowth and superinfection. Administer within 24 h of preparation, or 48 h if refrigerated. May be used concomitantly with aminoglycosides, but never to be mixed in same syringe or infusate. To avoid danger of phlebitis, rotate IV site carefully and ensure patency of vessel.

Precautions

Safety for infants under 3 mo of age has not been established; use with caution in pregnancy. Contains 2.3 mEq sodium per gram; may contribute to electrolyte imbalance and cardiac irregularities.

Contraindications

Known sensitivity to cephalosporins or penicillins.

Side Effects

Gastrointestinal: Nausea, vomiting.

Hematologic: Leukopenia, neutropenia, and transient elevation of BUN, SGOT, SGPT, and alkaline phosphatase.

Other: Thrombophlebitis, pseudomembranous colitis, false-positive for urine glucose except with Tes-Tape or Keto-Diastix, pain at injection site.

Patient/Caregiver Teaching

Instruct patient (1) to report all side effects immediately; (2) to provide accurate drug profile; (3) to learn principles of home self-administration; and (4) to recognize signs and symptoms of impending phlebitis.

Home Care
Appropriate; administer initial dose in inpatient environment.

Administration in Other Clinical Settings
Appropriate; administer initial dose in inpatient environment.

Nursing Interventions
The physician should be notified of all side effects immediately. Resuscitative equipment should be readily available.

Ceftazidime
US: Fortax, Tazidime, Tazicef

Third-generation cephalosporin   pH 5–8

ACTION
A third-generation cephalosporin antibiotic; bactericidal to selected gram-positive, gram-negative, and anaerobic organisms. Excreted in the urine; also crosses the placental barrier and may be secreted in breast milk.

INDICATIONS/USES
Used in the treatment of serious infections of the lower respiratory tract, urinary tract, skin and skin structures, bone and joint, abdomen, and CNS.

USUAL DOSE
Adults: 1 g every 8–12 h to maximum of 6 g/day, based on severity of illness; continue for at least 2 days; maximum dose 6 g/day.
Children
- 1 mo–12 yr: 30–50 mg/kg body wt every 8 h not to exceed 6 g/24 h.
- Newborn to 1 mo: 30 mg/kg every 12 hours.

PREPARATION/RECONSTITUTION

Reconstitute 0.5 g with 5 ml sterile water for injection and shake well (will generate CO_2). Vent with needle attached to syringe barrel prior to drawing up dose; do not inject air into the vial.

INCOMPATIBILITIES

Incompatible in syringe or solution with many other bacteriostatic agents and all aminoglycosides; compatible with cefuroxime, heparin, potassium chloride.

RATE/MODE OF ADMINISTRATION

IV push: Yes, over 3–5 min.
Intermittent: Yes, 500 mg in 25 ml or 1 g in 50–100 ml of infusate over 30 min by Y-site or piggyback administration set.
Continuous: Not recommended; may be utilized if indicated.
Filter: Applicable; use consistent with institutional guidelines.

NURSING CONSIDERATIONS

Nursing Diagnoses

1. Potential for alteration in nutrition, related to drug side effects.
2. Potential for alteration in patient comfort, related to phlebitis and discomfort associated with drug.

Acute Care

Sensitivity studies should be obtained prior to administration of this drug. Avoid prolonged use to avoid superinfection and drug overgrowth. Administer within 18 h of preparation, or refrigerate for maximum of 7 days. May be frozen for up to 3 mo after initial dilution; thaw at room temperature after frozen and do not refreeze. Solution may be light yellow or amber and is safe to use. Rotate IV site with care to avoid phlebitis.

Precautions

Avoid concurrent administration of bacteriostatic agents; sometimes ordered in antibiotic regimen with aminoglycosides, vancomycin, or clindamycin. Each gram contains 2.3 mEq of sodium and may contribute to electrolyte imbalance and cardiac irregularities. Cross-sensitivity may occur in penicillin-sensitive patients; use with extreme caution.

Contraindications

Known sensitivity to ceftazidime, cephalosporins, or penicillins.

Side Effects

Hematologic: Elevated alkaline phosphatase, SGOT, SGPT, and BUN.
Gastrointestinal: Nausea, vomiting, diarrhea.
Other: Pseudomembranous colitis, burning, and discomfort at injection site.

Patient/Caregiver Teaching

Instruct patient (1) to report all side effects immediately; (2) to provide accurate history of allergic reactions and drug sensitivities; (3) to report discomfort at injection site; and (4) to learn principles of home self-administration.

Home Care

Appropriate; administer initial dose in inpatient environment.

Administration in Other Clinical Settings

Appropriate; administer initial dose in inpatient environment.

Nursing Interventions

The physician should be notified of all side effects. Resuscitative equipment should be readily available. Hemodialysis may counteract overdose. Mild cases of colitis may respond to discontinuation of ceftazidime.

Ceftizoxime sodium
US: Cefizox

Third-generation cephalosporin   pH 6–8

ACTION

A third-generation cephalosporin antibiotic bactericidal to gram-negative, gram-positive, and anaerobic organisms. Excreted in the urine; also crosses the placental barrier and is secreted in breast milk.

INDICATIONS/USES

Used in the treatment of serious infections of the lower respiratory tract, urinary tract, abdomen, skin and skin structure, and bone and joint, and septicemia and gonorrhea.

USUAL DOSE

Adults: 500 mg–4 g every 8–12 h.
Children over 6 mo: 50 mg/kg body wt/every 6–8 h; up to 200 mg/kg has been used. Maximum dose 12 g/day.

PREPARATION/RECONSTITUTION

Reconstitute each gram with 10 ml sterile water for injection or 0.9% sodium chloride for injection.

INCOMPATIBILITIES

Incompatible in syringe or solution with all other bacteriostatic agents and all aminoglycosides.

RATE/MODE OF ADMINISTRATION

IV push: As a single dose over 3–5 min.
Intermittent: Yes, by Y-site or piggyback administration set in 50–100 ml of infusate over 30 minutes.
Continuous: No.
Filter: Applicable; use consistent with institutional guidelines.

NURSING CONSIDERATIONS

Nursing Diagnoses

1. Potential for alteration in comfort, related to drug side effects.
2. Potential for injury, related to development of bleeding disorders.

Acute Care

Sensitivity studies should precede administration of this drug. Administer within 8 h of preparation, or within 48 h if refrigerated. Avoid concurrent administration of bacteriostatic agents. May cause phlebitis; rotate IV sites carefully consistent with institutional policy.

Precautions

Contains 2.6 mEq sodium per gram; may contribute to electrolyte imbalance and cardiac irregularities. Monitor patient carefully for development of same. Use in pregnancy only if absolutely necessary. Adverse interaction may occur with promethazine, procainamide, quinidine, muscle relaxants, potent diuretics, and aminoglycosides.

Contraindications

Known sensitivity to cephalosporins or penicillins. Do not give to children under 6 mo of age.

Side Effects

Hematologic: Decreased hemoglobin or hematocrit; decreased PT and platelet function; elevated SGOT, SGPT, total bilirubin, alkaline phosphatase, LDH, and BUN (transient); thrombocytopenia; leukopenia.

Gastrointestinal: Oral thrush, vomiting, diarrhea, nausea.

Other: Pseudomembranous colitis, vaginitis, dyspnea, false-positive reaction for urine glucose except with Tes-Tape or Keto-Diastix.

Patient/Caregiver Teaching

Instruct patient (1) to report all side effects immediately; (2) to provide accurate history of allergic reactions and drug sensitivities; and (3) to learn principles of home self-administration.

Home Care

Appropriate; administer initial dose in inpatient environment.

Administration in Other Clinical Settings

Appropriate; administer initial dose in inpatient setting.

Nursing Interventions

The physician should be notified of all side effects immediately. Resuscitative equipment should be readily available. Hemodialysis may reverse overdose.

Ceftriaxone sodium

US: Rocephin

Third-generation cephalosporin   pH 6.7

ACTION

A third-generation cephalosporin antibiotic bactericidal to selected gram-positive, gram-negative, and anaerobic organisms. Excreted through bile and urine; also crosses the placental barrier and is secreted in breast milk.

INDICATIONS/USES

Used in the treatment of serious infections of the lower respiratory tract, urinary tract, skin and skin structure, bone and joint, and abdomen; bacterial septicemia; meningitis. Also used in perioperative prophylaxis.

USUAL DOSE

Adults: 1–2 g as a single dose every 24 h or in equally divided doses every 12 h; not to exceed 4 g/24 h.
  • Perioperative prophylaxis: 1 g IV 30–120 min before incision.
Children: 50–75 mg/kg body wt/24 h in divided doses every 12 hours; not to exceed 2 g/24 h except for meningitis.
Infants: 50 mg/kg/day every 24 h. *Note: Buildup of cephalosporins in neonates may increase half-life of drug, resulting in less frequent dosing for young infants.*

PREPARATION/RECONSTITUTION

Dilute each 250 mg of drug with 2.4 ml of sterile water, 0.9% sodium chloride solution, or 5% or 10% dextrose in water. A single dose may be further diluted in 50–100 ml of compatible infusate.

INCOMPATIBILITIES

Incompatible in syringe or solution with all other bacteriostatic agents and all aminoglycosides.

RATE/MODE OF ADMINISTRATION
IV push: Yes, over 2–4 min.
Intermittent: Yes, over 30 min in 50–100 ml of solution.
Continuous: No.
Filter: Applicable; use consistent with institutional guidelines.

NURSING CONSIDERATIONS
Nursing Diagnoses
1. Potential for injury, related to tendency toward bleeding disorders.
2. Potential for alteration in comfort level, related to pain at the injection site.
3. Potential for alteration in cardiac output, related to excessive sodium level of drug.

Acute Care
Sensitivity studies should be performed prior to administration of ceftriaxone sodium. Monitor PT and administer vitamin K if needed. May cause bleeding episodes when used with anticoagulants. Avoid prolonged use of this drug and subsequent development of overgrowth and superinfection. Drug is stable at room temperature for 24 h in appropriate diluent, or for up to 10 days if refrigerated. Solution may be yellow, depending on concentration and diluent. Thaw frozen solution at room temperature prior to use and do not refreeze.

Precautions
Adverse interactions may occur with concomitant use of promethazine, procainamide, quinidine, muscle relaxants, potent diuretics, and aminoglycosides. May be used with aminoglycosides to treat severe infections but must never be mixed in same syringe or infusate. Avoid concurrent administration of bacteriostatic agents. Monitor cardiac function due to high level of sodium (3.6 mEq/g) in drug.

Contraindications
Known sensitivity to ceftriaxone or other cephalosporins.

Side Effects

Hematologic: Bleeding episodes; eosinophilia; elevated alkaline phosphatase, bilirubin, BUN, creatinine, SGOT, and SGPT; leukopenia; prolonged PT.

Gastrointestinal: Diarrhea, pseudomembranous colitis.

Other: Burning, discomfort, pain at injection site; casts in urine; dizziness.

Patient/Caregiver Teaching

Instruct patient (1) to report all side effects immediately; (2) to provide accurate history of allergic reactions and drug sensitivities; and (3) to learn principles of home self-administration.

Home Care

Appropriate; administer initial dose in inpatient environment.

Administration in Other Clinical Settings

Appropriate; administer initial dose in inpatient environment.

Nursing Interventions

The physician should be notified of all side effects immediately. Resuscitative equipment should be readily available. Mild cases of colitis may respond to discontinuation of the drug. Vitamin K may be helpful in reversing bleeding episodes. Hemodialysis may counteract overdose.

Cefuroxime sodium

US: Zinacef

Second-generation cephalosporin   pH 6.0–8.5

ACTION

A second-generation cephalosporin antibiotic bactericidal to selected gram-positive, gram-negative, and anaerobic organisms. Excreted in the urine; also crosses the placental barrier and is secreted in breast milk.

INDICATIONS/USES

Used in the treatment of serious infections of the lower respiratory tract, urinary tract, skin, and skin structures, and of septicemia, meningitis, gonorrhea. Also used to provide perioperative prophylaxis.

USUAL DOSE

Adults: 750 mg–3 g every 8 h for 5–10 days.
- Perioperative prophylaxis: 1.5 g IV 30–60 min before incision; then 750 mg every 8 h for 24 h or 1.5 g every 12 h for a total dose of 6 g in patients of open heart surgery.

Children over 3 mo: 50–100 mg/kg body wt/24 h in equally divided doses every 6–8 h; increase to 200–240 mg/kg/24 h to treat bacterial meningitis.

PREPARATION/RECONSTITUTION

Reconstitute 750 mg in 9 ml sterile water, 5% dextrose in water, or saline solution and shake well. May further dilute as needed.

INCOMPATIBILITIES

Incompatible in syringe or solution with all other bacteriostatic agents and all aminoglycosides.

RATE/MODE OF ADMINISTRATION

IV push: Yes, over 3–5 min.
Intermittent: Yes, in 50–100 ml of solution by Y-site or piggyback administration set; temporarily discontinuing other fluids at the same site is recommended.
Continuous: Yes, in 500–1000 ml of compatible infusate by electronic flow control device if available.
Filter: Applicable; use consistent with institutional guidelines.

NURSING CONSIDERATIONS

Nursing Diagnoses

1. Potential for alteration in cardiac output, related to extremely high sodium content of this drug.
2. Potential for alteration in comfort, related to drug side effects.

Acute Care

Sensitivity studies should be performed prior to administration of this drug. Avoid prolonged use of this drug to avoid superinfection and drug overgrowth. May cause phlebitis; select IV site carefully and rotate consistent with institutional guidelines. Administer within 24 h of preparation, or within 48 h if refrigerated.

Precautions

Safety for use in pregnancy has not been established. Contains 2.4 mEq sodium per gram; monitor electrolyte imbalance and cardiac function carefully. Adverse interactions may occur with promethazine, procainamide, quinidine, muscle relaxants, potent diuretics, and aminoglycosides. May be used concomitantly with aminoglycosides, but never to be mixed in same syringe or infusate.

Contraindications

Known sensitivity to cephalosporins and penicillins.

Side Effects

Hematologic: Decreased hemoglobin, hematocrit, PT, platelet function; elevated SGOT, SGPT, total bilirubin, alkaline phosphatase, LDH, and BUN (transient); eosinophilia; leukopenia; neutropenia.
Gastrointestinal: Vomiting, oral thrush, diarrhea.
Respiratory: Dyspnea.
Other: False-positive reaction for urine glucose except with Tes-Tape or Keto-Diastix, pain at injection site, vaginitis.

Patient/Caregiver Teaching

Instruct patient (1) to report all side effects immediately; (2) to report accurate history of drug sensitivities; and (3) to learn principles of home self-administration.

Home Care

Appropriate; administer initial dose in inpatient environment.

Administration in Other Clinical Settings

Appropriate; administer initial dose in inpatient environment.

Nursing Interventions
The physician should be notified of all side effects immediately. Resuscitative equipment should be readily available. Hemodialysis may reverse overdose.

Cephalothin sodium
US: Keflin

First generation cephalosporin   pH 6.0–8.5

ACTION
A broad-spectrum first-generation cephalosporin antibiotic that is bactericidal against some gram-negative and gram-positive organisms. Excreted in the urine; also crosses the placental barrier and is secreted in breast milk.

INDICATIONS/USES
Used in the treatment of serious infections of bone, joints, skin, soft tissue, bloodstream, cardiovascular system, respiratory tract, GU system, and gastrointestinal tract. Also used to treat peritonitis, septic abortion, and staphylococcal and pneumococcal meningitis.

USUAL DOSE
Adults: 1–2 g every 4–6 h; not to exceed 12 g/24 h.
- Perioperative prophylaxis: 1–2 g 30–60 min prior to surgery; may repeat in operating room and every 6 h for 24 additional hours.

Children: 80 to 160 mg/kg body wt/24 h in equally divided doses.
- Perioperative prophylaxis: 20–30 mg/kg; give initial dose 30–60 min preoperatively and repeat if necessary every 6 h for 24 h.

Neonates: Safety not established for infants less than 1 mo old; aminoglycosides preferred.

PREPARATION/RECONSTITUTION

Reconstitute each gram in 10 ml sterile water for injection; further dilution in 50 ml or more of 5% dextrose in water, 0.9% sodium chloride solution, or other compatible infusate may prevent incidence of thrombophlebitis.

INCOMPATIBILITIES

Alkaline earth metals, amikacin, aminophyllin, amobarbital, bleomycin, calcium chloride, calcium gluceptate, calcium gluconate, cimetidine, dopamine, doxorubicin, epinephrine, erythromycin, gentamicin, heparin sodium, kanamycin, penicillin G potassium or sodium, phenytoin, tetracycline.

RATE/MODE OF ADMINISTRATION

IV push: Over 3–5 min or longer.
Intermittent: Preferred method by Y-site or piggyback administration system.
Continuous: Yes.
Filter: Applicable; use consistent with institutional guidelines.

NURSING CONSIDERATIONS

Nursing Diagnoses

1. Potential for alteration in comfort: pain, related to side effects of drug and possible development of thrombophlebitis.
2. Potential for infection, related to hematologic side effects of drug.

Acute Care

Sensitivity studies should be performed prior to administration of this drug. *Note: Sometimes given to penicillin-sensitive patients.* Administer within 24 h of preparation and warm to body temperature if precipitate forms on refrigeration. Agitate to dissolve. Rotate IV sites carefully to avoid thrombophlebitis; use large veins whenever possible.

Precautions

Adverse interaction may occur with promethazine, procainamide, quinidine, muscle relaxants, aminoglycosides, and potent diuretics. Reduce total daily dose in the nephrotoxic patient. Avoid prolonged use to prevent superinfection caused by overgrowth.

Contraindications

Known penicillin or cephalothin sensitivity.

Side Effects

Hematologic: Neutropenia, hemolytic anemia.
Gastrointestinal: Diarrhea, pseudomembranous colitis.
Other: False-positive reaction for urine glucose except with Tes-Tape and Keto-Diastix; local site pain and redness.

Patient/Caregiver Teaching

Instruct patient (1) to report all side effects immediately and (2) to learn principles of home self-administration.

Home Care

Appropriate; administer initial dose in inpatient environment.

Administration in Other Clinical Settings

Appropriate; administer initial dose in inpatient environment.

Nursing Interventions

The physician should be notified of all side effects immediately. Resuscitative equipment should be readily available.

Cephapirin sodium

US: Cefadyl

First-generation cephalosporin   pH 6.5–8.5

ACTION

A first-generation cephalosporin antibiotic that is bactericidal through inhibition of cell wall synthesis to some gram-negative and gram-positive organisms. Excreted in the urine; also crosses the placental barrier and is secreted in breast milk.

INDICATIONS/USES

Used in the treatment of moderate to severe infections of skin, soft tissue, respiratory tract, GU system. Also used to provide perioperative prophylaxis.

USUAL DOSE

Adults: 500–1000 mg every 4–6 h; 8–12 g/24 h is appropriate in severe infections.
  • Perioperative prophylaxis: 1–2 g 30–60 min before surgery; may repeat in operating room and every 6 h for 24 h, up to maximum of 5 days. Refer to manufacturer's recommendations for use.
Children: 40–80 mg/kg body wt/24 h in 4 equally divided doses.
Neonates: Safety not established for infants less than 1 mo old; aminoglycosides preferred.

PREPARATION/RECONSTITUTION

Reconstitute 1 g in 10 ml sterile water for injection. May be further diluted in 50–100 ml of 5% dextrose in water, 0.9% sodium chloride solution, or other compatible infusate to prevent thrombophlebitis.

INCOMPATIBILITIES

Amikacin, aminophylline, epinephrine, gentamicin, kanamycin, mannitol, phenytoin, tetracycline, thiopental.

RATE/MODE OF ADMINISTRATION

IV push: Over 5 min or longer.
Intermittent: Preferred method by Y-site or piggyback administration set.
Continuous: No.
Filter: Applicable; use consistent with institutional guidelines.

NURSING CONSIDERATIONS

Nursing Diagnoses

1. Potential for alteration in comfort: pain, related to drug side effects.
2. Potential for infection, related to hematologic properties of drug.

3. Potential for alteration in bowel elimination: diarrhea, related to drug side effects.

Acute Care

Sensitivity studies are needed prior to administration of this drug. Administer within 24 h of preparation. Avoid prolonged use of drug to avoid superinfection caused by overgrowth.

Precautions

Monitor patient for signs of possible allergic reaction. Reduce total daily dose if signs of nephrotoxicity occur. Adverse interaction possible with promethazine, procainamide, muscle relaxants, aminoglycosides, and potent diuretics. Avoid concurrent administration of bacteriostatic agents.

Contraindications

Safety for use in infants less than 3 mo old not established. Known sensitivity to cephalosporins or penicillins.

Side Effects

Hematologic: Neutropenia; leukopenia; transient elevation of SGOT, SGPT, BUN, and alkaline phosphatase; anemia.
Gastrointestinal: Jaundice, diarrhea, pseudomembranous colitis.
Other: False-positive reaction for urine glucose except with Tes-Tape or Keto-Diastix; local site pain, thrombophlebitis.

Patient/Caregiver Teaching

Instruct patient (1) to provide accurate drug profile and (2) to learn principles of home self-administration.

Home Care

Appropriate; administer initial dose in inpatient environment.

Administration in Other Clinical Settings

Appropriate; administer initial dose in inpatient environment.

Nursing Interventions

The physician should be notified of all side effects immediately. Resuscitative equipment should be readily available.

Cephradine

US: Velosef

First-generation cephalosporin   pH 8.5–9.5

ACTION

A first-generation cephalosporin antibiotic that is bactericidal through inhibition of cell wall synthesis to gram-negative and gram-positive organisms. *Note: Pseudomonas is resistant to this drug.* Excreted in the urine; also crosses the placental barrier and is secreted in breast milk.

INDICATIONS/USES

Used in the treatment of serious infections of bone, joint, skin, soft tissue, GI and GU systems, respiratory tract, and bloodstream. Also used to treat peritonitis and meningococcal meningitis and for perioperative prophylaxis.

USUAL DOSE

Adults: 500–1000 mg every 4–6 h; not to exceed 8 g/24 h.
- Perioperative prophylaxis: 1 g 30–90 min before surgery; repeat in 4–6 h and every 6 h thereafter for 24 h.

Children: 50–100 mg/kg body wt/24 h in divided doses every 6 h.
Neonates: Safety not established for infants less than 1 mo old; aminoglycosides preferred.

PREPARATION/RECONSTITUTION

Reconstitute each 500 mg in 5 ml sterile water for injection. May be further diluted in additional quantity of 5% dextrose in water, 0.9% sodium chloride solution, or other compatible infusate; refer to manufacturer's recommendations for use.

INCOMPATIBILITIES

Do not mix in syringe or solution with any other antibiotic. Calcium salts, epinephrine, lidocaine, Ringer's injection, tetracycline.

RATE/MODE OF ADMINISTRATION

IV push: Over 3–5 min or longer.

Intermittent: Yes, by Y-site or piggyback administration set.

Continuous: Not recommended due to potential for development of phlebitis.

Filter: Applicable; use consistent with institutional guidelines.

NURSING CONSIDERATIONS

Nursing Diagnoses

1. Potential for alteration in comfort: pain, related to thrombophlebitis properties of drug.
2. Potential for alteration in bowel elimination: diarrhea, related to drug side effects.

Acute Care

Sensitivity studies should be performed prior to administration of this drug. Administer within 2 h of preparation; stability of drug ensured for 10 h in compatible infusates and 24 h if refrigerated. Protect solution from direct exposure to sunlight. Rotate IV sites carefully, selecting large veins if possible.

Precautions

Adverse interaction may occur with promethazine, procainamide, quinidine, muscle relaxants, aminoglycosides, and potent diuretics. Avoid concurrent administration of bacteriostatic agents. Avoid prolonged use to avoid superinfection caused by overgrowth. Total daily dose should be reduced in the nephrotoxic patient.

Contraindications

Infants less than 1 mo old. Known sensitivity to cephalosporins or penicillins.

Side Effects

Hematologic: Transient leukopenia and neutropenia; transient elevated SGOT, SGPT, total bilirubin, alkaline phosphatase, LDH, BUN, serum creatinine.

Gastrointestinal: Vomiting, diarrhea, pseudomembranous colitis.

Respiratory: Dyspnea.

Circulatory: Edema.

Neurologic: Paresthesias, dizziness, headache.
Other: Vaginitis, joint pains, monilial overgrowth, false-positive
urine glucose reaction except with Tes-Tape, Clinitest, or Diastix.

Patient/Caregiver Teaching

Instruct patient (1) to report all side effects immediately and (2) to
learn principles of home self-administration.

Home Care

Appropriate; administer initial dose in inpatient environment.

Administration in Other Clinical Settings

Appropriate; administer initial dose in inpatient environment.

Nursing Interventions

The physician should be notified of all side effects immediately.
Resuscitative equipment should be readily available.

Chloramphenicol sodium succinate

US: Chloromycetin

Bactericidal   pH 6.4–7.0

ACTION

Bacteriostatic and bactericidal; acts by inhibiting protein synthesis.
Excreted in the urine, bile, and feces; also crosses the placental
barrier and is secreted in breast milk.

INDICATIONS/USES

Used in the treatment of serious infections including salmonella-
type infection, meningeal infections, bacteremia, Rocky Mountain
spotted fever. Also used in cystic fibrosis regimens.

USUAL DOSE

Adults and children: 50 mg/kg body wt/24 h in equally divided doses every 6 h; refer to manufacturer's recommendations relevant to increasing dose.

Neonates

- Under 2 kg: 25 mg/kg/once daily.
- Over 2 kg and less than 1 wk old: 50 mg/kg/once daily.
- Over 7 days: 50 mg/kg/24 h in equally divided doses every 12 h.

PREPARATION/RECONSTITUTION

Reconstitute each gram in 10 ml of sterile water or 5% dextrose in water to prepare a 10% solution. Can be further diluted in 50–100 ml of 5% dextrose in water, if desired.

INCOMPATIBILITIES

Ampicillin, amobarbital, ascorbic acid, carbenicillin, erythromycins, oxacillin, pentobarbital, phenytoin, procaine, prochlorperazine, promazine, promethazine, solutions with a pH below 5.5, solutions with a pH above 7, tetracyclines, thiopental, vancomycin.

RATE/MODE OF ADMINISTRATION

IV push: Over 1 min of at least a 10% solution.

Intermittent: Preferred method, diluted in 50–100 ml of compatible solution and infused over 30–60 min by Y-site or piggyback administration set.

Continuous: No.

Filter: Applicable; use consistent with institutional guidelines.

NURSING CONSIDERATIONS

Nursing Diagnoses

1. Potential for infection, related to severe bone marrow depression.
2. Potential for alteration in sensory-perceptual function: auditory, related to drug side effects.
3. Potential for alteration in nutrition: less than body requirements, related to possible development of diarrhea, stomatitis, vomiting.

Acute Care

Monitor baseline blood levels every 2–3 days during therapy; desired blood level range is 5–20 µg/ml. For IV use only; do not administer IM. This is a lethal drug and its use should be carefully monitored.

Precautions

Potentiates action of chlorpropamide, cyclophosphamide, phenytoin, oral anticoagulants, phenobarbital. Can have a cumulative potency effect in those with impaired or immature liver and kidney metabolic functions. Superinfection related to overgrowth is possible. Inhibits the action of iron dextran.

Contraindications

Known chloramphenicol sensitivity; pregnancy, labor, delivery, and lactation.

Side Effects

Hematologic: Aplastic anemia, bone marrow depression, granulocytopenia, hypoplastic anemia, leukemia, thrombocytopenia.
Gastrointestinal: Diarrhea, nausea, stomatitis, vomiting.
Neurologic: Headache, confusion, depression, optic and peripheral neuritis.
Other: Anaphylaxis; this is a potentially lethal drug.

Patient/Caregiver Teaching

Instruct patient (1) to report all side effects immediately (stressing danger) and (2) to provide accurate drug sensitivity profile.

Home Care

Not recommended.

Administration in Other Clinical Settings

Not recommended.

Nursing Interventions

The physician should be notified of all side effects immediately. Resuscitative equipment must be readily available when chloramphenicol is to be given.

Chromium

Refer to trace elements

Chlordiazepoxide hydrochloride

US: Librium

CNS depressant   pH 2.5–3.5

ACTION

A CNS depressant that produces a calming effect and relaxes skeletal muscle. Slowly metabolized and slowly excreted in the urine.

INDICATIONS/USES

Used in the treatment of acute or severe agitation, tremors, anxiety, or acute alcoholism withdrawal.

USUAL DOSE

50–100 mg; follow with 25–100 mg in 2–4 h if needed. Alternative therapy: 25–50 mg every 6–8 h to a maximum of 300 mg in 6–24 h.

PREPARATION/RECONSTITUTION

Reconstitute 100 mg in 5 ml of saline solution or sterile water for injection for a concentration of 20 mg/ml. *Note: The diluent provided by the manufacturer is for IM administration only.*

INCOMPATIBILITIES

Ascorbic acid, benzquinamide, heparin sodium, pentobarbital, phenytoin, promethazine, Ringer's injection, 0.9% sodium chloride.

127

RATE/MODE OF ADMINISTRATION

IV push: Over 1 min.
Intermittent: No; do not mix with infusates.
Continuous: No.
Filter: Not applicable in less than 1-ml dose.

NURSING CONSIDERATIONS

Nursing Diagnoses

1. Potential for alteration in cardiac output: decreased, related to drug side effects.
2. Potential for impairment of skin integrity, related to drug side effects.
3. Potential for injury, related to possibility of syncope.

Acute Care

Use only freshly prepared solutions and discard unused portion. Maintain a minimum of 3 h of bed rest following IV injection. Use with caution in depressed patients; may lead to development of suicidal tendencies.

Precautions

Potentiates or is potentiated by narcotics, phenothiazines, prochlorperazine, antihistamines, barbiturates, MAO inhibitors, alcohol, cimetidine, phenytoin. Reduce dosing parameters for children, the elderly, and the debilitated. Reduce dosing parameters in renal or hepatic dysfunction.

Contraindications

Known hypersensitivity to chlordiazepoxide, known psychoses, pregnancy, childbirth, lactation, children under age 12, shock, coma.

Side Effects

Hematologic: Blood dyscrasias.
Dermatologic: Urticaria, skin eruptions.
Gastrointestinal: Constipation, nausea, hiccoughs.
Cardiovascular: Hypotension, EEG changes, tachycardia.
Genitourinary: Urinary retention, menstrual irregularities.
Overdose: Caused by too rapid injection and evidenced by apnea,

ataxia, bradycardia, cardiovascular collapse, coma, diminished reflexes, hypotension, somnolence.

Patient/Caregiver Teaching

Instruct patient (1) to report all side effects immediately; (2) to provide accurate drug profile and medication history; and (3) to avoid concomitant use of alcohol.

Home Care

Not recommended for IV use.

Administration in Other Clinical Settings

Not recommended for IV use.

Nursing Interventions

The physician should be notified of all side effects immediately. Do not treat with barbiturates or CNS stimulants. Dopamine is the drug of choice to counteract hypotension. Administer osmotic diuretics to enhance excretion; hemodialysis may be required. Physostigmine 0.5–4.0 mg administered at 1 mg/min may be used to reverse neurologic symptoms (may also contribute to development of seizures and should be used with caution). Resuscitative equipment should be readily available.

Chlorothiazide sodium

US: Diuril

Nonmercurial diuretic   pH 9.2–10.0

ACTION

Related to the sulfonamides, chlorothiazide sodium is a nonmercurial diuretic and antihypertensive agent with carbonic anhydrase inhibitor and thiazide effects. Acts within 15 min of administration in the renal tubules to excrete electrolytes, water, and, in high doses, bicarbonate. Excreted unchanged in the urine.

INDICATIONS/USES
Used in the treatment of edema, toxemia of pregnancy, diabetes insipidus.

USUAL DOSE
0.5–1.0 g once or twice daily as indicated.

PREPARATION/RECONSTITUTION
Dilute each 0.5 g in 18–20 ml sterile water for injection; may be further diluted in 5% dextrose in water or 0.9% sodium chloride solution for infusion.

INCOMPATIBILITIES
Amikacin, ascorbic acid, chlorpromazine, hydralazine, methadone, morphine, Normosol solutions, prochlorperazine, promazine, promethazine, protein hydrolysates, tetracycline, vancomycin, vitamin B with C.

RATE/MODE OF ADMINISTRATION
IV push: Over 5 min. *Note: IV use should be reserved for patients unable to take oral medications or for emergency use only.*
Intermittent: No.
Continuous: No.
Filter: Not applicable in less than 1-ml concentration.

NURSING CONSIDERATIONS
Nursing Diagnoses
1. Potential for alteration in nutrition: decreased, related to drug side effects.
2. Potential for injury, related to paresthesias, orthostatic hypotension, and vertigo.

Acute Care
Discard reconstituted solution after 24 h. Determine patency of vein to avoid extravasation. Monitor electrolyte panels carefully. May alter laboratory test results, including potassium, BUN, uric acid, glucose, and protein-bound iodine.

Precautions

Reduce dosage when used with other antihypertensive drugs. Effect is increased by alcohol, barbiturates, narcotics. Discontinue drug 48 h prior to elective surgery. Use with caution in patients with hepatic or renal dysfunction. Use with caution in patients with bronchial asthma. Potentiates action of amantadine, calcium salts, lithium, muscle relaxants, other diuretics, MAO inhibitors. Inhibits action of methotrexate, norepinephrine.

Contraindications

Anuria, oliguria, known sulfonamide sensitivity, children, pregnancy (unless patient is preeclamptic), lactation.

Side Effects

Gastrointestinal. Diarrhea, nausea, vomiting, weakness.
Neurologic: Dizziness, fatigue, paresthesias, vertigo.
Dermatologic: Rash, urticaria.
Other: Blood volume reduction, circulatory collapse, dehydration, excessive diuresis, hematuria, hypokalemia, vascular thrombosis.

Patient/Caregiver Teaching

Instruct patient (1) to report all side effects immediately; (2) to provide accurate drug profile and medication history; (3) to recognize signs and symptoms of adverse reaction to drug; (4) to ensure adequate fluid intake.

Home Care

Not generally recommended.

Administration in Other Clinical Settings

Appropriate in well-monitored settings.

Nursing Interventions

The physician should be notified of all side effects immediately. Resuscitative equipment should be readily available.

Chlorpromazine hydrochloride

US: Chlorzine, Ormazine, Thorazine

Phenothiazine   pH 4.0–4.3

ACTION
Acts on the central, autonomic, and peripheral nervous systems to decrease anxiety and tension, relax muscles, and sedate and tranquilize the patient. Excreted slowly through the kidneys; quick onset in IV route.

INDICATIONS/USES
Used in the treatment of severe nausea, vomiting, hiccoughs, restlessness, retching. Used to deter nausea during operative procedures; to provide preoperative sedation of a psychotic patient; to treat drug-induced hypertension.

USUAL DOSE
Adults
- Nausea, vomiting, perioperative prophylaxis: 1 mg; may repeat at 2-min intervals as needed, not to exceed 0.5 mg/kg.
- Intractable hiccoughs: 25–50 mg in 500–1000 ml of 0.9% sodium chloride solution.
- Tetanus: 0.5 mg/kg every 6–8 h.

Children: IV route is rarely used; refer to manufacturer's recommendations for use.

PREPARATION/RECONSTITUTION
Reconstitute each 25 mg (1 ml) in 24 ml of normal saline to produce a 1:1 solution.

INCOMPATIBILITIES
Aminophylline, amphotericin B, ampicillin, atropine, caffeine and sodium benzoate, cephalothin, chloramphenicol, chlorothiazide, dimenhydrinate, epinephrine, folic acid, kanamycin, magnesium

sulfate, methicillin, penicillin G potassium, sodium bicarbonate, tetracycline, thiopental.

RATE/MODE OF ADMINISTRATION

IV push: Yes, over 3–5 min (1 mg/min).

Intermittent: No.

Continuous: In 500–1000 ml of normal saline by electronic infusion device.

Filter: Not applicable for push administration in less than 1-ml volume; applicable, consistent with institutional guidelines for continuous infusion.

NURSING CONSIDERATIONS

Nursing Diagnoses

1. Potential for injury, related to drug side effects.
2. Potential for alteration in cardiac output: decreased, related to development of distorted Q and T waves and tachycardia.
3. Potential for activity intolerance, related to excitement, weakness, and other symptoms.

Acute Care

This drug is sensitive to the light; slightly yellow color does not alter potency. Discard drug if marked discoloration is evident. Maintain patient in supine position and monitor blood pressure and pulse before administration and between doses.

Precautions

May depress cough reflex; use with caution in the patient with cardiovascular, hepatic, or respiratory disease. May discolor urine pink to reddish brown and cause photosensitivity of skin. May mask diagnosis of brain tumor, drug intoxication, intestinal obstruction. Potentiates the action of CNS depressants, MAO inhibitors, anticholinergics, antihistamines, antihypertensives, hypnotics, and muscle relaxants.

Contraindications

Bone marrow depression, cerebral arteriosclerosis, children less than 6 mo old, circulatory collapse, coma, severe depression, hypersensitivity to phenothiazines, lactation, pregnancy, hypo- or hypertension, coronary diseases.

Side Effects

Cardiopulmonary: Cardiac arrest, distorted Q and T waves, hyper- or hypotension, tachycardia.

Neurologic: Pseudoparkinsonism, restlessness, weakness of extremities.

Other: Anaphylaxis, hallucinations, convulsions, death.

Patient/Caregiver Teaching

Instruct patient (1) to report all side effects immediately and (2) to provide accurate history of allergic reactions and drug sensitivities.

Home Care

Not recommended for routine use.

Administration in Other Clinical Settings

Appropriate in well-monitored settings.

Nursing Interventions

The physician must be notified of all side effects immediately. Hypotension may be countered with administration of dopamine or phenylephrine and IV fluids. Extrapyramidal symptoms may be reversed by administration of benztropine or diphenhydramine. Administration of diazepam may reverse convulsions and hyperactivity. Treat ventricular dysrhythmias with phenytoin. Resuscitative equipment should be readily available.

Cimetidine

US: Tagamet
CAN: Apo-cimetidine (Apotex), Tagamet (SK & F)

Histamine hydrogen antagonist   pH 3.8–6.0

ACTION

Inhibits day and nocturnal basal gastric acid secretion. Excreted in the urine; also crosses the placental barrier and is secreted in breast milk.

INDICATIONS/USES

Used in the short-term treatment of active duodenal ulcers, active benign gastric ulcers, and other hypersecretory conditions.

USUAL DOSE

300 mg every 6 h; may increase frequency not to exceed 2400 mg/day.

Prevention of aspiration pneumonitis: 300 mg 60–90 min prior to administration of anesthetic agent.

PREPARATION/RECONSTITUTION

Reconstitute 300 mg in 20 ml of normal saline for injection for direct injection.

INCOMPATIBILITIES

Aminophylline, amphotericin B, cephalothin. Do not add any other drugs to premixed cimetidine in plastic IV containers.

RATE/MODE OF ADMINISTRATION

IV push: 300 mg over 2 min. *Caution: May precipitate instances of cardiac dysrhythmias, hypotension, death.*

Intermittent: Yes; dilute 300 mg in 50–100 ml of 5% dextrose in water or other compatible infusate and administer by Y-site or piggyback administration set over 15–20 min.

Continuous: Not recommended.

Filter: Applicable consistent with institutional guidelines.

NURSING CONSIDERATIONS

Nursing Diagnoses

1. Potential for alteration in cardiac output: decreased, related to drug side effects.
2. Potential for injury, related to development of hallucinations and delirium.

Acute Care

Bolus administration by IV route has precipitated rare cases of cardiac dysrhythmias, hypotension, and death. Use with extreme caution. Stable at room temperature for 48 h following dilution. Clinical effect is reversed by cigarette smoking. To avoid danger of air embolism, do not use premixed plastic containers in series connections.

Precautions

Monitor bleeding parameters carefully. Potentiates effects of benzodiazepines, beta blockers, caffeine, calcium channel blockers, hydantoins, lidocaine, metronidazole, tricyclic antidepressants, theophyllines. May precipitate apnea, confusion, and muscle twitching when used in conjunction with morphine sulfate.

Contraindications

Known hypersensitivity to dimetidine; pregnant and lactating women; and possibly children under age 16.

Side Effects

Cardiopulmonary: Bradycardia, cardiac dysrhythmias, hypotension, respiratory failure, tachycardia, fever.
Neurologic: Dizziness, delirium, confusion, hallucinations, muscular pain.
Hematologic: Elevated SGOT.
Dermatologic: Rash.

Patient/Caregiver Teaching

Instruct patient (1) to report all side effects immediately; (2) to provide accurate history of drug sensitivities; and (3) to learn principles of home self-administration by intermittent infusion.

Home Care

Appropriate.

Administration in Other Clinical Settings

Appropriate.

Nursing Interventions

The physician should be notified of all side effects immediately. Resuscitative equipment should be readily available. CNS toxicity may be countered by administration of physostigmine.

Cisplatin
US: CDDP, Platinol

Cell-cycle—nonspecific
antineoplastic   pH 3.5—5.5

ACTION
A heavy metal complex with platinum and chloride atoms; cell cycle nonspecific and similar in composition to alkylating agents. One quarter to one half of the dose is excreted in the urine by the end of 5 days.

INDICATIONS/USES
Used to suppress or retard neoplastic growth of metastatic tumors of ovaries, bladder, testes.

USUAL DOSE
Metastatic testicular tumors: 20 mg/m^2 daily for 5 days every 3 wk for 3 sequences; given in combination with bleomycin and vinblastine.

Metastatic ovarian tumors: 50 mg/m^2 once every 3 wk; given in combination with doxorubicin.

Single-agent treatment: 50—70 mg/m^2 once every 3—4 wk; all doses require adjustment based on prior radiation therapy or antineoplastic administration.

PREPARATION/RECONSTITUTION
Specific techniques are required; refer to Appendix 14 for further information. Reconstitute each 10 (50)-mg vial with 10 (50) ml of sterile water for injection for a concentration of 1 mg/ml. After withdrawing desired dose, dilute half of a single dose in 1000 ml of 5% dextrose in 0.2% sodium chloride or 0.45% sodium chloride with 37.5 g mannitol; the chloride ion is needed to avoid decomposition of the drug.

INCOMPATIBILITIES

Considered incompatible in syringe or solution with any other drug except mannitol. Inactivated by alkaline solutions (eg, sodium bicarbonate, sodium bisulfite, sodium thiosulfate).

RATE/MODE OF ADMINISTRATION

IV push: No.
Intermittent: No.
Continuous: Yes; requires hydration before and after use; administer total dose of 2000 ml over 6–8 h by electronic infusion device.
Filter: Applicable consistent with institutional guidelines.

NURSING CONSIDERATIONS

Nursing Diagnoses

1. Potential for impaired swallowing, related to development of nausea and vomiting, which may be severe and lengthy.
2. Potential for alteration in patterns of urinary elimination, related to drug toxicity and need for excessive hydration.
3. Potential for alteration in nutrition: less than body requirements, related to drug side effects.
4. Potential for injury, related to hypotension.

Acute Care

Administered under the supervision of a specialist physician. Hydrate patient wth 1–2 L of infusate for 8–12 h prior to injection, and maintain hydration and urinary output for 24 h following each dose of cisplatin. Monitor kidney function, blood counts, and electrolytes on a regular basis. Hold repeat dose unless serum creatinine is below 1.5 mg/100 ml or BUN is below 25 mg/100 ml; platelets should be at least 100,000 mm^3 and leukocyte count should be 4000/mm^3. Reconstituted solutions must be kept at room temperature and discarded after 20 h. Cisplatin interacts with aluminum alloys; do not use needles or tubing with aluminum parts to administer this drug.

Precautions

Will produce teratogenic effects on the fetus and has mutagenic potential. Prophylactic administration of antiemetics (metoclopramide, dexamethasone, droperidol) recommended to relieve severity of nausea and vomiting. Potential ototoxicity is increased in children and may be potentiated with concurrent administration of aminoglycosides. May inhibit phenytoin.

Contraindications

Hypersensitivity to cisplatin or other platinum-containing compounds; myelosuppressed patients; those with preexisting renal dysfunction or hearing deficit.

Side Effects

Side effects occur frequently, possibly with the first dose, and become more severe as treatment proceeds.

Gastrointestinal: Nausea, vomiting.
Neurologic: Peripheral neuropathy, hearing loss in high-frequency range, tinnitus.
Cardiopulmonary: Anaphylaxis, facial edema, hypotension, tachycardia, wheezing.
Hematologic: Bone marrow suppression.
Genitourinary: Nephrotoxicity, hyperuricemia.

Patient/Caregiver Teaching

Instruct patient (1) to report all side effects immediately and (2) to remain hydrated both before and after treatment.

Home Care

Appropriate in well-monitored settings.

Administration in Other Clinical Settings

Appropriate in well-monitored settings.

Nursing Interventions

The physician should be notified of all side effects immediately. It may be necessary to discontinue cisplatin permanently or until recovery occurs. Anaphylaxis may be treated with epinephrine, corticosteroids, oxygen, and antihistamines.

Clindamycin phosphate
US: Cleocin phosphate

Antibiotic   pH 6.0–6.3

ACTION

A semisynthetic antibiotic that inhibits protein synthesis in the bacterial cell, producing irreversible changes in protein-synthesizing ribosomes. Excreted in the urine and in small amounts in the stool. Clindamycin crosses the placental barrier and is secreted in breast milk.

INDICATIONS/USES

Used in the treatment of serious infections caused by anaerobic bacteria or aerobic bacterial infections in penicillin-sensitive patients; also used to treat infections that do not respond to less potent antibiotics and to treat pelvic inflammatory disease.

USUAL DOSE

Adults: 600–2700 mg/24 h in 2–4 equally divided doses; a maximum dose of 4.8 g has been reported in extenuating circumstances.

- Acute pelvic inflammatory disease: 600 mg every 6 h for 4 days. May administer gentamicin concurrently.

Children over 1 mo: 15–25 mg/kg body wt/24 h (350 mg/m²/24 h) in 3 or 4 equally divided doses; up to 40 mg/kg/24 h (450 mg/m²/24 h) may be used if necessary.

PREPARATION/RECONSTITUTION

Dilute each 300 mg or fraction thereof in 50 ml of 5% dextrose in water, normal saline for injection, or other compatible infusate.

- Acute pelvic inflammatory disease: Further dilute in 1000 ml compatible solution and administer as continuous infusion.

INCOMPATIBILITIES

Aminophylline, ampicillin, calcium gluconate, magnesium sulfate, phenytoin, Ringer's solution.

140

RATE/MODE OF ADMINISTRATION

IV push: No.
Intermittent: 300 mg over minimum of 10 min; not to exceed 1200 mg in 60 min.
Continuous: Yes.

- Acute pelvic inflammatory disease: Administer initial dose at 10 mg/min over 30 min; follow with maintenance infusion at 0.75 mg/min to maintain serum level at 4. Refer to product literature for manufacturer's recommendations for use.

Filter: Applicable consistent with institutional guidelines.

NURSING CONSIDERATIONS

Nursing Diagnoses

1. Potential for alteration in comfort: pain, related to drug side effects.
2. Potential for alteration in bowel elimination: diarrhea, related to drug side effects.

Acute Care

Sensitivity studies must be on file prior to administration of this drug. Avoid prolonged use to prevent superinfection caused by overgrowth. Potential for development of fatal colitis is severe; observe patient for evidence of diarrhea carefully. Monitor organ system function in infants and newborns.

Precautions

Each ml contains 9.45 mg benzyl alcohol. Too rapid injection may cause severe hypotension and cardiac arrest. Antagonized by erythromycin. Use with caution in patients with history of renal or hepatic dysfunction or gastrointestinal disease.

Contraindications

Known hypersensitivity to clindamycin, lincomycin; pregnant and lactating women and newborns.

Side Effects

Gastrointestinal: Abdominal pain, colitis, diarrhea, jaundice, nausea, vomiting.
Other: Thrombophlebitis.

Patient/Caregiver Teaching

Instruct patient (1) to report all side effects immediately and (2) to learn principles of home self-administration.

Home Care

Appropriate in well-monitored settings; administer initial dose in inpatient environment.

Administration in Other Clinical Settings

Appropriate in well-monitored settings; administer initial dose in inpatient environment.

Nursing Interventions

The physician must be notified of all side effects immediately. Discontinue drug for evidence of colitis, diarrhea, or allergic reaction. Resuscitative equipment should be readily available. Colitis may be reversed following administration of fluid, electrolyte, and protein supplements, systemic corticosteroids, and corticoid retention enemas.

Colistimethate sodium
US: Coly-Mycin M

Antibiotic   pH 7–8

ACTION

Bactericidal against specific gram-negative bacilli. Excreted through the kidneys; also crosses the placental barrier.

INDICATIONS/USES

Used in the treatment of acute and chronic infections of the urinary tract and other body systems caused by gram-negative bacilli, for example, *Pseudomonas aeruginosa, Aerobacter aerogenes, Escherichia coli*, and others.

USUAL DOSE

2.5–5.0 mg/kg body wt/24 h in 2 equally divided doses every 12 h; patient must have normal renal function prior to administration of this dose, not to exceed 5 mg/kg/24 h.

PREPARATION/RECONSTITUTION

Reconstitute 150-mg vial with 2 ml sterile water for injection; 1 ml equals 75 mg. May further dilute each single dose with 20 ml sterile water for injection prior to direct IV administration; additional infusate is needed for infusion purposes.

INCOMPATIBILITIES

Administer this drug separately. Incompatible with cefazolin, cephalothin, erythromycin, hydrocortisone, hydroxyzine, kanamycin.

RATE/MODE OF ADMINISTRATION

IV push: Yes; 75 mg, or half of the total daily dose, given over 5 min.
Intermittent: Yes, in 50 ml or more of 5% dextrose in water, isotonic saline, lactated Ringer's solution, or 10% invert sugar solution by Y-site or piggyback administration set.
Continuous: Administered 1–2 h following initial dose at rate of 5–6 mg/h, use electronic infusion device to control accuracy of infusion.
Filter: Applicable consistent with institutional guidelines.

NURSING CONSIDERATIONS

Nursing Diagnoses

1. Potential for injury, related to side effects resulting from average dose of drug.
2. Potential for disturbance in sensory-perceptual alteration: visual, tactile, and olfactory, related to drug side effects.

Acute Care

Use only the IV form of the drug for IV use; read label carefully. Sensitivity studies are indicated prior to administration. Daily dose is reduced for renal dysfunction and calculated according to intensity of impairment. Monitor patient for evidence of decreased urinary output, increased BUN, and increased serum creatinine. Store reconstituted drug in refrigerator for up to 7 days; discard solutions after 24 h.

Precautions

Potentiated by anesthetics, other neuromuscular blocking antibiotics, and muscle relaxants. Watch for signs/symptoms of apnea and report such symptoms immediately. Avoid superinfection caused by overgrowth associated with prolonged use of drug. May cause impaired motor function. Do not use in pregnancy unless absolutely necessary.

Contraindications

Known sensitivity to multiple allergens; known colistimethate sensitivity. Do not use in pregnancy unless absolutely necessary.

Side Effects

Average dose, neurologic: Circumoral paresthesia, dizziness, numbness of extremities, slurred speech, tingling of extremities, vertigo.
Overdose, neurologic: Muscle weakness.
Other: Anaphylaxis, apnea, decreased urine output, renal insufficiency.

Patient/Caregiver Teaching

Instruct patient (1) to report all side effects immediately and (2) to provide accurate drug profile and sensitivity history.

Home Care

Not recommended.

Administration in Other Clinical Settings

Not recommended.

Nursing Interventions

The physician should be notified of all side effects immediately, regardless of the dose provided. Symptoms will be alleviated following reduction in dose. If symptoms of overdose are evident, discontinue the drug and notify physician. Maintain adequate airway and provide artificial ventilation as needed. Allergic symptoms may be relieved by administration of antihistamines or pressor amines.

Conjugated estrogens
US: Premarin intravenous

Antithrombin decreaser   pH 6.8–7.4

ACTION
Conjugated estrogens produce an increase in circulating prothrombin and accelerator globulin and resultant decrease in antithrombin activities. Coagulability is enhanced.

INDICATIONS/USES
Used in the treatment of dysfunctional uterine bleeding related to hormonal imbalance in absence of organic pathologic condition.

USUAL DOSE
25 mg as a single injection; may repeat in 6–12 h as needed.

PREPARATION/RECONSTITUTION
Add contents of ampule of sterile diluent (provided) to vial of powder, directing flow against the interior side of the vial. Mix by rotating vial between the palms of the hands and do not shake to ensure thorough reconstitution of powdered drug.

INCOMPATIBILITIES
Ascorbic acid, lactated Ringer's, protein hydrolysate, Ringer's injection, $1/6$ molar sodium lactate solution, any acidic solution.

RATE/MODE OF ADMINISTRATION
IV push: Yes, 5 mg over 1 min; give as close to IV site as possible if using sideport method; use compatible infusate only.
Intermittent: No.
Continuous: No.
Filter: Not applicable in less than 1-ml dose.

NURSING CONSIDERATIONS
Nursing Diagnoses
1. Potential for alteration in nutrition: less than body requirements, related to drug side effects.

2. Potential for ineffective thermoregulation, related to flushing.

Acute Care

Direct IV administration is preferred method. Refrigerate before and after reconstitution of drug; stable for up to 60 days if protected from light. Do not use solution if discolored or if there is evidence of precipitate.

Precautions

Etiology of bleeding condition must be determined and appropriate long-term therapy provided. May increase blood glucose levels. Use with caution in patients with epilepsy, migraine, asthma, or cardiac or renal disease. May increase neuromuscular blocking effects of succinylcholine.

Contraindications

Breast cancer (other than selected metastatic disease), pregnancy, thrombophlebitis or other thromboembolic disorder, undiagnosed abnormal genital bleeding.

Side Effects

Gastrointestinal: Nausea, vomiting.
Other: Flushing.

Patient/Caregiver Teaching

Instruct patient to report all side effects immediately.

Home Care

Appropriate in well-monitored settings.

Administration in Other Clinical Settings

Appropriate in well-monitored settings.

Nursing Interventions

No evidence of toxicity has been reported.

Copper

Refer to trace elements.

Corticotropin injection
US: ACTH, Acthar

Hormonal agent   pH 2.5–6.0

ACTION

Anterior pituitary hormone effective only when the adrenal glands are normal and able to respond to stimulation. Excreted in the urine.

INDICATIONS/USES

Used in the diagnosis of adrenocortical function and treatment of idiopathic thrombocytopenic purpura.

USUAL DOSE

10–25 U/24 h as initial dose; may administer up to 80 U as single injection for diagnostic purposes.

PREPARATION/RECONSTITUTION

Dilute powder with 2 ml water or sodium chloride for injection. Further dilute in 500 ml of 5% dextrose in water; isotonic saline solution may be used if patient's sodium intake is unrestricted.

INCOMPATIBILITIES

Aminophylline, sodium bicarbonate.

RATE/MODE OF ADMINISTRATION

IV push: No.
Intermittent: No.
Continuous: Yes, over an 8-h period.
Filter: Applicable; use consistent with institutional guidelines.

NURSING CONSIDERATIONS

Nursing Diagnoses

1. Potential for fluid volume deficit: actual, related to electrolyte imbalance.
2. Potential for injury, related to bleeding episodes.

Acute Care

Sensitivity testing required prior to administration. Use vial that states "for IV use." Observe patient for initial 30 min and frequently during administration. Monitor vital signs frequently. Refrigerate remaining medication after preparation/reconstitution.

Precautions

May increase insulin needs in the diabetic patient. Use with caution in cirrhosis and hypothyroidism. Do not vaccinate for smallpox during treatment. Patient may require additional doses of anticoagulants and hemorrhagic episodes may occur.

Contraindications

Do not use in ocular herpes simplex, acute psychoses, scleroderma, osteoporosis, systemic fungal infections, or recent surgical intervention. May also be contraindicated in congestive heart failure, diabetes mellitus, hypertension, pregnancy, psychotic tendencies, renal insufficiency, thromboembolic tendencies.

Side Effects

Note: Side effects of this drug are usually reversible.

Cardiovascular: Electrolyte imbalance, increased blood pressure, hyperglycemia, negative nitrogen balance.
Gastrointestinal: Pancreatitis.
Other: Moon face, suppression of growth, anaphylaxis.

Patient/Caregiver Teaching

Instruct patient (1) to report all side effects immediately; (2) to provide accurate medical history and drug profile; and (3) that potential side effects are usually reversible.

Home Care

Not recommended.

Administration in Other Clinical Settings

Not recommended.

Nursing Interventions

The physician should be notified of all side effects immediately. Resuscitative equipment should be readily available.

Cosyntropin
US: Cortrosyn

Hormonal agent   pH 5.5–7.5

ACTION
A synthetic adrenocorticotropic hormone (ACTH) that stimulates the adrenal cortex to secrete cortisol, corticosterone, androgenic agents, and aldosterone.

INDICATIONS/USES
Used as a diagnostic aid for adrenocortical insufficiency.

USUAL DOSE
Adults: 250 µg (0.25 mg).
Children over age 2: 250 µg (0.25 mg).

PREPARATION/RECONSTITUTION
Dilute using solution provided and administer as is; 250 µg/250 ml equals 1 µg/ml solution.

INCOMPATIBILITIES
Information unavailable.

RATE/MODE OF ADMINISTRATION
IV push: Yes, as a single dose over 2 min.
Intermittent: No.
Continuous: At 40 µg/h over 6-h period by electronic infusion device.
Filter: Applicable for continuous infusion.

NURSING CONSIDERATIONS
Nursing Diagnoses
1. Potential for alteration in cardiac output, related to drug side effects.
2. Potential for alteration in skin integrity, related to drug side effects.

Acute Care

Drug is stable following reconstitution for 24 h at room temperature and 21 days if refrigerated. Infusion is stable for 12 hours at room temperature. Preferable to ACTH because it is less likely to cause allergic reactions.

Precautions

May be used in those who have had a past allergic reaction to ACTH; less antigenic than corticotropin.

Contraindications

Use with caution in pregnancy and lactation.

Side Effects

Circulatory: Bradycardia.
Respiratory: Dyspnea.
Neurologic: Fainting, dizziness, seizures.
Other: Urticaria, irritability.

Patient/Caregiver Teaching

Instruct patient to report all side effects immediately.

Home Care

Not recommended.

Administration in Other Clinical Settings

Not recommended.

Nursing Interventions

Notify the physician of any side effects immediately. Emergency treatment with epinephrine or diphenhydramine may be needed.

Cyclophosphamide

US: Cytoxan, Neosar
CAN: Procytox (Horner), Cytoxan
(Bristol)

Alkylating agent   pH 5.05

ACTION

An alkylating agent of the nitrogen mustard family; cyclophosphamide has antitumor activity and is cell cycle nonspecific
(most effective in "S" phase). Excreted in the urine.

INDICATIONS/USES

Used to suppress or retard neoplastic growth in Hodgkin's disease,
leukemia, multiple myeloma, and solid malignancies of the breast
and ovary. Investigational use for rheumatologic conditions.

USUAL DOSE

Initial: Dose may reach 40–50 mg/kg body wt in divided doses over
    2–5 days time. Dose is reduced by one third to one half if
    hematologic system is affected or in case of extensive radiation.
Maintenance: Varies from 3–5 mg/kg twice weekly to 10–15 mg/kg
    every 7–10 days.

PREPARATION/RECONSTITUTION

Precautions and specific technique involved in preparation of this
antineoplastic agent; refer to Appendix 14 for further information.
Reconstitute each 100 mg in 5 ml sterile water or bacteriostatic
water for injection (paraben-preserved only). Shake vial gently and
allow to stand until solution is clear. May add additional diluent (to
a maximum of 250 ml 5% dextrose in water or 0.9% sodium
chloride solution) to reduce severity of side effects.

INCOMPATIBILITIES

Administer separately and consider incompatible with all other
drugs in syringe or solution.

RATE/MODE OF ADMINISTRATION

IV push: 100 mg over 1 min by Y-site or sideport of glucose or saline infusion.

Intermittent: No.

Continuous: As above to minimize severity of side effects.

Filter: Not applicable in less than 1-ml dose.

NURSING CONSIDERATIONS

Nursing Diagnoses

1. Potential for infection, related to immunosuppressive qualities of drug.
2. Potential for alteration in urinary elimination patterns, related to possible cystitis.

ACUTE CARE

Do not store in temperatures over 37°C. Diluted solution is unstable and must be used within 24 h. Solution is stable for 6 days if refrigerated. Dosage is based on average weight in presence of ascites or edema. Administer dose before 4 pm to decrease amount of drug remaining in the bladder overnight, and encourage adequate fluid intake to prevent cystitis.

Precautions

Used under the direction of a licensed physician specialist. Marked leukopenia occurs after the initial dose; recovery is usually evident within 7–10 days. Maintenance doses are regulated by adequate leukocyte count (2500–4000 cells/mm^3) and absence of serious known side effects. Use the maximum effective maintenance dose. Use with caution in patients with leukopenia, thrombocytopenia, bone marrow infiltrated with malignant cells, hepatic or renal dysfunction. May be used in combination with other antineoplastic agents in reduced doses to achieve tumor remission. A mutagenic drug that may produce teratogenic effects on the fetus; breast-feeding should be discontinued.

Contraindications

None reported.

Side Effects

Hematologic: Leukopenia, bone marrow depression.
Genitourinary: Amenorrhea, gonadal suppression, sterile hemorrhagic cystitis (*Caution: Potentially fatal*).
Gastrointestinal: Nausea, Vomiting, Mucosal ulcerations.
Other: Pulmonary fibrosis, darkened skin and fingernails, susceptibility to infection, alopecia.

Patient/Caregiver Teaching

Instruct patient (1) to report all side effects immediately; (2) to provide accurate drug profile; and (3) to increase fluid intake and frequency of voiding to prevent cystitis.

Home Care

Appropriate.

Administration in Other Clinical Settings

Appropriate.

Nursing Interventions

The physician should be notified of all side effects immediately; minor side effects may be treated symptomatically if needed. Report hematuria immediately and discontinue the drug; responds to hemodialysis.

Cyclosporine
US: Sandimmune

Immunosuppressant

ACTION

A potent immunosuppressive agent. Excreted in bile and urine; crosses the placental barrier and is secreted in breast milk.

INDICATIONS/USES

Used in conjunction with adrenal corticosteroids as prophylactic treatment for organ rejection in kidney, liver, and heart allogeneic transplants. Used in treatment of chronic rejection in those treated previously with other immunosuppressive agents. Investigationally used as a prophylaxis of organ rejection in pancreas, bone marrow, and heart/lung transplantation.

USUAL DOSE

5–6 mg/kg body wt as a single dose 4–12 h prior to transplantation; may repeat once daily until patient is able to tolerate oral dosing.

PREPARATION/RECONSTITUTION

Dilute 50 mg immediately prior to use with 20–100 ml of 0.9% sodium chloride solution of 5% dextrose in water.

INCOMPATIBILITIES

Unknown; administer separately in solution. Use glass containers only; may leach plasticizers (phthalate) from polyvinylchloride containers.

RATE/MODE OF ADMINISTRATION

IV push: No.
Intermittent: No.
Continuous: Yes, by electronic infusion device over 2–6 h.
Filter: Applicable; use consistent with institutional guidelines.

NURSING CONSIDERATIONS

Nursing Diagnoses

1. Potential for alteration in nutrition: decreased, related to drug side effects.
2. Potential for infection, related to drug side effects.

Acute Care

Dilute immediately prior to use and discard unused portion of drug. Protect diluted solution from direct light. Adequate laboratory and supportive medical services must be available. Monitor bone marrow function, RBC and WBC counts, platelet count. Monitor timing and amount of increase in BUN and creatinine, serum bilirubin, and liver enzymes. Observe patient for signs of infection.

Precautions

Do not administer any other immunosuppressive agent. Given concomitantly with adrenal corticosteroids only. Safety for use in pregnancy has not yet been established. Potentiated by other nephrotoxic agents, for example, amphotericin B, gentamicin, ethacrynic acid.

Contraindications

Known hypersensitivity to cyclosporine or polyoxyethylated castor oil.

Side Effects

Gastrointestinal: Diarrhea, cramps, nausea, vomiting.
Hematologic: Leukopenia.
Neurologic: Paresthesias, tremor, convulsions.
Other: Hypertension, hirsutism, lymphoma, renal dysfunction.

Patient/Caregiver Teaching

Instruct patient (1) to report all side effects immediately; (2) to provide accurate drug profile; and (3) to report possible pregnancy.

Home Care

Inappropriate.

Administration in Other Clinical Settings

Inappropriate.

Nursing Interventions

The physician should be notified of all side effects immediately. Incidence of nephrotoxicity, hepatotoxicity, or hematopoietic depression may require temporary decrease in dosing; dialysis not effective to reverse overdose.

Cytarabine

US: Cytosine arabinoside,
ARA-C, Cytosar-U
CAN: Cytosar (Upjohn)

Antimetabolite   pH 5

ACTION
Intereferes with synthesis of DNA and RNA; cell cycle specific for S phase. Metabolized in the liver and excreted in the urine.

INDICATIONS/USES
Used to induce remission in acute myelocytic leukemia of adults and children and other acute leukemias in adults and children.

USUAL DOSE
(Dose is disease-state specific and dependent on regimen or protocol.)
100 mg/m^2/24 h in divided doses every 12 h; may repeat for 7–10 days.
Acute myelocytic leukemia remission/induction: 200 mg/m^2/24 h for 5 days (continuous infusion) for a total dose of 1000 mg/m^2; repeat every 2 wk.

PREPARATION/RECONSTITUTION
Extreme care is required in handling this antineoplastic agent; refer to Appendix 14 for further information. Reconstitute each 100-mg vial in 5 ml of sterile water for injection with benzyl alcohol 0.9% preservative for a concentration of 20 mg/ml. May be further diluted as needed.

INCOMPATIBILITIES
Fluorouracil, methylprednisolone sodium succinate.

RATE/MODE OF ADMINISTRATION
IV push: Yes, sideport through freely flowing infusion.
Intermittent: Yes, in 50–100 ml or more of 0.9% sodium chloride solution or 5% dextrose in water.

Continuous: Yes.
Filter: Not applicable in less than 1-ml dose.

NURSING CONSIDERATIONS

Nursing Diagnoses

1. Potential for injury, related to drug side effects.
2. Potential for alteration in nutrition: decreased, related to gastrointestinal symptoms.
3. Potential for alteration in comfort, related to stomatitis and pain.

Acute Care

Refrigerate until after dilution; solution is then stable at room temperature for 48 h (use clear solutions only). Monitor leukocyte and platelet counts daily. Cytarabine therapy should be discontinued for platelet count under 50,000 or polymorphonuclear granulocytes under 1000 cells/mm^3. Prophylactic administration of antiemetics recommended. Dosage is based on average weight in presence of ascites or edema.

Precautions

Monitor patient for evidence of bone marrow depression. Monitor uric acid levels and maintain hydration. May produce teratogenic effects on fetus during first trimester of pregnancy. Use only under direct supervision of licensed physician specialist.

Contraindications

First trimester pregnancy; known hypersensitivity to cytarabine; preexisting drug-induced bone marrow depression.

Side Effects

Gastrointestinal: Abdominal pain, diarrhea, esophagitis, hepatic dysfunction, nausea, oral ulceration, stomatitis, vomiting.
Hematologic: Megaloblastosis, bone marrow depression, anemia, leukopenia, thrombocytopenia.
Other: Conjunctivitis, thrombophlebitis, fever, chest pain, bone pain.

Patient/Caregiver Teaching

Instruct patient (1) to report all side effects immediately and (2) to provide accurate drug profile and sensitivity history.

Home Care
Appropriate in well-monitored setting.

Administration in Other Clinical Settings
Appropriate in well-monitored setting.

Nursing Interventions
The physician should be notified of all side effects immediately. Treat cytarabine syndrome (fever, myalgia, bone pain, chest pain, rash, conjunctivitis, and malaise) with corticosteroid therapy; may occur in 6–12 h following administration.

Dacarbazine
US: DTIC, DTIC-Dome, Imidazole carboxamide
CAN: DTIC (Miles)

Antineoplastic   pH 3–4

ACTION
An alkylating agent, cell cycle phase nonspecific; thought to inhibit DNA and RNA synthesis. Excreted in the urine.

INDICATIONS/USES
Used in the induction of remission of malignant melanoma with metastasis following surgical excision; in the treatment of Hodgkin's disease; and for soft tissue sarcomas.

USUAL DOSE
Malignant melanoma: 2.0–4.5 mg/kg body wt/24 h for 10 days; may repeat at 4-wk intervals. 250 mg/m² for 5 days; repeat in 3 wk.
Hodgkin's disease: 150 mg/m² for 5 days; repeat every 4 wk. Used in combination with other drugs in specific treatment regimes.

PREPARATION/RECONSTITUTION

Reconstitute each 100 mg with 9.9 ml sterile water for injection diluted to 10 mg/ml.

INCOMPATIBILITIES

Hydrocortisone sodium succinate, hydrocortisone sodium phosphate, lidocaine hydrochloride. Incompatible in syringe or solution with all other drugs owing to high incidence of toxicity and side effects.

RATE/MODE OF ADMINISTRATION

IV push: Over 1 min by Y-site or sideport of a freely flowing infusion.
Intermittent: No.
Continuous: Diluted in 50–250 ml of 5% dextrose in water or 0.9% sodium chloride solution over 15–30 min.
Filter: Not applicable by push mode of administration; refer to institutional guidelines.

NURSING CONSIDERATIONS

Nursing Diagnoses

1. Potential for injury related to hematologic properties of the drug.
2. Potential for alteration in self-concept, disturbance in body image and self-esteem related to alopecia and skin necrosis.
3. Potential for alteration in thought processes related to malaise.

Acute Care

Special handling of this cytotoxic agent is needed; follow recommendations provided in Appendix 14. Administer in the inpatient environment under the direction of a specialist physician. Determine patency of vein to avoid extravasation, cellulitis, and tissue necrosis. Diluted solution is stable for 72 h if refrigerated; discard in 6–8 h if maintained at room temperature. Monitor bone marrow function and hematologic parameters regularly.

Precautions

Dosage is based on average weight in presence of edema or ascites. Do not administer vaccines or chloroquine to patients receiving dacarbazine. Inhibited by phenobarbital and phenytoin. Monitor patient for evidence of bleeding or infection.

Contraindications

Known hypersensitivity to dacarbazine.

Side Effects

Hematologic: Leukopenia, thrombocytopenia.
Gastrointestinal: Nausea, vomiting, anorexia, hepatotoxicity.
Neurologic: Tingling, facial paresthesias, myalgia, malaise.
Other: Skin necrosis, alopecia, anaphylaxis.

Patient/Caregiver Teaching

Instruct patient (1) to report all side effects immediately and (2) to be aware of the possibility of photosensitivity skin reaction.

Home Care

Appropriate in well-monitored environment.

Administration in Other Clinical Settings

Appropriate in well-monitored environment.

Nursing Interventions

The physician should be notified of all side effects immediately. Resuscitative equipment should be readily available. Long-acting dexamethasone or hyaluronidase may be used to counteract extravasation; refer to antidote chart in Appendix 15.

Dactinomycin

US: ACT, Actinomycin D, Cosmegen

Antibiotic antineoplastic   pH 5.5–7.0

ACTION

An antibiotic antineoplastic agent, cell-cycle-phase nonspecific, that is found in high concentrations in the kidney, spleen, and liver.

INDICATIONS/USES

Used to suppress or retard neoplastic growth in Wilms' tumor, rhabdomyosarcoma, Ewing's sarcoma, carcinoma of the testis and uterus, and choriocarcinoma.

USUAL DOSE

Adults: 0.5 mg/24 h for 5 days; may repeat after 3 wk if no evidence of toxicity. Do not exceed 15 μg/kg body wt/day in adults and children.

Children: 0.015 mg/kg/24 h for 5 days; may repeat after 3 wk if no evidence of toxicity is present.

PREPARATION/RECONSTITUTION

0.5 mg with 1.1 ml of sterile water for injection without preservatives for a concentration of 0.5 mg/ml (to avoid precipitation).

INCOMPATIBILITIES

Considered incompatible in syringe or solution with any other drug.

RATE/MODE OF ADMINISTRATION

IV push: Each 0.5 mg or fraction thereof over 2 min.
Intermittent: No.
Continuous: As a single dose over 10–15 min.
Filter: Not usually used; dictated by institutional policy.

NURSING CONSIDERATIONS

Nursing Diagnoses

1. Potential for injury, related to drug side effects.
2. Potential for alteration in nutrition, related to stomatitis, vomiting, and gastrointestinal ulceration.

Acute Care

Follow recommendations in Appendix 14 for handling this highly toxic drug. Administer under the care of a qualified physician specialist. Determine patency of vein to avoid extravasation, cellulitis, and tissue necrosis. Use sterile two-needle technique for direct IV administration (one needle to inject into vein and rinse with blood before removing). Monitor renal, hepatic, and bone marrow function.

Precautions
Dosage is based on average weight in presence of edema or ascites. Drug is light sensitive if not reconstituted. Side effects (other than nausea and vomiting) may be delayed. Do not administer vaccines or chloroquine to patients receiving dactinomycin. Radiation therapy potentiates action of dactinomycin. Inhibits action of penicillin. To reduce uric acid levels, increase fluid intake and alkalinization of urine.

Contraindications
Exposure to chickenpox; known sensitivity to the drug; infants less than 6 mo old.

Side Effects
Gastrointestinal: Abdominal pain, anorexia, cheilitis, diarrhea, dysphagia, esophagitis, gastrointestinal ulceration, nausea, pharyngitis, proctitis, ulcerative stomatitis, vomiting.
Neurologic: Malaise, myalgia, fatigue.
Hematologic: Thrombocytopenia, leukopenia.
Other: Erythema flare-up, hypocalcemia, alopecia.

Patient/Caregiver Teaching
Instruct patient (1) to report all side effects immediately; (2) to report exposure to chickenpox; and (3) to be aware of the danger of delayed reactions to drug.

Home Care
Appropriate in well-monitored settings.

Administration in Other Clinical Settings
Appropriate in well-monitored settings.

Nursing Interventions
The physician should be notified of all side effects immediately. Resuscitative equipment should be readily available. Long-acting dexamethasone or hyaluronidase may be used to counteract extravasation; refer to Appendix 15.

Daunorubicin hydrochloride

US: Cerubidine, DNR
CAN: Cerubidine (Rhone-Poulenc)

Antibiotic antineoplastic   pH 4.5−6.5

ACTION

An antibiotic antineoplastic agent that is rapidly cleared from plasma and inhibits synthesis of DNA. Cell-cycle specific for "S" phase. Slowly excreted in bile and urine.

INDICATIONS/USES

Used to induce remission of acute nonlymphocytic leukemia in adults and as combination therapy for acute lymphocytic leukemia in children.

USUAL DOSE

Adults: 60 mg/m^2/day for 3 days; repeat in 3−4 wk. Dose is reduced in combination chemotherapy for remission induction in acute myelogenous leukemia. Refer to manufacturer's recommendations for dosing parameters and concurrent use with other antineoplastic agents.

Children

- Acute lymphocytic anemia: 25 mg/m^2 on day 1 of each week, vincristine 1.5 mg/m^2 on day 1 each week, and prednisone 40 mg/m^2 by mouth daily; remission probable in 4−6 wk.

PREPARATION/RECONSTITUTION

Reconstitute each 20 mg with 4 ml sterile water for injection for concentration of 5 mg/ml; agitate gently to completely dissolve. May further dilute each dose with 10−15 ml of normal saline. Do not add to IV solutions.

INCOMPATIBILITIES

Dexamethasone, heparin sodium. Considered incompatible with any drug because of extreme toxicity.

RATE/MODE OF ADMINISTRATION

IV push: As a single dose over 3–5 min by sideport of freely flowing infusion of 5% dextrose in water or 0.9% sodium chloride solution.

Intermittent: No.

Continuous: No.

Filter: Not applicable in less than 1-ml dose.

NURSING CONSIDERATIONS

Nursing Diagnoses

1. Potential for alteration in nutrition: decreased, related to drug side effects.
2. Potential for alteration in cardiac output: decreased, related to acute congestive heart failure and cardiac toxicities.

Acute Care

A cytotoxic drug; refer to recommendations in Appendix 14 for preparation to avoid toxicity. Administer under the direction of a skilled physician specialist. Determine patency of vein to avoid extravasation and subsequent cellulitis and tissue necrosis. Diluted solution is stable for 24 h at room temperature, 48 h if refrigerated. Protect solution from sunlight. Monitor hematologic functions and observe patient for signs and symptoms of infection.

Precautions

May produce teratogenic effects on fetus. Use caution in preexisting drug-induced bone marrow suppression, existing heart disease, or previous treatment with doxorubicin or radiation therapy (involving the heart). Total cumulative dose of 550 mg/m^2 may produce congestive heart failure. Reduce dose up to half if hepatic or renal dysfunction occurs. Monitor uric acid levels. Maintain hydration; dosage is based on average weight if edema or ascites present.

Contraindications

Preexisting bone marrow suppression; impairment of cardiac function; preexisting infection.

Side Effects

Cardiovascular: Acute congestive heart failure, decreased systolic ejection fraction, depressed QRS voltage, myocarditis, pericarditis.
Gastrointestinal: Vomiting, nausea, mucositis, diarrhea.
Dermatologic: Skin rash.
Other: Bone marrow suppression.

Patient/Caregiver Teaching

Instruct patient (1) to report all side effects immediately; (2) to provide accurate health history; and (3) to be aware of the possibility of urine turning reddish from dye.

Home Care

Appropriate in well-monitored settings.

Administration in Other Clinical Settings

Appropriate in well-monitored settings.

Nursing Interventions

The physician must be notified of all side effects. Extravasation may be counteracted by flushing site with normal saline and injecting long-acting dexamethasone or hyaluronidase; refer to Appendix 15 for specific recommendations.

Deferoxamine mesylate
US: Desferal

Iron chelating agent

ACTION

An iron-chelating agent that combines with iron to form ferrioxamine thus preventing the iron from entering into further chemical reactions. Metabolized by plasma enzymes, it removes iron from free serum iron, ferritin, and transferrin, but not from hemoglobin or cytochromes.

INDICATIONS/USES

Used to facilitate removal of iron in treatment of acute iron intoxication or chronic iron overload following multiple transfusions. Investigationally used to manage accumulation of aluminum in bone of renal failure patients and in aluminum-induced dialysis encephalopathy.

USUAL DOSE

Adults
- Acute iron intoxication: Initial dose of 2 g may be followed by doses of 500 mg every 4 h as needed; not to exceed 6 g/24 h.
- Chronic iron overload: 2 g with each unit of packed cells; administered concurrently in separate veins.

Children: 50 mg/kg body wt up to 2 g every 6 h; not to exceed 6 g/24 h.

PREPARATION/RECONSTITUTION

Dilute each 500 mg in 2 ml sterile water for injection; further dilute in IV solution of 0.9% sodium chloride solution, 5% dextrose in water, or lactated Ringer's solution.

INCOMPATIBILITIES

Do not mix with any IV medication or solution other than those listed.

RATE/MODE OF ADMINISTRATION

IV push: No.

Intermittent: No.

Continuous: Yes, 2 g in 1000 ml infusate by electronic infusion device set to administer 15 mg/kg/h.

Filter: Not applicable; protect from light.

NURSING CONSIDERATIONS

Nursing Diagnoses

1. Potential for injury, related to blurring of vision and leg cramps.
2. Potential for alteration in nutrition, related to drug side effects.

Acute Care

May be stored at room temperature for 7 days if diluted with sterile water for injection under sterile conditions. Protect solution from light.

Precautions

IV route used only in state of cardiovascular shock or chronic iron overload. Initiate blood transfusion simultaneously with deferoxamine infusion in opposite extremities. Check for cataract development following long-term use.

Contraindications

Severe renal disease or anuria.

Side Effects

Neuromuscular: Leg cramps, blurring of vision.
Gastrointestinal: Abdominal discomfort, diarrhea.
Other: Shock, tachycardia, urticaria, anaphylaxis.

Patient/Caregiver Teaching

Instruct patient to report all side effects immediately.

Home Care

Appropriate in well-monitored environment.

Administration in Other Clinical Settings

Appropriate in well-monitored environment.

Nursing Interventions

Decrease rate of administration at first sign of side effects. Resuscitative equipment must be readily available.

Deslanoside injection

US: Cedilanid-D

Lanotoside C derivative   pH 5.9–6.5

ACTION
Increases strength of myocardial contraction and alters myocardial automaticity, conduction velocity, and refractory periods. Excreted in the urine.

INDICATIONS/USES
Used in the treatment of congestive heart failure, atrial fibrillation, atrial flutter, paroxysmal tachycardia, cardiogenic shock, and ventricular dysrhythmias with congestive heart failure.

USUAL DOSE
Adults
- Digitalization: 1.2–1.6 mg as a single dose or in equally divided doses over 12 h.
- Maintenance: Usually one quarter of the digitalizing dose; half is given every 12 h.

Children
- Digitalization: *Newborns,* total dose of 0.022 mg/kg body wt; *2 wk–3 yr,* total dose of 0.025 mg/kg. *3 yr and over,* 0.022 mg/kg. Administer in divided doses every 3–4 h; may be administered as a single dose if needed.

PREPARATION/RECONSTITUTION
May be administered undiluted; may further dilute with 10 ml compatible diluent.

INCOMPATIBILITIES
Acids, alkalis, calcium chloride, calcium disodium edetate, calcium gluceptate, calcium gluconate.

RATE/MODE OF ADMINISTRATION
IV push: By sideport of IV administration set; do not mix with IV fluids.

Intermittent: No.
Continuous: No.
Filter: Inappropriate in less than 1-ml dose.

NURSING CONSIDERATIONS

Nursing Diagnoses

1. Potential alteration in nutrition: decreased, related to drug side effects.
2. Potential alteration in cardiac output, related to action of drug on myocardium.

Acute Care

Potassium depletion causes the heart to be more sensitive to possible digitalis intoxication. Monitor patient's electrolyte levels during treatment. Use with extreme caution in patient with hypercalcemia or renal/hepatic disease. Monitor ECG regularly.

Precautions

Potentiated by phenytoin sodium, thyroid preparation, veratrum alkaloids, reserpine, quinidine, propranolol, verapamil, and diuretics. Inhibited by potassium salts and others. Do not give digitalized patients calcium; death has been reported.

Contraindications

Digitalis toxicity; ventricular tachycardia; known hypersensitivity to this drug.

Side Effects

Cardiovascular: AV block, dysrhythmias. First clinical signs of toxicity relate to other body systems.
Gastrointestinal: Diarrhea, anorexia, nausea, salivation, vomiting.
Neurologic: Blurred vision, confusion, disturbed color vision, headache.

Patient/Caregiver Teaching

Instruct patient (1) to report all side effects immediately, including evidence of visual disturbances and (2) to provide accurate medical history and drug profile.

Home Care

Inappropriate.

Administration in Other Clinical Settings
Inappropriate.

Nursing Interventions
The physician must be advised of all side effects immediately; dosage may need to be decreased or discontinued. Digoxin immune FAB is a specific antidote for severe symptoms.

Desmopressin acetate
US: Vasopressin

Hormonal agent   pH 3.5–4

ACTION
A synthetic analogue of human ADH used to promote reabsorption of water in the renal tubular epithelium; increases levels of clotting factor VIII.

INDICATIONS/USES
Used in the treatment of neurogenic diabetes insipidus and hemophilia A and for von Willebrand's disease.

USUAL DOSE
Adults
- Diabetes insipidus: 0.5–1.0 ml/day IV, divided into 2 doses.
- Hemophilia A or von Willebrand's disease: 0.3 μg/kg diluted in 50 ml sterile physiologic saline infused over 15–30 min.

Children
- Diabetes insipidus: Parenteral administration not determined to be safe.
- Hemophilia A or von Willebrand's disease: 0.3 μg/kg diluted in 10 ml sterile physiologic saline over 15–30 min.

PREPARATION/RECONSTITUTION
Dilute per manufacturer's directions in sterile physiologic saline prior to administration by parenteral route.

INCOMPATIBILITIES
Unknown.

RATE/MODE OF ADMINISTRATION
IV push: Applicable, usually sideport with ongoing infusion over 15–30 min.

Intermittent: Applicable, usually sideport with ongoing infusion over 15–30 min.

Continuous: No.

Filter: Applicable.

NURSING CONSIDERATIONS
Nursing Diagnoses
1. Potential alteration in comfort, related to GI and local effects.
2. Potential alteration in fluid volume, related to water retention.
3. Potential alteration in cardiac output, related to increased intravascular volume.
4. Potential knowledge deficit regarding drug therapy.

Acute Care
Monitor patients with cardiovascular disease carefully. Monitor pulse and blood pressure during infusion for hemophilia A and von Willebrand's disease.

Precautions
Monitor clinical response and laboratory reports to determine effectiveness of treatment and need for additional medication.

Contraindications
Known allergy to desmopressin acetate; type II von Willebrand's disease; vascular disease or hypertension; pregnancy, lactation.

Side Effects
Circulatory: Headache, elevation of blood pressure, facial flushing, fluid retention, water intoxication, hyponatremia.

Dermatologic: Burning pain at site of injection, local erythema.

Patient/Caregiver Teaching
Instruct patient (1) to report all side effects immediately; (2) to report use of this medication to caregiver; and (3) to learn principles of nasal self-administration.

Home Care
Appropriate.

Administration in Other Clinical Settings
Appropriate.

Nursing Interventions
Individualize dosage to establish a diurnal pattern of water turnover; estimate response by adequate duration of sleep and adequate, not excessive, water turnover. Notify physician of all side effects immediately.

Dexamethasone sodium phosphate
US: Decadron phosphate, Decadrol, Decaject, Dexasone, Dexone, Dezone, Hexadrol phosphate

Antiinflammatory agent   pH 7.0–8.5

Betamethasone sodium phosphate
US: Betameth, Celestone phosphate, selestoject

Antiinflammatory agent   pH 8.5

ACTION
Inflammatory glucocorticoid that is seven times as potent as pred-

nisolone and 20 to 30 times as potent as hydrocortisone. Excreted in the urine and secreted in breast milk.

INDICATIONS/USES

Used as supplemental therapy for severe allergic reactions; reduction of cerebral edema and acute exacerbations of disease for patients receiving steroid therapy; viral hepatitis; thyroid crisis; antineoplastic therapy; and as an antiemetic for cisplatin-induced vomiting.

USUAL DOSE

Dexamethasone: 0.5–9.0 mg daily.
Betamethasone: Up to 12 mg daily; may be divided into 2–4 equal doses. Larger doses may be indicated consistent with patient's clinical condition; not to exceed 80 mg/24 h.

PREPARATION/RECONSTITUTION

May be administered undiluted or added to 5% dextrose in water or 0.9% sodium chloride solutions.

INCOMPATIBILITIES

Amikacin, daunorubicin, doxorubicin, metaraminol, prochlorperazine, vancomycin. Other drugs may be administered concurrently; consult manufacturer's literature relevant to administration.

RATE/MODE OF ADMINISTRATION

IV push: Over 1 min or less.
Intermittent: No.
Continuous: May be administered as a continuous infusion by electronic flow control device.
Filter: Not recommended for dose less than 1 ml.

NURSING CONSIDERATIONS

Nursing Diagnoses

1. Potential for injury, related to drug side effects.
2. Potential for fluid volume deficit: actual, related to electrolyte disturbances.

Acute Care

Use diluted solutions within 24 h; solution is sensitive to heat exposure. Protect solution from freezing. Withdrawal from therapy should be gradual; patient should be weaned to avoid symptoms of adrenal insufficiency and to prevent elevation of body temperature. Insulin needs in diabetics may be increased.

Precautions

Use with caution in patients with hypothyroidism and cirrhosis. Altered protein-binding capacity will affect effectiveness of drug. Administer as a single dose prior to 9 am to reduce suppression of individual's own adrenocortical activity. Salt and potassium replacement may be needed; monitor electrolyte status regularly. Inhibits anticoagulants, isoniazids, and salicylates. Potentiates action of theophyllines and cyclosporine.

Contraindications

Known hypersensitivity to any component including sulfites; systemic fungal infections. Others may include active or latent peptic ulcer, acute or healed tuberculosis, acute or chronic infection, acute psychoses, diabetes mellitus, diverticulitis, osteoporosis, pregnancy, septic shock.

Side Effects

Cardiovascular: Electrolyte imbalance, embolism, hyperglycemia, hypersensitivity, hypertension, thromboembolism.
Neurologic: Weakness, tingling.
Other: Menstrual irregularities, Cushing's syndrome.

Patient/Caregiver Teaching

Instruct patient (1) to report all side effects immediately; (2) to provide accurate medical history and drug profile; and (3) to learn principles of home self-administration.

Home Care

Appropriate in well-monitored settings.

Administration in Other Clinical Settings

Appropriate in well-monitored settings.

Nursing Interventions

The physician should be notified of all side effects immediately. Resuscitative equipment (epinephrine) must be readily available.

Dextran 40, low molecular weight

US: Gentran 40, L.M.D. 10%, Rheomacrodex

Plasma volume expander   pH 3–7

ACTION

A low molecular weight, short-acting plasma volume expander. Increases plasma volume by once or twice its own volume and helps to restore normal circulatory dynamics. Mobilizes water from body tissues and increases urinary output. Each gram of dextran holds 25 ml of water in the vascular space.

INDICATIONS/USES

Used as adjunctive therapy in treatment of shock caused by hemorrhage, trauma, burns, or surgery. Prophylaxis during surgical procedures with a high incidence of venous thrombosis and pulmonary embolism.

USUAL DOSE

20 ml/kg body wt over first 24 h; 10 ml/kg over each succeeding 24 h. Drug should be discontinued after 5 days of treatment.

Prophylaxis: 20 mg/kg on surgical day; 500 ml daily for 2–3 days; 500 ml every 2–3 days for up to 2 wk.
As priming fluid: 10–20 ml/kg; do not exceed.

PREPARATION/RECONSTITUTION

Available as a 10% concentration in 500-ml containers ready for use.

INCOMPATIBILITIES

Ascorbic acid, chlortetracycline, promethazine. Do not add any drug to this infusate.

RATE/MODE OF ADMINISTRATION

IV push: No.
Intermittent: No.
Continuous: Only method of administration; electronic infusion device may be used to monitor rate of infusion. Initial 5 ml may be administered over 15–30 min. *Note: Promit should be administered before every initial dose.* Monitor patient carefully for signs of impending anaphylaxis. Remainder of any dose should be evenly distributed over 8–24 h.
Filter: 1.2 μ may be used consistent with institutional policies.

NURSING CONSIDERATIONS

Nursing Diagnoses

1. Potential for alteration in fluid volume, related to action fo drug.
2. Potential for injury, related to bleeding tendencies.

Acute Care

Monitor patient carefully; anaphylaxis has been documented following administration of small amounts of dextran 40. For IV use only. Monitor vital signs every 5–15 min for the first hour and hourly thereafter. Maintain patient's hydration with additional IV fluids. Change IV tubing or flush well with 0.9% sodium chloride solution before administering blood transfusion. Crystallization may occur at low temperatures; may need to submerge in warm water and dissolve crystals prior to administration. Use only a clear solution; partially used solutions should be discarded.

Precautions

If anuric or oliguric after 500 ml of dextran, discontinue the infusate and notify physician. Mannitol may help to increase urinary output. Avoid overhydration with dilution of electrolyte balance. May reduce coagulability of circulatory blood slightly. Maintain patient's hematocrit level above 30%.

Contraindications

Severe bleeding disorders; extreme hemostatic defects; known hypersensitivity to dextran; lactation and pregnancy; severe congestive heart failure; renal failure.

Side Effects

Hematologic: Bleeding, wound hematoma, wound seroma, wound bleeding, distant bleeding (melena).

Cardiopulmonary: Wheezing, severe anaphylaxis (death), dehydration, fever, hypotension, overhydration, tightness of chest.

Gastrointestinal: Nausea.

Other: Joint pain.

Patient/Caregiver Teaching

Instruct patient: (1) to report all side effects immediately and (2) to provide accurate medical history and drug profile.

Home Care

Inappropriate.

Administration in Other Clinical Settings

Inappropriate except in well-monitored setting (ambulatory care only).

Nursing Interventions

The physician must be notified of all side effects immediately. Keep resuscitative equipment readily available. Discontinue the drug at first sign of allergic reaction. Epinephrine may be administered as indicated. Factor VIII infusion may counteract excessive bleeding.

Dextran, high molecular weight

US: Dextran 75, Dextran 70, Gentran 75, Macrodex

Plasma volume expander   pH 3–7

ACTION
A plasma volume expander that provides hemodynamically significant plasma volume expansion in excess of the amount infused for approximately 24 h. Dilutes total serum proteins and hematocrit values; excreted in the urine.

INDICATIONS/USES
Used in the treatment of shock or impending shock caused by surgery, hemorrhage, burns, or trauma.

USUAL DOSE
Dose varies according to amount of fluid loss and existing hemoconcentration. Usually 500 ml is given initially; total dose not to exceed 20 ml/kg body wt/24 h for adults and children.

PREPARATION/RECONSTITUTION
Administer as is.

INCOMPATIBILITIES
Ascorbic acid, chlortetracycline, promethazine. Do not add any drug to this solution.

RATE/MODE OF ADMINISTRATION
IV push: No.
Intermittent: No.
Continuous: 500 ml at 20–40 ml/min by electronic infusion device. Flow should then be reduced to lowest possible rate to maintain hemodynamic status.
Filter: 1.2 μ may be used consistent with institutional policy.

NURSING CONSIDERATIONS

Nursing Diagnoses

1. Potential for injury, related to bleeding tendencies.
2. Potential alteration in cardiac output, related to drug action.

Acute Care

Administer IV only; use when whole blood or blood components are not readily available. Monitor vital signs constantly, including every 5–15 min for first hour and hourly thereafter. Maintain hydration with other IV fluids; avoid overhydration with dilution of electrolyte balance. Draw venous sample for type and crossmatch prior to administration of dextran. Crystallization may occur; submerge solution in warm water to dissolve all crystals prior to administration. Use only clear solution; store at constant temperatures, not to exceed 25°C. Discard partially used solutions. Change IV tubing or flush thoroughly with 0.9% sodium chloride solution prior to administration of blood.

Precautions

Use with caution in heart/renal diseases. May reduce coagulability of circulating blood. Maintain hematocrit level above 30%. May alter blood sugar and total bilirubin levels. Monitor hemoglobin, hematocrit, electrolyte, and serum protein levels during therapy.

Contraindications

Severe bleeding disorders, marked hemostatic disorders, known hypersensitivity, lactation, pregnancy, cardiac or renal disease.

Side Effects

Hematologic: Bleeding, wound hematoma, seroma, distant bleeding.
Cardiopulmonary: Wheezing, dehydration, fever, hypotension, overhydration, tightness of chest, anaphylaxis, pulmonary edema.
Gastrointestinal: Nausea, vomiting.
Other: Joint pain, urticaria.

Home Care

Not recommended.

Administration in Other Clinical Settings

Inappropriate except in well-monitored setting (ambulatory care only).

Nursing Interventions

The physician must be notified of all side effects immediately. Discontinue the drug immediately at signs/symptoms of allergic reaction. Epinephrine may relieve symptoms; factor VIII infusion may counteract excessive bleeding. Resuscitative equipment should be readily available.

Dextran 1

US: Promit

Prophylactic

ACTION

Binds to one of two available sites on dextran-reacting antibodies; prevents formation of immune complexes with polyvalent clinical dextrans and helps to prevent anaphylaxis. Excreted in the urine.

INDICATIONS/USES

Used as prophylaxis for serious anaphylactic reactions associated with administration of clinical dextran solutions.

USUAL DOSE

Adults: 20 ml.
Children: 0.3 ml/kg body wt.

PREPARATION/RECONSTITUTION

May be administered undiluted by sideport of an ongoing infusion (not coadministered with dextran solution).

INCOMPATIBILITIES

Dextran 40, low molecular weight; dextran, high molecular weight.

RATE/MODE OF ADMINISTRATION

IV push: As a single dose over 1 min; administer 1–2 min before clinical IV dextran infusion. If 15 or more min pass before initiation of clinical dextran, dose will need to be repeated.

Intermittent: No.
Continuous: No.
Filter: Not applicable in less than 1-ml dosage.

NURSING CONSIDERATIONS

Nursing Diagnoses

1. Potential for alteration in cardiac output, related to drug side effects.
2. Potential for alteration in comfort, related to side effects.

Acute Care

Administer IV only; will not prevent allergic reactions associated with dextran infusates.

Precautions

If patient experiences a reaction to dextran 1, do not administer clinical dextran solution. May cause severe and rapid hypotension and bradycardia.

Contraindications

Severe bleeding disorders, marked hemostatic defects, lactation, pregnancy, congestive heart failure, renal failure.

Side Effects

Cardiopulmonary: Bradycardia, hypotension, pallor, shivering.
Gastrointestinal: Nausea.
Other: Cutaneous reactions.

Home Care

Not recommended.

Administration in Other Clinical Settings

Not recommended.

Nursing Interventions

The physician should be notified at first sign of allergic reaction or side effect. Epinephrine may be needed to reverse effect. Resuscitative equipment must be readily available.

Dextrose
US: Glucose

Monosaccharide   pH 3.5–6.5

ACTION

Provides glucose calories for metabolic needs, lowers excess ketone production, protects body proteins. Hypertonic solutions (20%–50%) act as diuretics and reduce CNS edema. Excreted by the kidneys, producing diuresis.

INDICATIONS/USES

Used to provide calories, singularly or in combination with amino acids (by central vein); to treat insulin hypoglycemia (50% solution), cerebral and meningeal edema (50% solution), shock (10%–70% solution), hyperkalemia (20% solution), diuresis (20%–50% solution); and as a diluent for administration of IV medications (2.5%–10% solution).

USUAL DOSE

Adults: Depends on use, age, weight, clinical condition of patient.
- 50–1000 ml of 2.5% (25 g/L) and 5% (50 g/L) solutions.
- 5 ml of 10% dextrose; repeat as necessary.
- 500–1000 ml of 10% dextrose (100 g/L) solution once or twice every 24 h as needed.
- 500 ml of 20% dextrose (200 g/L) solution once or twice every 24 h as needed.
- 50 ml of 50% dextrose (25 g) solution; 10–25 g for insulin-induced hypoglycemia; repeat as needed.
- 500–1500 ml/24 h of 30% (300 g/L), 60% (60 g/L), 70% (700 g/L) as a component of nutritional support formula.

Children
- Acute symptomatic hypoglycemia: 250–500 mg/kg body wt of 25% dextrose solution.

PREPARATION/RECONSTITUTION

May be administered undiluted.

INCOMPATIBILITIES

Cyanocobalamin, kanamycin, sodium bicarbonate, whole blood.

RATE/MODE OF ADMINISTRATION

IV push: Yes, consistent with following guidelines:
- 10% solution: 5 ml over 10–15 sec.
- 50% solution: 10 ml over 1 min.

Intermittent: Yes, as follows:
- 20% solution: 500 ml over 30–60 min.

Continuous: Yes, consistent with following guidelines:
- 10% solution: 1000 ml over 3 h.
- 30%–70% solution: 500 ml over 4–12 h, depending on body weight. *Note: A rate of 0.5 g/kg/h will not cause glycosuria. At 0.8 g/kg/h 95% is retained and will cause glycosuria.*

NURSING CONSIDERATIONS

Nursing Diagnoses

1. Potential for alteration in fluid volume, related to drug side effects.
2. Potential for alteration in cardiac output, related to drug side effects.

Acute Care

Dextrose causes hemolysis of red blood cells; do not administer simultaneously with blood products. Do not use unless solution is clear and vial is sterile. Hypertonic solutions in excess of 12.5% should be administered by central vein. Confirm patency of vein and avoid extravasation.

Precautions

Use with caution in infants of diabetic mothers. Can cause fluid or solute overload. May result in solution of serum electrolyte concentration, overhydration, congestion, or pulmonary edema. Rapid administration of hypertonic solutions will cause hyperglycemia and may cause hyperosmolar syndrome. Do not withdraw concentrated dextrose solutions abruptly, or rebound hypoglycemia will result. If nutritional support formula is not readily available, replace solution with a like solution that most nearly approximates existing dextrose concentration.

Contraindications

Delirium tremens with dehydration; diabetic coma while blood sugar is high; intracranial or intraspinal hemorrhage; glucose-galactose malabsorption.

Side Effects

Circulatory: Fluid overload, hyperglycemia, hyperosmolar syndrome, hypokalemia, hypoglycemic alkalosis, acidosis.
Other: Thrombosis.

Patient/Caregiver Teaching

Instruct patient (1) to report all side effects immediately and (2) to provide accurate medical history and drug profile.

Home Care

Appropriate for administration by peripheral or central vein.

Administration in Other Clinical Settings

Appropriate for administration by peripheral or central vein.

Nursing Interventions

The physician should be notified of all side effects immediately.

Diazepam

US: Valium

Nervous system depressant   pH 6.2–6.9

ACTION

Depresses the autonomic, central, and peripheral nervous systems. Provides a sedative, hypnotic effect; acts as an amnesic, anticonvulsant, skeletal muscle relaxant. Diminishes patient recall. Excreted very slowly in the urine; also crosses the placental barrier and is secreted in breast milk.

INDICATIONS/USES

Used in the treatment of moderate to severe psychoneurotic reactions, acute alcohol withdrawal, acute stress reactions, muscle spasm, status epilepticus, severe recurrent convulsive seizures, preoperative medication, pre-endoscopic procedure sedation, cardioversion.

USUAL DOSE

Adults: 2–10 mg every 3–4 h; may repeat in 1 h up to maximum of 30 mg in 8 h.

- Status epilepticus: 5–10 mg; repeat at intervals of 5–10 min up to total dose of 30 mg (maximum dose is 100 mg/24 h).
- Cardioversion: 5–15 mg before procedure.
- Endoscopy: Up to 20 mg before procedure begins if a narcotic is not being used; titrate to desired degree of sedation.

Children

- Tetanus in infants over 30 days old: 1–2 mg every 3–4 h.
- Tetanus in children 5 yr or older: 5–10 mg every 3–4 h.
- Status epilepticus in infants over 30 days old: 0.2–0.5 mg every 2–5 min up to maximum of 10 mg.
- Status epilepticus in children 5 yr or older: 0.5–2 mg every 2–5 min up to maximum of 10 mg.

PREPARATION/RECONSTITUTION

Stable only in its own diluent; do not dilute or mix and do not add to any IV solution.

INCOMPATIBILITIES

Any other drug or solution in syringe or solution (causes precipitation).

RATE/MODE OF ADMINISTRATION

IV push: 5 mg or fraction thereof over 1 min; in children and infants, administer total dose over a minimum of 3 min.

Intermittent: No.

Continuous: No.

Filter: Not applicable in less than 1-ml dose.

NURSING CONSIDERATIONS
Nursing Diagnoses
1. Potential for alteration in comfort: decrease in pain, related to sedative qualities of drug.
2. Potential for injury, related to blurred vision and diminished reflexes.
3. Potential for disturbance in sleep pattern, related to drug side effects.
4. Potential for ineffective breathing pattern, related to drug side effects.

Acute Care
Administer directly into the vein; avoid smaller veins to prevent incidence of thrombophlebitis. Do not extravasate. Resuscitative equipment must be readily available. Bed rest is required for at least 3 h following IV administration of this drug.

Precautions
Respiratory assistance should be immediately available. Potentiates narcotics, phenothiazines, MAO inhibitors and tricyclic antidepressants for up to 48 h. Potentiated by cimetidine, alcohol, and other CNS depressants. Inhibits antiparkinsonian effects of levodopa. Reduce dosage accordingly for administration to elderly patients and those with renal/hepatic dysfunction.

Contraindications
Acute narrow-angle glaucoma; infants and children under age 12 (except in tetany and status epilepticus); known psychoses; pregnancy, childbirth, and lactation; shock; coma; acute alcohol intoxication with depression of vital signs.

Side Effects
Respiratory: Apnea, depressed respirations, dyspnea, hyperventilation, laryngospasm, coughing.
Cardiovascular: Bradycardia, cardiac arrest, cardiovascular collapse.
Neurologic: Ataxia, blurred vision, coma, confusion, depression, diminished reflexes, drowsiness, headache, hyperexcited states, syncope.
Other: Venous thrombosis, phlebitis, nystagmus.

Patient/Caregiver Teaching

Instruct patient (1) to report all side effects immediately; (2) to report use of alcohol; and (3) to report incidence of venous spasm or irritation.

Home Care

Inappropriate because of potential for respiratory arrest.

Administration in Other Clinical Settings

Inappropriate unless full resuscitative support is readily available.

Nursing Interventions

The physician must be notified of all side effects immediately. Resuscitative equipment must be readily available. Maintain adequate airway and ventilation; promote excretion of drug through fluid resuscitation. Caffeine and sodium benzoate may counteract CNS depression of diazepam overdose. Dopamine, levarterenol, or metaraminol may be used to reverse hypotensive effects of drug. Physostigmine 0.5–4 mg at 1 mg/min may counteract symptoms of anticholinergic overdose (may also potentiate seizures).

Diazoxide

US: Hyperstat IV

Antihypertensive   pH 11.6

ACTION

A potent, rapid-acting antihypertensive agent that produces vasodilation by relaxing smooth muscle of peripheral arterioles. Cardiac output is increased within 1–5 min. Crosses the placental barrier and is secreted in breast milk.

INDICATIONS/USES

Used in the treatment of malignant and nonmalignant hypertensive emergencies. *Note: This drug should be reviewed for administration by professional nurses and, on approval of the institution's Pharmacy and Therapeutics Committee, added to the list of IV drugs that a nurse may administer safely.*

USUAL DOSE

Adults: 150 mg; to calculate exact dose preferred, use 1–3 mg/kg body wt. May repeat dose in 5–15 min if appropriate response has not been achieved; repeat as needed at 4- to 24-hour intervals to maintain blood pressure reading. (For short-term use only.)

Children: 1–3 mg/kg, not to exceed 150 mg.

PREPARATION/RECONSTITUTION

Administer undiluted as liquid in ampule.

INCOMPATIBILITIES

Do not mix in syringe or solution with any other drug.

RATE/MODE OF ADMINISTRATION

IV push: Rapid administration over 30 sec or less.
Intermittent: No.
Continuous: No.
Filter: Not recommended.

NURSING CONSIDERATIONS

Nursing Diagnoses

1. Potential for alteration in comfort, related to abdominal pain, flushing.
2. Potential for hyperthermia, related to drug side effects.
3. Potential for sensory-perceptual alteration: visual or tactile, related to drug side effects.
4. Potential for injury, related to weakness.

Acute Care

Administer directly into the vein; avoid extravasation. Patient should be maintained in recumbent position during injection and for 30 min following injection. Monitor blood pressure every 5 min until stable, and hourly thereafter. Record blood pressure reading with patient in standing position prior to ambulation. Do not use for more than 10 days. Diazoxide is sensitive to light and temperature; protect from freezing.

Precautions

May cause hyperglycemia; use with caution in diabetes mellitus. Use with caution in those with impaired cerebral or cardiac circulation. A reduced dose of anticoagulant may be needed; monitor carefully. Potentiated by thiazides and other diuretics. Profound hypotension results if used with peripheral vasodilators (eg, nitroprusside sodium, hydralazine).

Contraindications

Compensatory hypertension; known sensitivity to thiazides; pheochromocytoma; pregnancy and lactation. Safety for use in children not yet established.

Side Effects

Gastrointestinal: Abdominal discomfort, ileus, nausea, vomiting.
Neurologic: Confusion, convulsions, flushing, headache, lightheadedness, paralysis.
Circulatory/cardiovascular: Cerebral ischemia, congestive heart failure, edema, hyperglycemia, hypotension, myocardial ischemia, orthostatic hypotension, palpitations.

Patient/Caregiver Teaching

Instruct patient (1) to report all side effects immediately; (2) to report sensations of warmth immediately; (3) to provide accurate drug and medical profiles; and (4) to remain in supine position for at least 30 min after administration.

Home Care

Inappropriate.

Administration in Other Clinical Settings

Inappropriate.

Nursing Interventions

The physician must be notified of all side effects immediately. Treat sensitivity reactions as needed. Resuscitative equipment must be readily available. Insulin may counteract excessive hyperglycemia. Hemodialysis or peritoneal dialysis may reverse overdose.

Diethylstilbestrol diphosphate

US: Stilphostrol
CAN: Honvol (Horner)

Estrogen hormone   pH 9.0–10.5

ACTION
An estrogen hormone that decreases the percentage of cells actively proliferating in a tumor mass.

INDICATIONS/USES
Used as palliative treatment of prostatic carcinoma in advanced stage.

USUAL DOSE
Initial: 0.5 g/24 h; increase to 1 g/24 h beginning with second day of treatment and continue for 5 days or as needed.
Maintenance: 0.25–0.5 g once or twice weekly.

PREPARATION/RECONSTITUTION
Dilute single daily dose in 300 ml of 5% dextrose in water or 0.9% sodium chloride solution.

INCOMPATIBILITIES
Calcium gluconate.

RATE/MODE OF ADMINISTRATION
IV push: No.
Intermittent: 20 drops/min for initial 15 min; then increase rate to complete infusion within 60 min of starting time.
Continuous: No.
Filter: Appropriate for use consistent with institutional guidelines.

NURSING CONSIDERATIONS
Nursing Diagnoses
1. Potential for alteration in comfort, related to drug side effects.

2. Potential for disturbance of self-concept: body image, related to decreased libido.

Acute Care

Use with care in those with cardiac, renal, or hepatic disease and diabetes.

Precautions

As above. IV route is used when oral route is ineffective or unavailable. Monitor patient for salt and water retention.

Contraindications

Liver dysfunction; past history of or active thrombophlebitis, thromboembolic disease, or cerebral apoplexy; estrogen-dependent neoplasias.

Side Effects

Gastrointestinal: Abdominal cramps, nausea, vomiting.
Neurologic: Headache, dizziness.
Other: Short-lived burning and pain in perineal area and metastatic sites to be expected; decreased libido, elevated PT, hypercalcemia, painful swelling of breasts, pulmonary embolism, thrombophlebitis.

Patient/Caregiver Teaching

Instruct patient (1) to report all side effects immediately and (2) that burning and pain will subside.

Home Care

Appropriate; monitor weight and encourage a low-salt diet.

Administration in Other Clinical Settings

Appropriate; monitor weight and encourage a low-salt diet.

Nursing Interventions

The physician should be notified of all side effects. Hypercalcemia may be reversed by appropriate intervention with regime of increased fluids, ambulation, limited oral calcium intake.

Digoxin

US: Lanoxin

Cardiac glycoside   pH 6.6–7.4

ACTION

A crystalline cardiac glycoside with onset of action 5–10 min following administration and lasting 2–3 days. Increases myocardial contraction and decreases venous pressure. Rapidly excreted in the urine.

INDICATIONS/USES

Used in the treatment of congestive heart failure, atrial fibrillation, atrial flutter, cardiogenic shock, ventricular dysrhythmias with congestive heart failure, paroxysmal tachycardia, and preoperatively, intraoperatively, and postoperatively for stress on the heart muscle.

USUAL DOSE

Adults
- Digitalization: Administer 0.25–0.5 mg as initial dose, followed by 0.25–0.5 mg at 4–6-h intervals.
- Maintenance: 0.125–0.5 mg daily.

Children (Note: Use 0.1-mg/ml pediatric injection only.)
- Birth to 2 yr: 0.04–0.06 mg/kg body wt/24 h.
- Over 2 yr: 0.02–0.04 mg/kg/24 h; half of total dose initially, then quarter of daily dose 2 times at 8-h intervals.
- Maintenance: 20%–35% of total loading dose divided; administer every 12 h.

PREPARATION/RECONSTITUTION

May be administered undiluted; each 1 ml may be diluted in 4 ml sterile water, normal saline, or 5% dextrose in water (use solution immediately).

INCOMPATIBILITIES

Acids, alkalies, calcium chloride, calcium disodium edetate, calcium gluceptate, calcium gluconate.

RATE/MODE OF ADMINISTRATION
IV push: Yes.
Intermittent: No.
Continuous: No.
Filter: Inappropriate in less than 1-ml dose.

NURSING CONSIDERATIONS
Nursing Diagnoses
1. Potential for alteration in cardiac output, related to drug action.
2. Potential for injury, related to drug side effects.

Acute Care
Do not administer calcium products to digitalized patients. Monitor electrolyte levels regularly; potassium depletion increases sensitivity to digitalis intoxication. Monitor ECG.

Precautions
Use with caution in patients with hypercalcemia or renal/hepatic dysfunction. Dose may require adjustment downward. Potentiated by aminoglycosides, phenytoin, tetracyclines, thyroid preparations, veratrum alkaloids, propranolol, verapamil, diuretics, pressor agents. Inhibited by antineoplastic agents, potassium salts.

Contraindications
Digitalis intoxication.

Side Effects
Cardiovascular: Partial or AV block, dysrhythmias (note evidence of ST segment sag, prolonged PR interval, bigeminal rhythm).
Clinical signs of toxicity: Abdominal discomfort, blurred vision, confusion, diarrhea, nausea, vomiting.

Patient/Caregiver Teaching
Instruct patient (1) to report all side effects immediately and (2) to expect side effects to subside within a few days or on withdrawal of drug.

Home Care
Appropriate in well-monitored setting.

Administration in Other Clinical Settings
Appropriate in well-monitored setting.

Nursing Interventions
The physician should be notified of all side effects. Severe toxicity is treated with digoxin antidote (digoxin immune FAB).

Digoxin immune FAB (ovine)
US: Digibind

Digoxin antidote   pH 6—8

ACTION
FAB (fragment antigen binding) binds molecules of digoxin and makes them unavailable for binding at their site of action. Prompt onset of action and improvement within 30 min. Excreted in the urine.

INDICATIONS/USES
Used in the treatment of those with life-threatening digoxin intoxication or overdose; also given to relieve hyperkalemia with digitalis intoxication (potassium concentration above 5 mEq/L).

USUAL DOSE
Packaged 40 mg/vial (will bind 0.6-mg digoxin or deslanoside). If ingested dose is not available, administer 20 vials (800 mg); may repeat single dose if needed in several hours.

PREPARATION/RECONSTITUTION
Reconstitute each vial with 4 ml sterile water for injection and mix gently; may further dilute if needed.

INCOMPATIBILITIES

Unknown. Do not mix with any other drug in syringe or solution.

RATE/MODE OF ADMINISTRATION

IV push: Not recommended unless cardiac arrest is imminent.
Intermittent: No.
Continuous: Applicable.
Filter: Applicable.

NURSING CONSIDERATIONS

Nursing Diagnoses

1. Potential for impairment of potential skin integrity, related to drug side effects.
2. Potential for alteration in cardiac output, related to effects of drug.

Acute Care

Precautions are needed in those sensitive to ovine proteins or those who have previously received antibodies or FAB fragments produced from sheep; hypersensitivity testing is indicated. Dilute 0.1 ml of initially diluted solution with 10 ml sterile normal saline to produce a 1:100 solution (100 µg/ml) and perform scratch or skin test.

Scratch: ¼-inch skin scratch through a drop of 1:100 dilution; inspect in 20 min. Urticarial wheal surrounded by zone of erythema is a positive reaction.
Skin: Inject 0.1 ml of 1:100 dilution intradermally; inspect in 20 min. Urticarial wheal surrounded by zone of erythema is a positive reaction. Use reconstituted solution promptly or store in refrigerator for maximum of 4 h. Monitor vital signs, ECG, and potassium level frequently during and after administration.

Precautions

Obtain serum concentrations; wait 6–8 hours after last digitalis dose. Potassium may shift from inside to outside cell, causing increased renal excretion. Do not redigitalize patient until all FAB fragments have been eliminated from the body, which may take days. Use with caution in those with impaired cardiac function. Use only when clearly indicated in pregnancy, lactation, and infants.

Contraindications

None known when used as indicated.

Side Effects

Cardiopulmonary: Acute anaphylaxis, respiratory distress, vascular collapse.

Other: Hypokalemia (life-threatening).

Patient/Caregiver Teaching

Instruct patient (1) to report all side effects immediately and (2) to provide accurate medical history and drug profile.

Home Care

Inappropriate.

Administration in Other Clinical Settings

Inappropriate.

Nursing Interventions

If hypersensitivity exists and treatment is needed, preload with corticosteroids and diphenhydramine; prepare to treat anaphylaxis. The physician should be notified of all side effects immediately. Resuscitative equipment should be readily available. Treat hypokalemia with caution.

Dimenhydrinate

US: Dramamine, Dramanate, Dramilin, Dramocen, Dymenate, Hydrate, Marmine, Wehamine

Antihistamine   pH 6.8–7.2

ACTION

An antihistamine and CNS depressant. Excreted in the urine and secreted in breast milk.

INDICATIONS/USES
Used in the treatment of motion sickness, nausea and vomiting, vertigo, and Meniere's disease.

USUAL DOSE
Adults: 50–100 mg every 4 h.
Children: 5 mg/kg body wt divided into 4 equal doses over 24 h; not to exceed total dose of 300 mg.

PREPARATION/RECONSTITUTION
Dilute each 50 mg in 10 ml of sodium chloride injection.

INCOMPATIBILITIES
Alkaline solutions, aminophylline, ammonium chloride, amobarbital, chlorpromazine, diphenhydramine, heparin sodium, hydrocortisone, hydroxyzine, phenytoin, prednisolone, prochlorperazine, promazine, promethazine, tetracyclines.

RATE/MODE OF ADMINISTRATION
IV push: Inject each 50 mg or fraction thereof over 2 min.
Intermittent: No.
Continuous: No.
Filter: Not applicable in less than 1-ml dose.

NURSING CONSIDERATIONS
Nursing Diagnoses
1. Potential for injury, related to drug side effects.
2. Potential for activity intolerance, related to drug side effects.

Acute Care
Breast-feeding patients should be encouraged to discontinue. Induces drowsiness; patient should be protected from injury.

Precautions
Will cause irreversible ototoxicity when given in conjunction with some antibiotics such as gentamicin, kanamycin, neomycin, streptomycin, vancomycin. Reduce dosage for the debilitated or elderly patient. Alcohol and CNS depressants produce an additive effect. Use with caution in pregnancy, prostatic hypertrophy, bladder neck obstruction, glaucoma, cardiac dysrhythmias, asthma.

Contraindications
Known hypersensitivity; neonates.

Side Effects
Primary side effect is drowsiness.
Overdose: Convulsions, hallucinations, hyperpyrexia, marked irritability.

Patient/Caregiver Teaching
Instruct patient (1) to provide accurate medical history and drug profile and (2) to prevent injury related to drowsiness.

Home Care
Appropriate.

Administration in Other Clinical Settings
Appropriate.

Nursing Interventions
The physician should be notified of all side effects; diazepam may relieve convulsions initially. Exaggerated side effects should be reported; may require discontinuing the drug.

Diphenhydramine
US: Ban-Allergin-50, Benadryl, Benoject 10/50, Dihydrex, Nordryl, Wehdryl

Antihistamine   pH 5–6

ACTION
An antihistamine, anticholinergic, and antiemetic with sedative effects. Readily absorbed and easily metabolized; excreted unchanged in the urine and some secretion may occur in breast milk.

INDICATIONS/USES
Used to treat allergic reactions to blood or plasma; as supplemental therapy to epinephrine in anaphylaxis and angioneurotic edema; as preoperative sedation; and to reduce effects of severe nausea and vomiting.

USUAL DOSE
Adults: 10–50 mg; up to 100 mg may be administered, but not to exceed 400 mg/24 h.
Children: 5 mg/kg body wt/24 h; divide into 4 equal doses; not to exceed 300 mg/24 h.

PREPARATION/RECONSTITUTION
Administer undiluted.

INCOMPATIBILITIES
Amobarbital, amphotericin B, cephalothin, dexamethasone, furosemide, methylprednisolone, phenobarbital, phenytoin, secobarbital, thiopental.

RATE/MODE OF ADMINISTRATION
IV push: 25 mg or fraction thereof over 1 min.
Intermittent: No.
Continuous: No.
Filter: Not applicable in less than 1-ml dose.

NURSING CONSIDERATIONS
Nursing Diagnoses
1. Potential for injury, related to drowsiness.
2. Potential for pain, related to possible subcutaneous or perivascular injection.

Acute Care
IV route is used in emergency situations only; IM route is preferred. Avoid subcutaneous or perivascular injection.

Precautions
Use with extreme caution in infants, children, elderly, or debilitated patients. Use with caution in lactation and pregnancy, asthmatic

attack, glaucoma, lower respiratory tract infections. Increases effectiveness of epinephrine. Potentiates action of anticholinergics, alcohol, hypnotics, sedatives, tranquilizers, other CNS depressants. Inhibits effect of anticoagulants and corticosteroids.

Contraindications

Known hypersensitivity; those receiving MAO inhibitors; premature or newborn infants.

Side Effects

Neurologic: Blurred vision, confusion, diplopia, drowsiness, headache, nervousness, restlessness, tingling of hands, vertigo.

Gastrointestinal: Vomiting, nausea, epigastric distress, dry mouth and throat.

Other: Hemolytic anemia, hypotension, nasal stuffiness, photosensitivity.

Patient/Caregiver Teaching

Instruct patient (1) to provide accurate medical history and drug profile and (2) to avoid injury related to drowsiness.

Home Care

Appropriate as an emergency measure.

Administration in Other Clinical Settings

Appropriate as an emergency measure.

Antidote

The physician must be notified of all side effects immediately. If symptoms are extreme, discontinue drug and notify physician. Untreated hypotension may lead to cardiovascular collapse (epinephrine further enhances degree of hypotension). Propranolol is drug of choice for ventricular dysrhythmias; phenytoin will reverse convulsions. Resuscitative equipment should be readily available.

Dobutamine hydrochloride

US: Dobutrex

Inotropic agent   pH 2.5–5.5

ACTION

Induces short-term increase in cardiac output with minimal increase in rate and blood pressure; possesses beta stimulator activity. Half-life of dobutamine is about 2 min; peak effect is obtained in 2–10 min. Excreted in the urine.

INDICATIONS/USES

Used as a treatment to provide short-term inotropic support in cardiac decompensation resulting from depressed contractility. Investigationally used to increase cardiac output in children with congenital heart defects who are undergoing cardiac catheterization procedure.

USUAL DOSE

Initial: 2.5–10.0 µg/kg body wt/min to a maximum of 40 µg/kg/min.

Maintenance: Adjust according to patient's response as indicated by heart rate, blood pressure, urine flow, presence of ectopic heartbeats, and, whenever possible, by measurement of central venous or pulmonary wedge pressure and cardiac output.

PREPARATION/RECONSTITUTION

Dilute each 250-mg ampule with 10 ml sterile water or 5% dextrose in water. Must be further diluted to at least 50 ml (or more) of 5% dextrose in water, 0.9% sodium chloride solution, or sodium lactate.

INCOMPATIBILITIES

Alkaline solutions, bretylium, calcium chloride, calcium gluconate, cetamandole, cefazolin, cephalothin, diazepam, digoxin, furose mide, heparin sodium, hydrocortisone, insulin, magnesium sulfate, penicillin, phenytoin, potassium chloride and phosphate, sodium ethacrynate.

RATE/MODE OF ADMINISTRATION

IV push: No.

Intermittent: No.

Continuous: Applicable; start with recommended dosage for body weight and intensity of patient's condition. Infuse by electronic infusion device and titrate dose to patient's intended response.

Filter: Applicable; use consistent with institutional guidelines.

NURSING CONSIDERATIONS

Nursing Diagnoses

1. Potential for alteration in comfort, related to drug side effects.
2. Potential for alteration in cardiac output, related to effects of drug.
3. Potential for ineffective breathing pattern, related to development of shortness of breath.

Acute Care

Monitor patient carefully, observing heart rate, ectopic activity, vital signs, urine flow, and central venous pressure. Pulmonary wedge pressures are preferred measurement. Compatible through common IV administration set with dopamine, lidocaine, tobramycin, nitroprusside, potassium chloride, protamine sulfate. Refrigerate reconstituted solution up to 48 h or maintain at room temperature for 6 h; pink discoloration does not affect potency of admixed solution. As with all IV solutions, maximum hang time for infusate is 24 h.

Precautions

May be ineffective if beta-blocking agents have been administered. May produce higher cardiac output and lower pulmonary wedge pressure when given concomitantly with nitroprusside. May cause dysrhythmias in presence of cyclopropane or halogen anesthetics. Use with caution in patients taking MAO inhibitors. Concomitant administration of phenytoin may produce seizures and severe hypotension. Insulin requirements may be increased in diabetics.

Contraindications

Idiopathic hypertrophic subaortic stenosis.

Side Effects

Cardiovascular: Anginal pain, chest pain, increased ventricular ectopic activity, palpitations, tachycardia.
Other: Headache, shortness of breath, nausea.

Patient/Caregiver Teaching

Instruct patient (1) to report all side effects immediately and (2) to inform licensed caregiver of the principles of home administration and patient monitoring parameters (see *Home Care*).

Home Care

Safely administered in the home care environment under closely supervised conditions and only when subsequent solution is hung by a licensed caregiver (registered nurse, licensed physician). Only those home care agencies with certified IV nursing professionals and availability of constant patient monitoring should attempt to provide this intense level of IV care. *Note: Patient's treatment must have been initiated in the inpatient environment and patient must be considered stable before home treatment may be given.*

Administration in Other Clinical Settings

Not recommended.

Nursing Interventions

The physician should be notified of all side effects immediately. If number of PVCs increases or pulse rate increases dramatically (30 or more beats), notify physician and decrease infusion rate. Discontinuing medication counteracts accidental overdosage.

Dopamine hydrochloride

US: Dopastat, Intropin
CAN: Intropin (DuPont), Revimine
(Rorer)

Inotropic agent   pH 3.0–4.5

ACTION

Increases cardiac output with minimal increase in myocardial oxygen consumption. Short duration of action; promptly excreted in changed form in the urine.

INDICATIONS/USES

Used to correct hemodynamic imbalances such as hypotension (from shock syndrome associated with myocardial infarction, trauma, endotoxic septicemia, open heart surgery, renal failure).

USUAL DOSE

Initial: 2–5 µg/kg body wt; 5–10 µg/kg may be required to correct hypotension in the critically ill patient. Increase gradually by 5–10 µg/kg/min at 10–30-min increments and titrate to patient's specific needs.

Average: 20 µg/kg; over 50 µg/kg has been reported to have been administered.

PREPARATION/RECONSTITUTION

Reconstitute each 5-ml ampule in 250–500 ml of the following infusates: 0.9% sodium chloride solution, 5% dextrose in water, 5% dextrose in 0.9% sodium chloride solution, 5% dextrose in 0.45% sodium chloride solution, 5% dextrose in lactated Ringer's injection, 1/6 molar sodium lactate solution, lactated Ringer's injection.

Proportion: Dilution of 200 mg will result in 800 µg dopamine/ml in 250 ml; 400 µg dopamine/ml in 500 ml.

INCOMPATIBILITIES

Alkaline solutions, amphotericin B, cephalothin, gentamicin, sodium bicarbonate.

RATE/MODE OF ADMINISTRATION

IV push: No.

Intermittent: No.

Continuous: Applicable, by electronic infusion device; gradually increase by 5–10 µg/kg/min and titrate according to patient's response to treatment.

Filter: Applicable; use consistent with institutional guidelines.

NURSING CONSIDERATIONS

Nursing Diagnoses

1. Potential for alteration in cardiac output, related to action of drug.
2. Potential for ineffective breathing pattern, related to drug side effects.
3. Potential for alteration in nutrition, related to drug side effects.

Acute Care

Inactivated by alkaline solutions such as those containing sodium bicarbonate. Monitor blood pressure every 2 min until stabilized at desired level; check every 5 min thereafter. Monitor central venous pressure/pulmonary wedge pressures before administration and thereafter. Ensure patency of venous access; use large veins if possible to provide adequate hemodilution of drug. Avoid extravasation; may cause tissue necrosis and sloughing. Discard unused solution after 24 h.

Precautions

Correct hypovolemia, if possible, with administration of whole blood, plasma, and plasma volume expanders. Use with caution in children and pregnant women. Monitor urine output continuously. Dosage may require reduction to one tenth of calculated amount in those receiving MAO inhibitors and other sympathomimetics. Antagonizes effect of morphine. Potentiated by tricyclic antidepressants and diuretics. Concomitant use with phenytoin causes severe bradycardia and hypotension.

Contraindications

Pheochromocytoma, ventricular fibrillation, uncorrected tachyarrhythmias.

Side Effects

Cardiovascular: Aberrant conduction, anginal pain, chest pain, ectopic beats, hypertension, hypotension, tachycardia, vasoconstriction, widened QRS complex.

Patient/Caregiver Teaching

Instruct patient (1) to report all side effects immediately and (2) to provide accurate medical history and drug profile.

Home Care

Not recommended.

Administration in Other Clinical Settings

Not recommended.

Nursing Interventions

The physician must be notified of all side effects immediately. Decrease rate of infusion and notify physician of decreased urinary output, disproportionate rise in diastolic blood pressure, increasing degree of tachycardia, or development of new dysrhythmias. Reduction of dose may be required to counteract effect of accidental overdose. Extravasation should be treated with phentolamine regimen; refer to Appendix 14.

Doxapram hydrochloride
US: Dopram

CNS stimulant   pH 3.5–5.0

ACTION

An analeptic CNS stimulant that achieves maximum effect in 2 min and lasts 10–12 min with a single dose. Causes increase in blood pressure and heart rate; rapidly metabolized.

INDICATIONS/USES

Used to stimulate the respiratory system and to return laryngo-pharyngeal reflexes post anesthesia. Used to treat overdosage of CNS depressant drug (exceptions: muscle relaxant and narcotic). Used to treat COPD to prevent carbon dioxide retention.

USUAL DOSE

0.5–1.0 mg/kg body wt; up to 1.5 mg/kg may be given as a single dose or up to 2 mg/kg may be divided and administered as separate injections at 5-min intervals. Maximum dose is 2 mg/kg. Repeat dose every 1–2 h as needed or follow with continuous infusion. *Caution: Do not exceed 3 g/24 h.*

Chronic obstructive pulmonary disease: 400 mg in specific amount of diluent; administer over not more than 2 h. Infuse at 1–3 mg/min for maximum infusion time of 2 h.

PREPARATION/RECONSTITUTION

Administer undiluted or dilute with equal parts of sterile water for injection; may also dilute 250 mg in 250 ml of 5% or 10% dextrose in water or 0.9% sodium chloride solution and infused.

Chronic obstructive pulmonary disease: Dilute 400 mg in 180 ml infusate (2 mg/ml).

INCOMPATIBILITIES

Alkaline drugs, aminophylline, sodium bicarbonate, thiopental.

RATE/MODE OF ADMINISTRATION

IV push: Yes, according to manufacturer's guidelines and patient's clinical condition.
Intermittent: Applicable for COPD and management of drug-induced CNS depression.
Continuous: Applicable, by electronic infusion device.
Filter: Applicable; refer to institutional guidelines.

NURSING CONSIDERATIONS

Nursing Diagnoses

1. Potential for injury, related to drug side effects.
2. Potential for alteration in nutrition, related to drug side effects.

3. Potential for alteration in urinary retention, related to effects of drug.

Acute Care

Maintain an adequate airway at all times. Resuscitative equipment must be available, including oxygen and controlled ventilation support systems. Monitor patient continuously and for 1 h following discontinuation of drug. Arterial blood gas measurements are highly desirable. Adjust rate of infusion and oxygen concentrations consistent with arterial blood gas parameters and patient's response to treatment. Confirm patency of vein and avoid extravasation of infusate.

Precautions

Failure to respond to treatment may be indicative of CNS source for sustained coma; patient's neurologic system should be further evaluated. Does not inhibit depressant drug metabolism. Stimulates systemic epinephrine increase. Use with caution in agitation, asthma, cardiac dysrhythmias, cerebral edema, gastric surgery, increased intracranial pressure, pheochromocytoma, tachycardia. Potentiated by MAO inhibitors and inhalant anesthetics. Refer to manufacturer's recommendations for treatment of COPD.

Contraindications

Cerebrovascular accident, children under age 12, convulsions, head injury, coronary artery disease, hypertension, inadequate ventilation capacity, known hypersensitivity to the drug, pregnancy, pulmonary dysfunction.

Side Effects

Neurologic: Confusion, dizziness, hyperactivity.
Gastrointestinal: Hiccoughs, nausea, salivation, vomiting.
Respiratory: Diaphoresis, dyspnea.
Other: Warmth, fever.
Major: Bilateral Babinski sign, bronchospasm, convulsions, hypertension or hypotension, laryngospasm, PVCs, respiratory alkalosis, skeletal muscle spasms.

Patient/Caregiver Teaching

Instruct patient (1) to report all side effects immediately and (2) to provide accurate medical history and drug profile.

Home Care
Inappropriate.

Administration in Other Clinical Settings
Inappropriate.

Nursing Interventions
The physician must be notified of all side effects immediately. Doxapram should be discontinued at first evidence of hypotension or dyspnea. Diazepam or pentobarbital may counteract overdose. Resuscitative equipment should be readily available.

Doxorubicin hydrochloride
US: ADR, Adriamycin

Antineoplastic antibiotic   pH 3.8–6.5

ACTION
A cell cycle–specific (S phase) antibiotic antineoplastic agent. Rapidly cleared with plasma. Does not cross blood–brain barrier and is slowly excreted in bile and urine. Tissue levels remain constant for 7–10 days.

INDICATIONS/USES
Used in the suppression of neoplastic growth. Regression has been produced in osteogenic, soft tissue, and other sarcomas, Hodgkin's disease, non-Hodgkin's lymphomas, acute leukemias, and carcinomas of the breast, GU system, thyroid, lung, and stomach. Useful in treatment of neuroblastoma.

USUAL DOSE
Adults: 60–75 mg/m² as a single injection every 21 days.
- Other: 30 mg/m² as a single injection daily for 3 days; repeat

every 4 wk for a maximum total dose not greater than 550 mg/m^2 (normal kidney and liver function required).

- Elevated serum bilirubin: Administer 50% of above doses for serum bilirubin of 1.2–3.0 mg/ml and 25% for serum bilirubin above 3 mg/ml.

Children: 30 mg/m^2 as single injection daily for 3 days; repeat every 4 wk.

PREPARATION/RECONSTITUTION

Refer to *Precautions*. Reconstitute each 10 mg with 5 ml of sodium chloride for injection. An additional 5 ml of diluent is recommended by manufacturer to ensure reconstitution of drug. Shake to dissolve completely. *Caution: Do not use bacteriostatic diluent.*

INCOMPATIBILITIES

Aminophylline, cephalothin, dexamethasone, diazepam, fluorouracil, heparin sodium, methotrexate. Consider incompatible with other drugs due to high toxicities.

RATE/MODE OF ADMINISTRATION

IV push: As a single dose over a minimum of 3–5 min by sideport of a freely flowing infusion or 0.9% sodium chloride solution of 5% dextrose in water; use slow rate of injection to avoid erythematous streaking or facial flushing.

Intermittent: No.

Continuous: Applicable, by small volume ambulatory infusion pump.

Filter: Applicable; use consistent with institutional guidelines.

NURSING CONSIDERATIONS

Nursing Diagnoses

1. Potential for alteration in cardiac output, related to drug toxicities.
2. Potential for alteration in nutrition, related to drug side effects.
3. Potential for disturbance in self-concept: body image, related to hair loss.

Acute Care

Antineoplastic precautions are required to minimize exposure to drug; refer to Appendix 14 for further information. Must be administered under the care of a physician specialist. Use only large veins and ensure patency of vascular device prior to administration of this drug. Avoid extravasation. Avoid veins over joints or in compromised extremities. If stinging or burning sensation occurs, discontinue injection and use another vein. Prolonged infusion (48–96 h) and weekly administration have been found to reduce incidence of cardiotoxicities (administration must be by implanted port or tunneled catheter). Diluted solutions are stable for 24 h at room temperature, 48 h if refrigerated; then discard. Sensitive to sunlight; avoid exposure. Maintain adequate hydration.

Precautions

Refer to antineoplastic precautions to avoid exposure with skin. Use appropriate hazardous waste containers for disposal of drug related equipment. Urine turning reddish color for several days is drug-related. Monitor WBC and RBC counts, platelet count, uric acid level, kidney and liver functions, ECG, chest radiograph, and echocardiogram prior to therapy. Toxic to embryo with mutagenic potential. Use caution in those of childbearing age. May exacerbate cyclophosphamide-induced hemorrhagic cystitis or increase hepatotoxicities associated with administration of 6-mercaptopurine. Monitor patient for signs/symptoms of bone marrow depression, infection, or bleeding. Be aware of cumulative dose (550 mg/m^2) and manufacturer's recommendations for patient monitoring, including ECG, chest x-ray, echocardiogram, bone marrow, and systolic ejection fraction.

Contraindications

Impaired cardiac function; previous treatment with complete cumulative dose of doxorubicin or daunorubicin; myelosuppression resulting from other antineoplastic therapies.

Side Effects

Cardiovascular (may be dose-limiting): Cardiac failure, depressed QRS voltage.
Gastrointestinal: Diarrhea, esophagitis, nausea, stomatitis, vomiting.
Other: Alopecia (complete), bone marrow depression, hyperuricemia.

Patient/Caregiver Teaching

Instruct patient (1) to be aware of drug side effects, including discoloration of urine; (2) to remember that alopecia may be reversible; and (3) to learn principles of home self-administration of this drug, including disposal precautions.

Home Care

Appropriate under the direction of a physician specialist and by highly trained IV nurse specialists. Disposal precautions must be implemented to ensure proper handling of cytotoxic waste.

Administration in Other Clinical Settings

Appropriate under the direction of a physician specialist and by highly trained IV nurse specialists. Disposal precautions must be implemented to ensure proper handling of cytotoxic waste.

Nursing Interventions

The physician must be notified of all side effects; symptomatic treatment is advised. Hematopoietic toxicities may require dosage adjustment or cessation of treatment. Extravasation may be treated with long-acting dexamethasone or hyaluronidase; refer to Appendix 14.

Doxycycline hyclate

US: Doxy 100, Doxy 200, Vibramycin IV

Antibiotic   pH 2.8–4.0

ACTION

A broad-spectrum antibiotic that is bacteriostatic against many gram-negative and gram-positive organisms. Excreted through the bile to urine and feces; crosses the placental barrier and is secreted in breast milk.

INDICATIONS/USES

Used in the treatment of infections caused by susceptible strains or organisms, including rickettsiae and viruses. Used as a substitute for contraindicated penicillin or sulfonamide therapy.

USUAL DOSE

Adults and children over 45 kg: Initial dose of 200 mg in 1 or 2 infusions, followed by 100–200 mg/24 h.

Children under 45 kg and over 8 yr: 4.4 mg/kg body wt/24 h in 2 equally divided doses; follow with 2.2 mg/kg/24 h once daily or in 2 equally divided doses.

PREPARATION/RECONSTITUTION

Reconstitute each 100 mg in 10 ml sterile water or normal saline for injection for a concentration of 10 mg/ml. Further dilute with 100–1000 ml or compatible infusate such as 0.9% sodium chloride solution, 5% dextrose in water, lactated Ringer's, 10% invert sugar in water. *Note: Lactated Ringer's or 5% dextrose in lactated Ringer's may be used but may create compatibility problems with some drugs; use with caution.*

INCOMPATIBILITIES

Cephalothin.

RATE/MODE OF ADMINISTRATION

IV push: No.

Intermittent: Over 1–4 h in appropriate amount of diluent to avoid venous irritation (1 mg/ml solution must be given over 2 h); when lactated Ringer's injection with or without 5% dextrose is used as the infusate, administer within 6 h.

Continuous: May be administered with other infusates over 12-h period.

Filter: Applicable; doxycycline causes venous irritation, and filtration to 0.22-μ range may minimize effects.

NURSING CONSIDERATIONS

Nursing Diagnoses

1. Potential for alteration in nutrition: decreased, related to drug side effects.
2. Potential for injury, related to possible extravasation.

Acute Care

As with all drugs, shelf-life should be determined prior to use; administration of outdated medication will cause nephrotoxicity. Store away from heat and light; protect from direct sunlight during infusion. Following reconstitution, store at 2–8°C and use within 72 h. Sensitivity studies should be performed prior to administration of this drug. Avoid prolonged use and subsequent superinfection caused by overgrowth. Determine patency of vein and avoid extravasation.

Precautions

Initiate oral treatment as soon as feasible. Use with caution in those with liver dysfunction and in pregnant, postpartum, and lactating patients. May cause skeletal retardation in the fetus and infants; may cause permanent tooth discoloration in children under age 8. May be toxic with sulfonamides. May potentiate anticoagulants and digoxin; dosage reduction may be required. Potentiated by alcohol and hepatotoxic drugs and inhibited by alkalizing agents, including salts of calcium, magnesium and iron, and cimetidine.

Contraindications

Known hypersensitivity.

Side Effects

Gastrointestinal: Anorexia, diarrhea, dysphagia, enterocolitis, nausea, vomiting.
Other: Skin rashes, anogenital lesions, blood dyscrasias.
Major manifestations: Anaphylaxis, liver damage, photosensitivity.

Patient/Caregiver Teaching

Instruct patient (1) to report all side effects immediately; (2) to be aware of possibility of photosensitive skin reaction; (3) to provide accurate drug profile; (4) to learn principles of home self-administration.

Home Care

Appropriate.

Administration in Other Clinical Settings

Appropriate.

Nursing Interventions

The physician should be notified of all side effects immediately.

Droperidol
US: Inapsine

Antianxiety agent   pH 3.0–3.8

ACTION

An antianxiety agent with antiemetic action. Effective in 3–10 min with maximal results in 30 min. Usual effect lasts 2–4 h.

INDICATIONS/USES

Used as preoperative sedation, to induce and maintain general anesthesia, and as an antiemetic.

USUAL DOSE

Adults

- Antiemetic: 0.5 mg every 4 h; may increase as needed.
- Premedication: 2.5–10 mg 30–60 min prior to procedure or surgery; may repeat with 1.25–2.5 mg as needed. *Note: IM dosing information only.*
- Induction of anesthesia: 2.5 mg for every 10–12 kg body wt.
- Maintenance of anesthesia: 1.25–2.5 mg as needed.

Children 2–12 yr: 1–1.5 mg for every 10–12 kg, decrease if patient is receiving another CNS depressant.

PREPARATION/RECONSTITUTION

Administer undiluted; may be added to 5% dextrose in water, 0.9% sodium chloride solution, or lactated Ringer's injection (20 mg/1000 ml will provide 20 μg/ml or 2 mg/50 ml).

INCOMPATIBILITIES

Barbiturates, epinephrine.

RATE/MODE OF ADMINISTRATION

IV push: By sideport of an infusion set. ✻ over 1min
Intermittent: No.
Continuous: Follow preparation/dilution guidelines
Filter: Applicable; use according to institutional guidelines.

NURSING CONSIDERATIONS

Nursing Diagnoses

1. Potential for alteration in nutrition, related to side effects of drug.
2. Potential for alteration in cardiac output: reduced, related to action of drug.
3. Potential for ineffective breathing pattern, related to major side effects.

Acute Care

Usually used under the direction of an anesthesiologist. Monitor patient's vital signs and response to treatment carefully. Resuscitative equipment should be readily available. Follow manufacturer's guidelines for concomitant administration of CNS depressants. Physically compatible for 15 min in syringe with atropine, butorphanol, chlorpromazine, diphenhydramine, fentanyl, meperidine, morphine, promazine, promethazine, scopolamine.

Precautions

Reduce dose for the elderly or debilitated patient. Reduce dose for the poor-risk patients or those with renal/hepatic dysfunction. Move and position patient carefully; orthostatic hypotension has been reported frequently. If a narcotic has been used concurrently, a narcotic antagonist must be readily available along with appropriate IV infusion.

Contraindications

Known hypersensitivity; patients under age 2; pregnancy.

Side Effects

Neurologic: Dizziness, hallucinations, restlessness, abnormal EEG.
Cardiovascular: Shivering, hypotension, tachycardia.
Major manifestations: Apnea, hypotension, respiratory depression.

Patient/Caregiver Teaching

Instruct patient (1) to report all side effects immediately and (2) to keep in mind that minor side effects are transient.

Home Care

Not recommended.

Administration in Other Clinical Settings

Not recommended.

Nursing Interventions

The physician must be notified of all side effects immediately. Resuscitative equipment must be readily available. Vasopressors and fluid resuscitation may be needed. Extrapyramidal symptoms may be reversed with administration of benztropine or diphenhydramine.

Edetate disodium

US: EDTA disodium, Chealamide, Disotate

Calcium-chelating agent   pH 6.5–7.5

ACTION

A calcium-chelating agent that attracts calcium ions on injection, becoming calcium disodium edetate. Rapidly excreted in the urine.

INDICATIONS/USES

Used in the treatment of cardiac dysrhythmias caused by digitalis toxicity; to relieve symptoms of hypercalcemia; and to treat acute and chronic lead poisoning.

USUAL DOSE

Adults: 50 mg/kg body wt/24 h; total dose not to exceed 3 g/24 h. Administer for 5 days, then hold 2 days and repeat regime to a total of 15 doses.

Children: 35–40 mg/kg/24 h, not to exceed 70 mg/kg/24 h or adult dose, the lesser of the two.

PREPARATION/RECONSTITUTION

Available as a liquid ampule: 5-ml ampule equals 1 g (200 mg/ml). Dilute dose in 500 ml 5% dextrose in water or isotonic saline solution; use less diluent as needed in children (minimum concentration is a 3% solution).

INCOMPATIBILITIES

5% dextrose in 5% alcohol, any metals. Do not mix in syringe or solution with any other drug.

RATE/MODE OF ADMINISTRATION

IV push: No.
Intermittent: Administer over at least 1 h.
Continuous: Follow dilution recommendations and concentration levels.
Filter: Applicable; use consistent with institutional guidelines.

NURSING CONSIDERATIONS

Nursing Diagnoses

1. Potential for alteration in nutrition: decreased, related to drug side effects.
2. Potential for injury, related to drug side effects.

Acute Care

Monitor vital signs and ECG before, during, and following therapy. Monitor electrolyte panels. Obtain venous sample for serum calcium level before beginning a new infusion. Maintain patient in supine position during and after administration (15–30 min) to avoid postural hypotension.

Precautions

Use only when needed. May produce sudden hypocalcemia if used for other than chelating purposes. Magnesium deficiency may occur with prolonged period of use. Use with caution in those with cardiac disease, diabetes, renal, or hepatic dysfunction. Inhibits mannitol.

Contraindications

Known sensitivity to edetate disodium; anuria. Administration in the presence of lead encephalopathy may lead to increased intracranial pressure.

Side Effects

Gastrointestinal: Anorexia, nausea, thirst, vomiting.
Neurologic: Arthralgia, circumoral paresthesias, fatigue, headache.
Other: Urinary urgency, nasal congestion, fever.
Major manifestations: Anaphylaxis, anemia, hemorrhage, hypocalcemia tetany, prolonged QT interval, renal tubular destruction, death.

Patient/Caregiver Teaching

Instruct patient (1) to report all side effects immediately and (2) to provide accurate medical history and drug profile.

Home Care

Not recommended.

Administration in Other Clinical Settings

Not recommended.

Antidote

The physician must be notified of all side effects immediately. Calcium gluconate is the agent of choice and should be readily available and used with caution in the digitalized patient. Resuscitative equipment should be readily available.

Edrophonium chloride
US: Tensilon

Anticholinesterase   pH 5.4

ACTION

An antagonist of skeletal muscle relaxants and anticholinesterase, restores normal transmission of nerve impulses.

INDICATIONS/USES

Used in the diagnosis of myasthenia gravis; evaluation of adequacy of treatment; treatment of myasthenia crisis; as a curare antagonist; and for termination of supraventricular tachycardia.

USUAL DOSE

Adults: 1–10 mg; maximum not to exceed 40 mg (4 doses of 10 mg each)

- Myasthenia gravis diagnosis: 10 mg in tuberculin syringe. Administer 2 mg; if no reaction in 45 seconds, administer remaining 8 mg (may repeat test in 30 min).
- Myasthenia treatment evaluation: 1–2 mg 1 h after oral intake of drug being given for treatment.
- Myasthenia crisis evaluation: 2 mg in tuberculin syringe. Give 1 ml and, if patient's condition does not deteriorate, give 1 mg after 60 sec.
- Curare antagonist: 10 mg; may repeat as needed up to 4 doses.
- Antiarrhythmic: 5–10 mg; repeat once in 10 min if needed.

Children

- Myasthenia gravis diagnosis: *Infants,* 0.5 mg. *Under 34 kg,* 1 mg (if no response in 30–45 sec, give 1 mg every 30–45 sec up to a maximum of 5 mg). *Over 34 kg,* 2 mg (if no response in 30–45 sec, administer 1 mg evey 30–45 sec up to 10 mg).
- Antiarrhythmic: 2 mg administered very slowly.

PREPARATION/RECONSTITUTION

Administer undiluted. For treatment of myasthenia crisis, edrophonium chloride may be given as a continuous infusion (refer to mode of administration).

INCOMPATIBILITIES

Consider incompatible in syringe or solution with any other drug.

RATE/MODE OF ADMINISTRATION

IV push: As indicated in dosing guidelines.
Intermittent: No.
Continuous: For treatment of myasthenia crisis, administer by electronic infusion device.
Filter: Applicable; use consistent with institutional guidelines.

NURSING CONSIDERATIONS

Nursing Diagnoses

1. Potential for alteration in nutrition: decreased, related to drug side effects.
2. Potential for injury, related to drug side effects.
3. Potential for alteration in urinary elimination.

Acute Care

Use only under the direct supervision of a licensed physician. Monitor patient response continually.

Precautions

Atropine 1 mg must be readily available at all times. Respiratory support must be readily available. Use with caution in patients with bronchial asthma, myasthenia gravis treated with anticholinesterase drugs, and cardiac dysrhythmias. May be inhibited by magnesium or corticosteroids. Antagonizes anesthetics and aminoglycoside antibiotics. Prolongs muscle relaxant effect of succinylcholine chloride.

Contraindications

Known hypersensitivity; apnea; pregnancy; patients taking mecamylamine.

Side Effects

Gastrointestinal: Abdominal cramps, anorexia, diarrhea, dysphagia, increased salivation, nausea, vomiting.
Respiratory: Bronchial spasm, increased pulmonary secretions, laryngospasm, respiratory arrest.
Cardiovascular: Bradycardia, cold moist skin.
Other: Urinary frequency and incontinence, contraction of pupils, convulsions, fainting.

Patient/Caregiver Teaching

Instruct patient (1) to report all side effects immediately and (2) to provide accurate medical history and drug profile.

Home Care

Not recommended.

Administration in Other Clinical Settings
Not recommended.

Nursing Interventions
The physician should be notified of all side effects immediately. Discontinue the drug and notify physician. Atropine sulfate (0.4–0.5 mg IV) reverses most side effects; repeat in 3–10 min as needed. Pralidoxime chloride (50–100 mg/min, up to 1 g) may be used as a cholinesterase reactivator. Resuscitative equipment, including endotracheal intubation and artificial ventilation, must be readily available at all times. Epinephrine reverses allergic reactions to this drug.

Enalapril maleate
US: Vasotec

Antihypertensive agent

ACTION
An ACE inhibitor useful in lowering the blood pressure in those with severe hypertension.

INDICATIONS/USES
Used in the treatment of severe hypertension and congestive heart failure; most effective when pretreatment plasma renin levels are relatively elevated. Efficacy may be increased with concomitant use of diuretics.

USUAL DOSE
1.25 mg; repeat every 6 h as needed.

PREPARATION/RECONSTITUTION
Administer undiluted, or dilute with up to 50 ml of 5% dextrose or 0.9% sodium chloride.

INCOMPATIBILITIES
Unknown.

RATE/MODE OF ADMINISTRATION
IV push: Applicable, over 5 min.
Intermittent: No.
Continuous: No.
Filter: Not applicable in less than 1-ml dose.

NURSING CONSIDERATIONS
Nursing Diagnoses
1. Potential for alteration in urinary elimination patterns, related to drug side effects.
2. Potential for fluid volume deficit, related to drug actions.

Acute Care
Treatment of hypertensive crisis should be tailored to the patient's clinical needs. Monitor electrolyte levels regularly.

Precautions
As with other ACE inhibitors, avoid use in those with bilateral renal artery stenosis or unilateral renal artery stenosis with a solitary functioning kidney due to possibility that acute renal failure will develop. May provide hyperkalemia in patients who have a tendency toward elevated serum potassium levels.

Contraindications
Renal failure.

Side Effects
Minimal side effects reported.

Patient/Caregiver Teaching
Instruct patient (1) to provide accurate medical history and drug profile and (2) to report signs/symptoms of hyperkalemia.

Home Care
Inappropriate.

Administration in Other Clinical Settings
Inappropriate.

Nursing Interventions
The physician should be notified of all side effects.

Ephedrine sulfate

Sympathomimetic   pH 4.5–7.0

ACTION
A CNS stimulant and alkaloid sympathomimetic drug. Relaxes smooth muscle of bronchi and dilates the pupils. Increases metabolic and respiratory rates. Crosses the blood–brain barrier and is excreted in the urine and secreted in breast milk.

INDICATIONS/USES
Used as a pressor agent during spinal anesthesia; for treatment of Stokes-Adams syndrome; and to reverse allergic disorders. Helpful in treatment of narcotic, barbiturate, and alcohol poisoning.

USUAL DOSE
Adults: 25–50 mg; repeat in 3–4 h to a maximum of 150 mg/24 h (smaller doses of 10–25 mg are recommended for IV administration). May repeat doses in 5–10 min if needed.
Children: 3 mg/kg body wt/24 h divided into 4–6-hour doses; not usually given by IV route to children.

PREPARATION/RECONSTITUTION
Administer undiluted.

INCOMPATIBILITIES
Alkaline solutions, hydrocortisone, thiopental, phenobarbital.

RATE/MODE OF ADMINISTRATION
IV push: Applicable.
Intermittent: No.

Continuous: No.
Filter: Not applicable in less than 1-ml dose.

NURSING CONSIDERATIONS

Nursing Diagnoses

1. Potential for injury, related to drug side effects.
2. Potential for alteration in breathing pattern, related to drug side effects.

Acute Care

Monitor patient's blood pressure every 5 min during treatment. Ensure appropriateness of therapy for IV use by checking drug label. Ensure patency of vein to prevent extravasation and subsequent tissue sloughing.

Precautions

Interacts with many other drugs; monitor patient's response carefully. Potentiated by anesthetics, tricyclic antidepressants, antihistamines, and urinary alkalizers. Antagonized by β-adrenergic blockers. Inhibited by ergot alkaloids and phenothiazines. Inhibits action of insulin and oral hypoglycemia agents. Has a cumulative effect in the body. Hypertensive crisis may occur if used in conjunction with MAO inhibitors. Use with caution in patients with heart disease, diabetes mellitus, prostatic hypertrophy, and hyperthyroidism. Do not use to treat overdosage of phenothiazines (irreversible shock may result).

Contraindications

Known hypersensitivity; labor and delivery when maternal blood pressure is in excess of 130/80 mm Hg.

Side Effects

Gastrointestinal: Anorexia, nausea, vomiting.
Neurologic: Insomnia, headache, nervousness, vertigo, confusion, delirium, euphoria, hallucinations.
Cardiovascular: Cardiac dysrhythmias, palpitations, precordial pain, tachycardia.
Other: Dysuria, urinary retention.
Manifestations of overdosage: Convulsions, pulmonary edema, respiratory collapse.

Patient/Caregiver Teaching

Instruct patient (1) to report all side effects immediately, and (2) to remember that dysuria is transient and will be relieved when drug is discontinued.

Home Care

Not recommended.

Administration in Other Clinical Settings

Not recommended.

Nursing Interventions

The physician should be notified of all side effects immediately. Resuscitative equipment should be readily available, including IV fluids. Phentolamine may reverse hypertension; diazepam may counteract convulsions. Beta-blockers should be administered to reverse cardiac dysrhythmias.

Epinephrine hydrochloride

US: Adrenalin chloride
CAN: Adrenalin (Parke-Davis)

Sympathomimetic   pH 2.5–5.0

ACTION

A vasoconstrictor that delays absorption of many other drugs. Strengthens myocardial contraction and increases cardiac rate. Rapidly inactivated in the body by enzymes and excreted in changed form in the urine.

INDICATIONS/USES

Used as the drug of choice for anaphylactic shock and antidote of choice for histamine overdose and allergic reactions, including those associated with bronchial asthma, urticaria, angioneurotic edema. Used in cardiac resuscitation and in Stokes-Adams syndrome.

USUAL DOSE

Adults: 0.2–0.5 mg of 1:10,000 solution; repeat as needed.
- Cardiac arrest: 0.5–1.0 mg of 1:10,000 solution IV; repeat every 5 min. 1.0 mg of 1:10,000 solution may be administered by endotracheal tube before establishing an IV; 0.5 mg of 1:10,000 solution is administered intracardiac if no other route is available.
- Maintenance: 1–8 μg/min.

Children
- Cardiac arrest: 5–10 μg/kg body wt of 1:10,000 solution by IV; intracardiac route only if no other means available.

PREPARATION/RECONSTITUTION

Reconstitute each 1 mg of 1:1,000 solution in 10 ml normal saline for injection to produce a 1:10,000 solution. May be further diluted in 250 ml 5% dextrose in water for maintenance therapy to run at 1–4 μg/min.

INCOMPATIBILITIES

Any other drug in syringe. Unstable in any solution with a pH greater than 5.5.

RATE/MODE OF ADMINISTRATION

IV push: Applicable, in treatment of cardiac arrest.
Intermittent: No.
Continuous: As maintenance treatment; administer by electronic infusion device.
Filter: Applicable with infusion; not appropriate for less than 1-ml dose.

NURSING CONSIDERATIONS

Nursing Diagnoses
1. Potential for injury, related to drug side effects.
2. Potential for fluid volume deficit: actual, related to overdose.

Acute Care
IV effect is immediate; IM or subcutaneous route is preferred. Check appropriateness of solution for IV use; read label carefully. Monitor patient's blood pressure every 5 min. Ensure patency of

vein and avoid areas of limited blood supply (digits) due to potential for sloughing. Protect solution from light; do not use if brown color or sediment present.

Precautions

Intracardiac injection or IV injection in cardiac arrest must be accompanied by cardiac massage in order to perfuse drug into the myocardium and allow effective defibrillation. Use with extreme caution in the elderly, the debilitated, in patients with diabetes, in hypotension, in those with long-term emphysema or asthma. May not be used concurrently with isoproterenol; alternate use of these two drugs to maximize effect. Hypertensive crisis may result from simultaneous administration of oxytoxics or MAO inhibitors. Potentiated by anesthetics, antihistamines, urinary alkalizers. Antagonized by β- and α-adrenergic blockers. Often administered with corticosteroids in treatment of anaphylaxis.

Contraindications

Anesthesia containing inhalant anesthetic agents, hypertension, cerebral arteriosclerosis, labor, hyperthyroidism, glaucoma, organic brain damage.

Side Effects

Usually transitory and often occurring following average dosing.

Neurologic: Anxiety, dizziness.
Respiratory: Dyspnea.
Other: Palpitations, pallor.
Manifestations of overdosage: Cerebrovascular hemorrhage, collapse, fibrillation, severe headache, hypotension (irreversible), pulmonary edema, tachycardia, weakness, death.

Patient/Caregiver Teaching

Instruct patient (1) to report all side effects immediately and (2) to provide accurate medical history and drug profile.

Home Care

Appropriate as an emergency intervention to treat drug reaction only.

Administration in Other Clinical Settings

Appropriate as an emergency intervention to treat drug reaction only.

Nursing Interventions

The physician should be notified of all side effects immediately. In severe reactions, treat patient for shock and administer antihypertensive agent such as phentolamine or nitroprusside. Beta-blockers relieve cardiac dysrhythmias. Resuscitative equipment should be readily available.

Ergonovine maleate
US: Ergotrate maleate

Oxytocic agent   pH 2.7–3.5

ACTION

An oxytocic agent, causing contraction of uterus and vasoconstriction of uterine vessels. Effective within 1 min for period of 3 h. Excreted in bile and urine.

INDICATIONS/USES

Used to prevent or control postpartum or postabortal hemorrhage. Investigationally used in diagnosis of Prinzmetal's angina.

USUAL DOSE

0.2 mg or 1 ml; repeat in 2–4 h as needed. Investigationally used during coronary angiography in dose of 0.05–0.20 IV.

PREPARATION/RECONSTITUTION

Administer undiluted by Y-port of existing infusion.

INCOMPATIBILITIES

Amobarbital, ampicillin, cephalothin, chloramphenicol, epinephrine, heparin sodium, methicillin.

RATE/MODE OF ADMINISTRATION

IV push: 0.2 mg or fraction thereof over 1 min.
Intermittent: No.
Continuous: No.
Filter: Not applicable in less than 1-ml dose.

NURSING CONSIDERATIONS

Nursing Diagnoses

1. Potential for impaired fluid volume, related to bleeding.
2. Potential for injury, related to drug side effects.

IV route is for emergency use only; not recommended for use prior to delivery of placenta. Monitor patient's blood pressure. Refrigerate; do not store at room temperature in excess of 60 days (to do so will cause deterioration of properties of drug). Check expiration date prior to use.

Precautions

Use with caution in those with cardiac, renal/hepatic disease or those in febrile or septic condition. Potentiated by nitrates. Severe hypertension and cerebrovascular accidents may result in presence of regional anesthesia and with ephedrine, epinephrine, and other vasopressors. Chlorpromazine will reverse this hypertension.

Contraindications

Known hypersensitivity; pregnancy prior to third stage of labor.

Side Effects

With average dose
- Neurologic: Dizziness, blindness, confusion, dilated pupils, headache.
- Circulatory: Numbness/coldness of extremities, hypotension, hypertension.

With overdose: Abortion, convulsions, gangrene, hypercoagulability, uterine bleeding, shock.

Patient/Caregiver Teaching

Instruct patient (1) to report all side effects immediately and (2) to provide accurate medical history and drug profile.

Home Care
Not recommended, unless childbirth has occurred.

Administration in Other Clinical Settings
Not recommended, unless childbirth has occurred.

Nursing Interventions
The physician should be notified of all side effects immediately. Discontinue the drug. Heparin sodium may be administered to reverse hypercoagulability state.

Erythromycin lactobionate/ erythromycin gluceptate
US: Erythrocin IV, Ilotycin

Antibiotic   pH 6.5–7.5

ACTION
Antibiotic, bactericidal, and bacteriostatic as a substitute for penicillin or tetracycline preparations. Effective against some gram-negative and many gram-positive organisms. Excreted in urine and bile. Crosses the placental barrier and is secreted in breast milk.

INDICATIONS/USES
Used in the treatment of staphylococci, pneumococci, and streptococci infections. Used to provide prophylaxis against endocarditis preoperatively. Used to treat gonorrhea, syphilis in penicillin-sensitive patients and in Legionnaire's disease.

USUAL DOSE
Adults: 15–20 mg/kg body wt/24 h in divided doses every 6 h; maximum of 4 g/24 h has been administered.
Children: 10–20 mg/kg/24 h in divided doses every 6 h.

PREPARATION/RECONSTITUTION

Dilute each 500 mg or fraction thereof with 10 ml sterile water for injection without preservatives to form 5% solution. Further dilute in 100–250 ml compatible IV solution, such as 0.9% sodium chloride solution, 5% dextrose in water, or lactated Ringer's solution and add 1 ml neutralizing agent (Neut) if final dilution is less than 250 ml.

INCOMPATIBILITIES

Do not add to any drug. Incompatible with amikacin, aminophylline, ascorbic acid, carbenicillin, cephalothin, cephapirin, chloramphenicol, heparin sodium, lincomycin, phenytoin, prochlorperazine, sodium chloride solutions until after initial preparation/reconstitution, sodium salts, tetracycline, vancomycin, vitamin B complex with C.

RATE/MODE OF ADMINISTRATION

IV push: No.
Intermittent: Recommended; quarter of daily dose in 100–250 ml of diluent over 20–60 min.
Continuous: Applicable, at a concentration of 1 mg/ml by electronic infusion device, if available.
Filter: Applicable; use consistent with institutional guidelines (may minimize incidence of phlebitis).

NURSING CONSIDERATIONS

Nursing Diagnoses

1. Potential for alteration in comfort, related to possible venous irritation.
2. Potential for sensory-perceptual alteration, related to possible ototoxicity in high doses.

Acute Care

Sensitivity studies should precede administration of erythromycin. Not stable if final pH is less than 5.5. Administer within 4 h or use 1 ml sodium bicarbonate to neutralize and stabilize 100-ml solution. Refrigerate after dilution; remains stable for 7 days.

Precautions

Use with caution in those with hepatic dysfunction, pregnancy, lactation. Antagonized by clindamycin and lincomycin. Inhibits action of penicillins. Increases serum levels of cyclosporine, digoxin, methylprednisolone, and theophyllines; interpret results carefully.

Contraindications

Known sensitivity.

Side Effects

Urticaria and venous discomfort; may be minimized by proper dilution and use of a 0.22-μ filter.

Patient/Caregiver Teaching

Instruct patient (1) to report all side effects immediately and (2) to learn principles of home self-administration of this drug.

Home Care

Appropriate.

Administration in Other Clinical Settings

Appropriate.

Nursing Interventions

The physician should be notified of all side effects. Severe symptoms may require drug to be discontinued. Resuscitative equipment should be considered.

Esmolol hydrochloride

US: Brevibloc

Beta-blocker   pH 9.5

ACTION

Reduces ventricular response to atrial fibrillation, atrial flutter, and noncompensatory sinus tachycardia. Onset of action occurs within

1–2 min and has duration of 20–30 min. Metabolized in the urine; partially excreted in the urine.

INDICATIONS/USES

Used to treat myocardial infarction, angina, systolic hypertension, and supraventricular tachyarrhythmias. Valuable agent prior to, during, and after surgery.

USUAL DOSE

Individualized by titration.

Loading dose: 500 μg/kg body wt/min over 1 min; follow with 50 μg/kg/min for 4 min. If therapeutic results are not achieved after 5 min, repeat loading dose and increase 4-min infusions by 50 μg/kg/min increments.

Maintenance: Maximum infusion should not exceed 200 μg/kg/min.

PREPARATION/RECONSTITUTION

Reconstitute 5 g with 20 ml of one of the following solutions for a final concentration of 10 mg/ml (withdrawn from a 500-ml container): 5% dextrose in water, 5% dextrose in Ringer's injection, 5% dextrose in 0.9% sodium chloride solution, 5% dextrose in 0.45% sodium chloride solution, 0.45% sodium chloride solution, 0.9% sodium chloride solution, 5% dextrose in lactated Ringer's solution. Further dilute in remaining solution prior to administration.

INCOMPATIBILITIES

Sodium bicarbonate. Other drugs require compatibility testing prior to combining with this drug.

RATE/MODE OF ADMINISTRATION

IV push: No.
Intermittent: No.
Continuous: Applicable, by electronic infusion device.
Filter: Applicable; use consistent with institutional guidelines.

NURSING CONSIDERATIONS

Nursing Diagnoses

1. Potential for impaired tissue integrity, related to inflammation or induration of the infusion site.

2. Potential for urinary retention, related to drug side effects.
3. Potential for sensory-perceptual alteration: gustatory, related to drug side effects.

Acute Care

Monitor blood pressure; observe patient for cardiovascular, CNS, respiratory, and gastrointestinal symptoms. Monitor IV site carefully to avoid infusion phlebitis. Monitor ECG continuously; hypotension will reverse within 30 min after decreasing rate of infusion or discontinuing the drug. Stable at room temperature for 24 h.

Precautions

For short-term use only; follow manufacturer's recommendations for use of alternative agent and discontinuation of this drug. Antagonizes antihistamines, antiinflammatory agents, isoproterenol. Potentiated by general anesthetics, cimetidine, furosemide, phenothiazines, phenytoin (death may result). Use with caution in asthmatics, diabetics, and those with a history of hypoglycemia. Concomitant use of verapamil may result in potentiation of both drugs, severe myocardial depression, and AV conduction.

Contraindications

Not for use in chronic setting; not recommended for those with diabetes mellitus, bronchospastic disease, or hypotension.

Side Effects

Local: Induration of IV site.
Neurologic: Confusion, lightheadedness, paresthesias, speech disorders, taste disorders.
Other: Pallor, rhonchi, fever.

Patient/Caregiver Teaching

Instruct patient (1) to report all side effects promptly; (2) to report pain at IV site; and (3) to provide accurate medical profile.

Home Care

Not recommended.

Administration in Other Clinical Settings

Not recommended.

Nursing Interventions

The physician must be advised of all side effects immediately. Decreasing the dose or discontinuing infusion reverses hypotension within 30 min. Be prepared to administer IV fluids or vasopressors. Resuscitative equipment should be readily available.

Ethacrynic acid

US: Sodium Edecrin

Diuretic   pH 6.3–7.7

ACTION

A potent diuretic agent effective within 5–10 min; peak is noted 1–2 h following administration. Excreted in the urine.

INDICATIONS/USES

Used in the treatment of congestive heart failure, acute pulmonary edema, renal edema, hepatic cirrhosis accompanied by ascites, edema unresponsive to other agents.

USUAL DOSE

0.5–1.0 mg/kg body wt; 50 mg is appropriate for average adult, not to exceed 100 mg in a single dose.

PREPARATION/RECONSTITUTION

Add 50 ml sodium chloride injection or 5% dextrose in water to reconstitute.

INCOMPATIBILITIES

Any other drug in syringe, whole blood and derivatives, drugs and solutions with pH below 5, hydralazine, procainamide, reserpine.

RATE/MODE OF ADMINISTRATION

IV push: Applicable, through the sideport of a running infusion or directly over several minutes.

Intermittent: No.
Continuous: No.
Filter: Applicable if dose is greater than 1 ml in final concentration.

NURSING CONSIDERATIONS

Nursing Diagnoses

1. Potential for alteration in nutrition, related to drug side effects.
2. Potential for injury, related to weakness and muscle cramps.
3. Potential for fluid volume deficit, related to effect of drug.

Acute Care

Administer IV only; use new injection site for each dose to avoid danger of thrombophlebitis. Monitor electrolyte panel regularly to avoid hypokalemia. Do not administer simultaneously with blood components. Discard reconstituted solution after 24 h.

Precautions

Use with caution in patients with cirrhosis of the liver, electrolyte imbalance, hepatic encephalopathy. May cause permanent deafness if used concomitantly with other ototoxic drugs. Potentiates antihypertensive drugs. Inhibited by indomethacin. May cause cardiac dysrhythmias with digitalis or furosemide.

Contraindications

Anuria, pregnancy, lactation, infants, progressive renal disease, women during childbearing years, oliguria.

Side Effects

Gastrointestinal: Anorexia, dysphagia, nausea, thirst, vomiting, diarrhea, dehydration.
Neurologic: Weakness, muscle cramps, deafness (transient).
Major manifestations: Blood volume reduction, circulatory collapse, permanent deafness, vascular thrombosis, death.

Patient/Caregiver Teaching

Instruct patient (1) to report all side effects immediately; (2) to increase fluid intake; and (3) to provide accurate medical history and drug profile.

Home Care
Not recommended.

Administration in Other Clinical Settings
Usually not recommended.

Nursing Interventions
The physician should be notified of all side effects immediately; symptomatic treatment may be required. Resuscitative equipment should be readily available.

Etoposide
US: VePesid, VP-16-213

Antineoplastic   pH 3—4

ACTION
Cell-cycle–specific antineoplastic agent for the G_2 phase; half-life is from 3–12 h. Excreted through urine and feces.

INDICATIONS/USES
Used in suppression or retardation of neoplastic growth in refractory testicular tumors and small cell lung cancer. Also helpful in treatment of acute nonlymphocytic leukemias, Hodgkin's disease, non-Hodgkin's lymphoma, Kaposi's sarcoma, breast carcinoma.

USUAL DOSE
50–100 mg/m^2 daily for 5 days; alternative therapy is 100 mg/m^2 on days 1, 3, and 5. Repeat at 3–4-wk intervals.

PREPARATION/RECONSTITUTION
Dilute each 100 mg in 250 ml of 5% dextrose in water or 0.9% sodium chloride solution.

INCOMPATIBILITIES
All solutions other than the above. Consider incompatible with all other drugs in syringe or solution.

RATE/MODE OF ADMINISTRATION

IV push: No.

Intermittent: No.

Continuous: Applicable, by electronic infusion device; monitor flow for precipitation of drug.

Filter: Applicable; use consistent with institutional guidelines.

NURSING CONSIDERATIONS

Nursing Diagnoses

1. Potential for disturbance of self-concept, related to alopecia.
2. Potential for ineffective breathing pattern, related to drug side effects.
3. Potential for alteration in bowel elimination: diarrhea, related to drug side effects.
4. Potential for injury, related to immunosuppression.

Acute Care

This cytotoxic agent requires special handling; follow guidelines for disposal of cytotoxic waste materials. Determine patency of vein and avoid extravasation. Must be administered under the direction of a physician specialist by highly trained IV nursing personnel. Monitor patient's bleeding parameters carefully. Ensure adequate hydration.

Precautions

Withhold dosage if platelet count is less than 50,000/µL or absolute neutrophil count less than 500/µL. Dosage is based on average body weight in presence of edema or ascites. Monitor patient for signs of bone marrow depression or infection. Administer antiemetics as needed to ensure patient comfort.

Contraindications

Known hypersensitivity to this drug or its derivatives.

Side Effects

Gastrointestinal: Anorexia, diarrhea, nausea, oral lacerations, paralytic ileus, stomatitis, vomiting.

Neurologic: Neuritic pain.

Hematologic: Leukopenia, thrombocytopenia.
Other: Thrombophlebitis, alopecia, anaphylaxis.

Patient/Caregiver Teaching

Instruct patient (1) to report all side effects immediately; (2) to keep in mind that alopecia may be reversible; and (3) to avoid injury.

Home Care

Appropriate for administration by highly qualified personnel under the direction of a physician specialist.

Administration in Other Clinical Settings

Appropriate for administration by highly qualified personnel under the direction of a physician specialist.

Nursing Interventions

The physician must be notified of all side effects immediately. Rapid rate of infusion causes hypotension; administer at constant rate and discontinue if hypotension develops. Place patient in Trendelenburg position and administer IV fluids and vasopressors as needed. Discontinue infusion at first sign of allergic reaction.

Factor II, VII, IX, X complex (human)

US: Konyne HT, Proplex T, Proplex SX-T
CAN: Coagulation Factor IX (Winnipeg Plasma)

Coagulation factor   pH 7.0–7.4

ACTION

Human coagulation factor concentrate containing IX, II, VII, and X.

INDICATIONS/USES

Used to elevate demonstrated deficiency of one or more coagulation factors in such diseases as Christmas disease. Used to reverse coumarin effect and as prophylaxis to prevent spontaneous bleeding in those with congenital hemophilia B.

USUAL DOSE

Dosing is individualized, depending on specific factor needed, coagulation assays, and patient's clinical condition. Dosing is expressed in units of factor IX activity. The following calculations may be used to determine number of units required to elevate blood level percentages:

1 U/kg × kg body wt × desired increase (% of normal)

To maintain levels above 25%: Calculate dose to raise level to 40%–60% of normal. Range is 20–75 U/kg; may repeat in 12 h as needed.

Reversal of coumarin: 15 U/kg.

Prophylactic dose: 10–20 U/kg, 1 or 2 times weekly.

PREPARATION/RECONSTITUTION

1 ml sterile water for injection added to each 50 U (more dilute concentration is preferred); use diluent provided.

INCOMPATIBILITIES

All protein precipitants.

RATE/MODE OF ADMINISTRATION

IV push: No.
Intermittent: Not to exceed 10 min.
Continuous: No.
Filter: Not recommended.

NURSING CONSIDERATIONS

Nursing Diagnoses

1. Potential for alteration in comfort, related to drug side effects.
2. Potential for infection, related to risk of contracting AIDS and hepatitis.

Acute Care
Store lyophilized powder at 2–8 °C; do not freeze. Note shelf-life of drug and do not use after expiration date. Stable for 12 h following reconstitution; administer promptly to avoid bacterial contamination.

Precautions
Use with caution in newborns, infants, and those with hepatic dysfunction. Risk of AIDS increased with multiple administrations of this drug. Monitor coagulation factors before, between, and after administration; do not overdose.

Contraindications
Known hepatic disease, intravascular coagulation, fibrinolysis.

Side Effects
Cardiovascular: Chills, fever, flushing, disseminated intravascular coagulation.
Neurologic: Tingling.
Other: Risk of contracting AIDS and hepatitis, anaphylaxis.

Patient/Caregiver Teaching
Instruct patient (1) to report all side effects immediately; (2) to avoid injury; and (3) to be aware there is a risk of contracting AIDS and hepatitis; heat treatment greatly reduces transmission of AIDS and hepatitis.

Home Care
Appropriate.

Administration in Other Clinical Settings
Appropriate.

Nursing Interventions
The physician must be notified of all side effects. Disseminated intravascular coagulation and thrombosis may be reversed by anticoagulation with heparin sodium.

Famotidine
US: Pepcid IV

Histamine antagonist   pH 5–5.6

ACTION
A histamine hydrogen antagonist that inhibits gastric acid secretion. Eliminated by renal and other metabolic routes. Crosses the placental barrier and is secreted in breast milk.

INDICATIONS/USES
Used in the short-term treatment of active duodenal ulcer and pathologic hypersecretory conditions.

USUAL DOSE
20 mg every 12 h.

PREPARATION/RECONSTITUTION
Dilute 20 mg with 5–10 ml normal saline or other compatible infusate for direct administration. Add 20 mg to 100 ml of solution for intermittent infusion.

INCOMPATIBILITIES
Information not available.

RATE/MODE OF ADMINISTRATION
IV push: Applicable; 20 mg over 2 min; follow dilution requirements.
Intermittent: Applicable; 20 mg over 15–30 minutes; follow dilution requirements.
Continuous: No.
Filter: Applicable; use consistent with institutional guidelines.

NURSING CONSIDERATIONS
Nursing Diagnoses
1. Potential for alteration in nutrition, related to drug side effects.

2. Potential for disturbance of self-concept, related to alopecia.

3. Potential for injury, related to confusion and weakness.

Acute Care

Stable at room temperature for 48 h following reconstitution and dilution. Patient may experience recurrence of symptoms following discontinuation of drug.

Precautions

Concomitant use of antacids will relieve pain. Drug half-life may be in excess of 20 h if creatinine clearance level is less than 10 ml/min. Do not use in pregnancy unless clearly advised; discontinue breast-feeding.

Contraindications

Known hypersensitivity; children.

Side Effects

Gastrointestinal: Constipation, diarrhea, abdominal discomfort, anorexia, dry mouth, nausea, vomiting, taste disorder.

Neurologic: Dizziness, headache, agitation, anxiety, arthralgia, confusion, depression, hallucinations, insomnia, malaise, paresthesias, tinnitus.

Other: Orbital edema, alopecia, fever, thrombocytopenia.

Patient/Caregiver Teaching

Instruct patient (1) to use antacids to relieve pain associated with condition; (2) to discontinue nursing; and (3) to provide accurate drug profile.

Home Care

Appropriate.

Administration in Other Clinical Settings

Appropriate.

Nursing Interventions

The physician should be notified of all side effects immediately. Resuscitative equipment should be available. Hemodialysis or peritoneal dialysis may reverse symptoms of overdose.

Fluorouracil
US: Adrucil, 5-FU, 5-Fluorouracil

Antimetabolite   pH 9

ACTION
Antimetabolite antineoplastic agent, cell cycle phase nonspecific; interferes with synthesis of DNA and RNA. Excreted through the urine and as respiratory carbon dioxide.

INDICATIONS/USES
Used to suppress or retard neoplastic growth in carcinoma of the breast, colon, ovary, head and neck, rectum, urinary bladder, stomach, pancreas (often in combination with other drug treatments).

USUAL DOSE
12 mg/kg body wt/24 h for 4 days; total dose not to exceed 800 mg/24 h. If no toxicity occurs, a half dose is given on even days for 4 doses with no medication given on the odd days after the initial 4 doses.

Maintenance: Repeat entire course of therapy beginning 30 days after completion of previous course; may also give a single 10–15 mg/kg/wk dose; not to exceed 1 g/wk.

PREPARATION/RECONSTITUTION
Administer undiluted by sideport of free-flowing infusion.

INCOMPATIBILITIES
Incompatible with other drugs in syringe or solution; cytarabine; diazepam; doxorubicin; methotrexate.

RATE/MODE OF ADMINISTRATION
IV push: Applicable; over 1–3 min.
Intermittent: No.
Continuous: No.
Filter: Not applicable in less than 1-ml dose.

NURSING CONSIDERATIONS

Nursing Diagnoses

1. Potential for disturbance of self-concept, related to alopecia.
2. Potential for injury, related to drug side effects.
3. Potential for infection, related to drug toxicities.

Acute Care

Antineoplastic precautions are indicated in preparation of this drug agent; refer to Appendix 14 for further information on handling of cytotoxic waste. Should be administered by highly qualified professional nurse under the direction of a physician specialist. Confirm patency of vein and avoid extravasation. Slight discoloration of fluid does not affect potency. Dosage is based on average weight in presence of edema or ascites.

Precautions

Potentiates action of anticoagulants. Monitor patient for evidence of bone marrow depression or infection. Toxicities may be exacerbated by stress, bone marrow depression, poor nutrition. Monitor bleeding parameters, including WBC and platelet counts.

Contraindications

Bone marrow depression, poor nutritional state, serious infection.

Side Effects

Gastrointestinal: Diarrhea, esophagopharyngitis, mouth soreness/ulceration, stomatitis, vomiting, nausea.
Neurologic: Cerebellar syndrome, euphoria, photophobia.
Other: Thrombocytopenia, hemorrhage, alopecia, dermatitis, leukopenia.

Patient/Caregiver Teaching

Instruct patient (1) to report all side effects immediately; (2) to maintain adequate fluid intake; (3) to report injury or bleeding episodes; and (4) to bear in mind that alopecia is reversible.

Home Care

Appropriate for use by qualified professional.

Administration in Other Clinical Settings
Appropriate for use by qualified professional.

Nursing Interventions
The physician should be notified of all side effects immediately. Drug may be discontinued for presence of side effects, or if WBC is less than 3500 μl or platelets less than 100,000 μl.

Folic acid
US: Folvite

Vitamin   pH 8–11

ACTION
A part of the vitamin B complex; an important growth factor involved in synthesis of amino acids and DNA. Excreted in the urine and secreted in breast milk.

INDICATIONS/USES
Used in the treatment of megaloblastic anemias of malnutrition.

USUAL DOSE
1 mg daily; up to 5 mg may be given.

PREPARATION/RECONSTITUTION
Administer undiluted.

INCOMPATIBILITIES
Calcium salts, heavy metal ions, iron sulfate, oxidizing agents, reducing agents, vitamin B complex with C.

RATE/MODE OF ADMINISTRATION
IV push: 5 mg or fraction thereof over 1 min.
Intermittent: No.

Continuous: Applicable; may be added to standard infusate.
Filter: Applicable as infusion; refer to institutional guidelines.

NURSING CONSIDERATIONS

Nursing Diagnoses

1. Potential for injury, related to neurologic symptoms.
2. Potential for ineffective thermoregulation, related to drug side effects.

Acute Care

IV route is not used for children. Refrigerate solution and protect from light.

Precautions

May aggravate neurologic symptoms of disease. Inhibited by antimetabolites.

Contraindications

Children, pernicious anemia, aplastic anemia, iron-deficiency anemia.

Side Effects

Relatively nontoxic. Allergic reactions have been reported rarely and have included erythema, rash, itching, malaise.

Patient/Caregiver Teaching

Instruct patient (1) to report all side effects immediately and (2) to provide accurate drug profile.

Home Care

Appropriate.

Administration in Other Clinical Settings

Appropriate.

Nursing Interventions

The physician should be notified of all side effects. Resuscitative equipment should be readily available.

Furosemide

US: Lasix

Diuretic   pH 8.8–9.3

ACTION
A sulfonamide diuretic, antihypertensive, and antihypercalcemic drug related to thiazides. Excreted unchanged in the urine.

INDICATIONS/USES
Used in the treatment of congestive heart failure, acute pulmonary edema, cirrhosis of the liver with ascites, edema unresponsive to other diuretics, hypercalcemia, nephrotic syndromes.

USUAL DOSE
Adults: 20–40 mg; may repeat in 1–2 h as needed. In unresponsive adults, may be increased by 20 mg given at a minimum of every 2 h until desired effect is achieved. Maximum dosage is 600 mg/24 h.

Children: 1 mg/kg body wt; after 2 h, increase by 1 mg/kg increments to desired effect, not to exceed 5 mg/kg.

PREPARATION/RECONSTITUTION
Administer undiluted; 10 mg/ml ampules available. For continuous infusion, further dilute in equal volume of 5% dextrose in water, 5% dextrose in 0.9% sodium chloride, 10% dextrose in water, 0.9% sodium chloride, or lactated Ringer's injection.

INCOMPATIBILITIES
Acidic solutions, ascorbic acid, corticosteroids, diphenhydramine, dobutamine, epinephrine, gentamicin, meperidine, netilmicin, tetracyclines, any drug in a syringe.

RATE/MODE OF ADMINISTRATION
IV push: Applicable at rate of 20 mg/min or 1 mg/kg slowly over 1–2 min.

Intermittent: No.

Continuous: Applicable at rate of 4 mg/min by electronic infusion device.

Filter: Applicable in greater than 1-ml increment.

NURSING CONSIDERATIONS

Nursing Diagnoses

1. Potential for alteration in comfort, related to drug side effects.
2. Potential for fluid volume deficit, related to dehydration and excessive diuresis.
3. Potential for injury, related to drug side effects.

Acute Care

Discontinue drug at least 2 days prior to elective surgery. Monitor electrolyte studies regularly. Causes excessive potassium depletion when used with corticosteroids and spironolactone. Potentiates antihypertensive drugs. Discard after 24 h if diluted in compatible infusate such as 5% dextrose in water, 0.9% sodium chloride solution, lactated Ringer's solution.

Precautions

May cause transient deafness in doses exceeding the ordinary or when administered in conjunction with other ototoxic drugs. May increase blood glucose; inhibits oral anticoagulants.

Contraindications

Anuria, progressive renal disease with oliguria, children, pregnancy, lactation, known sensitivity.

Side Effects

Hematologic: Anemia, leukopenia.
Gastrointestinal: Vomiting, anorexia.
Neurologic: Tinnitus, weakness, leg cramps, lethargy, mental confusion, paresthesias, blurring of vision, reversible deafness.
Other: Urinary frequency, hypokalemia, hyperuricemia, hyperglycemia.

Patient/Caregiver Teaching

Instruct patient (1) to report all side effects immediately; (2) to increase fluid intake; and (3) to remember that hearing loss is reversible.

Home Care
Appropriate in well-monitored setting.

Administration in Other Clinical Settings
Appropriate in well-monitored setting.

Nursing Interventions
The physician should be notified of all side effects immediately. Discontinuing the drug may relieve minor side effects. Other treatment is symptomatic. Resuscitative equipment should be available.

Gentamicin sulfate
US: Garamycin, Janamicin
CAN: Cidomycin (Roussel)

Aminoglycoside antibiotic   pH 3.0–5.5

ACTION
An aminoglycoside antibiotic with neuromuscular blocking action. Bactericidal against specific gram-negative and gram-positive bacilli, such as *Escherichia coli, Klebsiella, Pseudomonas, Proteus*. Ineffective for viral and fungal infections. Half-life is usually 2 h; prolonged in infants, postpartum females, in presence of fever, hepatic disease and ascites, cystic fibrosis, the elderly, spinal cord injury. Shorter half-life is seen in burn patients. Crosses placental barrier. Excreted through the kidneys.

INDICATIONS/USES
Used in the treatment of infections of the GI, GU, and respiratory tracts, CNS, septicemia, skin, and soft tissue. Also used to treat infection in the immunocompromised patient; used concurrently with clindamycin to treat pelvic inflammatory disease.

USUAL DOSE

Adults: 3 mg/kg body wt/24 h in 3 or 4 equally divided doses; up to 5 mg/kg may be given if needed. Dosage is based on ideal weight of lean body mass (normal renal function recommended).

- Prevention of bacterial endocarditis in respiratory, GI, or GU surgery: 1.5 mg/kg 30 min prior to procedure; repeat in 8 h.
- Pelvic inflammatory disease: 2 mg/kg initial dose; then 1.5 mg/kg every 8 h for 2–4 days until improvement is seen.

Children under 40 kg: 6–7.5 mg/kg/24 h; divided into every 6–8 h.

Newborn: 5–7.5 mg/kg/24 h; divided into every 8 h.

- Premature infants and neonates less than 1 wk: 2.5 mg/kg every 12 h.

PREPARATION/RECONSTITUTION

Available in liquid form in vial. Prepared solutions available to equal 10 mg/ml or 100 mg/ml. Dilute each single dose in 50–200 ml of 5% dextrose in water or 0.9% sodium chloride solution to a 0.1% solution (1 mg/ml) or less. Commercially admixed solutions are readily available.

INCOMPATIBILITIES

Do not mix with any other drug in syringe or solution. Inactivated in solution with other penicillins, calcium gluconate, carbenicillin, cefazolin sodium, cephalosporins. Incompatible with amphotericin B, cefamandole, cephalothin, cephapirin, dopamine, heparin sodium, furosemide.

RATE/MODE OF ADMINISTRATION

IV push: No.
Intermittent: Applicable over 30–60 min; up to 2 h in children.
Continuous: No.
Filter: Applicable; use consistent with institutional guidelines.

NURSING CONSIDERATIONS

Nursing Diagnoses

1. Potential for alteration in nutrition: decreased, related to drug side effects.
2. Potential for ineffective breathing pattern, related to laryngeal edema.

3. Potential for sensory-perceptual alteration: auditory, related to ototoxicity of aminoglycoside preparations.

Acute Care

Monitor peak and trough concentrations to avoid peak serum levels above 12 µg/ml and trough levels above 2 µg/ml; a narrow range exists between toxic and therapeutic serum levels of gentamicin. Therapeutic level: 4–8 µg/ml. Sensitivity studies should be done prior to administration of gentamicin. Maintain good hydration.

Precautions

In renal impairment, intervals between doses should be extended. Potentiated by anesthetics, other neuromuscular blocking antibiotics, antineoplastics, cephalosporins, phenothiazines, sodium citrate, and procainamide; may produce apnea. Potentiated by other ototoxic drugs and all potent diuretics; may produce nephrotoxicity.

Contraindications

Known hypersensitivity, renal failure.

Side Effects

Gastrointestinal: Anorexia, nausea, vomiting, weight loss.
Renal: Oliguria.
EENT: Ototoxicity, tinnitus, roaring in ears.
Dermatologic: Rash, urticaria, itching, burning.
Neurologic: Headache, dizziness, lethargy, muscle twitching, numbness, tingling sensation, convulsions, neuromuscular blockade.
Cardiopulmonary: Hypotension, hypertension, fever, respiratory arrest.
Other: Blood dyscrasias, elevated bilirubin, BUN, serum creatinine, SGPT, SGOT.

Patient/Caregiver Teaching

Instruct patient (1) to report all side effects immediately; (2) to increase fluid intake; (3) to provide accurate drug profile; and (4) to learn principles of home self-administration of this drug.

Home Care
Appropriate.

Administration in Other Clinical Settings
Appropriate.

Nursing Interventions
The physician should be notified of all side effects immediately; the drug may need to be discontinued. Symptomatic treatment is preferred. Hemodialysis may reverse overdosage. Exchange transfusion is a consideration in the newborn. Neuromuscular blockade often is treated with calcium salts or neostigmine. Resuscitative equipment should be available.

Glucagon hydrochloride

Smooth muscle relaxant   pH 2.5–3.0

ACTION
Pancreatic extract that acts on liver glycogen producing relaxation of the smooth muscle of the stomach, duodenum, small bowel, and colon. Half-life is 3–6 min.

INDICATIONS/USES
Used in the treatment of hypoglycemia reactions during insulin therapy and in induced insulin shock (during psychiatric therapy). Also used to provide a hypotonic state in radiologic exams involving the GI tract.

USUAL DOSE
Hypoglycemia: 0.5–1.0 mg; repeat in 20 min for 2 doses if needed.
Diagnostic aid: 0.25 mg to 2 U

PREPARATION/RECONSTITUTION
1 U (1 mg) of powder is diluted with 1 ml of its own diluent; do not add to IV solutions. Use immediately.

INCOMPATIBILITIES

Do not mix with any other drug in syringe; do not mix with solutions containing sodium chloride, potassium chloride, calcium chloride. Unstable in any solution with a pH of 3.0–9.5.

RATE/MODE OF ADMINISTRATION

IV push: 1 U over 1 min.
Intermittent: No.
Continuous: No.
Filter: Not applicable.

NURSING CONSIDERATIONS

Nursing Diagnosis

1. Potential for alteration in nutrition: decreased, related to drug side effects.

Acute Care

Awaken the patient in 5–20 min. Patient should be expected to vomit upon awakening. Prevent aspiration by turning the patient face down. Administer oral sugars after arousing patient to prevent secondary hypoglycemia. Use immediately following reconstitution if possible; may refrigerate for a maximum of 48 h.

Precautions

May supplement with IV glucose (50%) to precipitate arousing. Potentiates oral anticoagulants. If patient does not awaken following administration of glucagon and glucose, coma may be related to another condition.

Contraindications

Known hypersensitivity to protein compounds.

Side Effects

Usually rare, but may occur.

Gastrointestinal: Nausea, vomiting.
Other: Anaphylaxis; hyperglycemia following excessive dosage; hypersensitivity reaction.

Patient/Caregiver Teaching

Instruct patient (1) to report all side effects immediately and (2) that vomiting is transient.

Home Care

Inappropriate.

Administration in Other Clinical Settings

Appropriate in well-monitored settings.

Nursing Interventions

The physician should be notified of all side effects other than nausea and vomiting, which are to be anticipated. Administration of insulin may reverse overdose.

Glycopyrrolate

US: Robinul

Anticholinergic   pH 2−3

ACTION

Synthetic anticholinergic agent that inhibits action of acetylcholine. Onset of action within 1 min; may last up to 2−3 h.

INDICATIONS/USES

Used as adjunctive therapy in peptic ulcer disease; to reverse neuromuscular blockade; and for intraoperative purposes.

USUAL DOSE

Adults

- Gastrointestinal disease: 0.1−0.2 mg every 4 h, 3 or 4 times daily.
- Reversal of neuromuscular blockade: 0.2 mg per 1 mg neostigmine or equivalent dose of pyridostigmine administered IV simultaneously (in same syringe).

- Intraoperative: 0.1 mg as needed; repeat every 2–3 min.

Children

- Reversal of neuromuscular blockade: Same as adult dose.
- Intraoperative: 0.004 mg/kg body wt; not to exceed 0.1 mg as single dose; may repeat every 2–3 min.

PREPARATION/RECONSTITUTION

Administer undiluted by sideport of IV.

INCOMPATIBILITIES

Alkaline solutions, chloramphenicol, diazepam, dexamethasone, dimenhydrinate, phenothiazines, sodium bicarbonate.

RATE/MODE OF ADMINISTRATION

IV push: 0.2 mg or fraction thereof over 1–2 min.
Intermittent: No.
Continuous: No.
Filter: Not applicable.

NURSING CONSIDERATIONS

Nursing Diagnoses

1. Potential for sensory-perceptual alteration: visual, related to drug side effects.
2. Potential for injury, related to weakness and paralysis.

Acute Care

For IV use only when an immediate effect is needed. Urinary retention may be avoided if the patient is asked to void prior to each dose.

Precautions

Use with caution in asthma, pregnancy, lactation, cardiac dysrhythmias, congestive heart failure, hepatic/renal dysfunction, coronary artery disease, hiatal hernia, hyperthyroidism, hypertension. Antagonized by histamine, reserpine, and others. Potentiated by alkalizing agents, MAO inhibitors, antihistamines, nitrates, and phenothiazines. Potentiates action of digoxin.

Contraindications

Known hypersensitivity, glaucoma, obstructive disease of the GI tract or obstructive uropathy, paralytic ileus, severe ulcerative colitis, megacolon, myasthenia gravis, unstable cardiovascular condition with acute hemorrhage.

Side Effects

EENT: Blurred vision, dry mouth, increased ocular tension, loss of taste.
Genitourinary: Urinary hesitancy, retention, impotence.
Cardiovascular: Tachycardia, decreased sweating, anaphylaxis.
Neurologic: Paralysis, nervousness, muscular weakness.

Patient/Caregiver Teaching

Instruct patient (1) to report all side effects immediately; (2) to void prior to each dose; and (3) to remember that dry mouth and related symptoms are reversible.

Home Care

Not recommended.

Administration in Other Clinical Settings

May be useful prior to outpatient procedures.

Nursing Interventions

The physician should be notified of all side effects. To counteract overdose, administer 1 mg neostigmine for each milligram of glycopyrrolate. Resuscitative equipment should be readily available.

Heparin sodium

US: Liquaemin sodium
CAN: Calciparine subcu calcium (Ang-Fr), Hepalean (Organon), Heparin Leo (Leo)

Anticoagulant   pH 5.0–7.5

ACTION

Heparin combines with other factors in the clotting cascade to inhibit conversion of prothrombin to thrombin and fibrinogen to fibrin. Reduces adhesiveness qualities of platelets. Duration of action 4–6 h; average half-life is 60–90 min. Metabolized in the liver and excreted in the kidneys.

INDICATIONS/USES

Used in the prevention and treatment of all thrombosis and emboli; used as a diagnostic and treatment aid in disseminated intravascular coagulation (DIC); used to prevent clotting in cardiac or vascular operative procedures and as an adjunctive treatment of coronary occlusion with acute myocardial infarction. Also used to maintain patency of vascular catheters, both intermittent and continuous therapies.

USUAL DOSE

Adults: Dose varies with use and clinical indications.

- Intermittent injection (minidose): 10,000 bolus; dosage adjusted according to PT levels and is usually 5,000–10,000 U every 4–6 h.
- Infusion: Administer bolus dose of 5000 U; then begin continuous infusion of 20,000–40,000 U/24 h in 500–1000 ml of 0.9% sodium chloride solution or other compatible infusate.
- Maintain patency of intermittent infusion device: 10–100 U in 0.5–1.0/ml normal saline (without bacteriostatics) after each use or as indicated in institutional policy; volume may need to be increased consistent with the requirement of the IV catheter being used.
- Maintain patency of arterial line: 1000–1500 U to each 1000 ml of infusate.

Children: Initial dose of 50 U/kg body wt followed by maintenance dose of 100 U/kg every 4 h.

- Alternate: 2000 U/m²/24 h as a continuous infusion.

PREPARATION/RECONSTITUTION

Administer undiluted or in appropriate quantity of 5% dextrose in water, isotonic saline, or Ringer's injection and administer as ordered.

INCOMPATIBILITIES

Most antibiotics, including amikacin, ampicillin, cephalothin, chlortetracycline, erythromycin, gentamicin, kanamycin, methicillin, oxytetracycline, penicillin G, polymyxin B, streptomycin, tobramycin, vancomycin. Also atropine, chlordiazepoxide, chlorpromazine, codeine, daunorubicin, dobutamine, hydrocortisone, insulin, meperidine, prochlorperazine, promazine, promethazine.

RATE/MODE OF ADMINISTRATION

IV push: Applicable.
Intermittent: Applicable.
Continuous: Applicable by electronic infusion device.
Filter: Applicable for intermittent and continuous infusions; use consistent with institutional guidelines.

NURSING CONSIDERATIONS

Nursing Diagnoses

1. Potential for injury, related to alteration of clotting parameters.
2. Potential for impairment of skin integrity: actual, related to drug side effects.

Acute Care

Read label carefully; determine appropriateness of treatment on an individual basis. Note that both bovine and pork solutions are available; obtain accurate allergy history. Exercise care to ensure accuracy of dose and avoid mixing heparin dose solution with heparin flush solution. Whole blood clotting time or activated PTT must be done prior to initial treatment and repeated thereafter for continuous or minidose treatment. Level should be maintained at 1.5 to 3 times control. Monitor other bleeding parameters, for example, platelet count. Do not discontinue treatment abruptly; to do so could increase patient's coagulability. Monitor stools for evidence of melena. To avoid precipitation and possible drug interaction, flush cannulas with saline to remove residual heparin prior to administration of drug. Administer drug, flush with saline, and reinstill heparin sodium solution (SASH technique). Use extreme caution if patient requires IM injections, subsequent venipuncture, or arterial punctures. Rotate IV sites carefully, applying firm pressure to avoid hematoma.

Precautions

Confirm desired control level with physician. Exercise caution in administering heparin in pregnancy; hemorrhage is most likely to occur during the last trimester or postpartum. Use extreme caution in any disease state in which hemorrhage is a risk, including subacute bacterial endocarditis; arterial sclerosis, aneurysm; during or immediately following spinal tap, spinal anesthesia, or major surgery; hemophilia; diverticulitis; threatened abortion; menstruation; visceral carcinoma; severe biliary, hepatic, or renal disorder. Decrease dosage gradually, weaning patient, to avoid increased coagulability. Discontinue heparin if platelet count falls below 100,000 or a thrombosis forms. May cause hyperkalemia in those with diabetes or renal insufficiency. Potentiated by chloramphenicol, dextran, ibuprofen, indomethacin, penicillin, salicylates. Inhibited by antihistamines, digitalis, calcium disodium edetate, hyaluronidase, nicotine, phenothiazines, tetracyclines, others. Potentiates oral anticoagulants, diazepam, phenytoin. IV administration of nitroglycerin may cause heparin resistance.

Contraindications

Active bleeding, blood dyscrasia, history of bleeding disorder, hypersensitivity (animal protein derivative), liver disease with hypoprothrombinemia.

Side Effects

Hematologic: Bleeding, prolonged coagulation time, tarry stools, thrombocytopenia, hematuria, bruising, epistaxis.
Vasospastic: Pain, ischemia locally.
Other: Arthralgia, chest pain, headache, hypertension; anaphylaxis is rare occurrence.

Patient/Caregiver Teaching

Instruct patient (1) to report all side effects immediately; (2) to provide accurate medical history and drug profile; (3) to avoid use of straight razor; (4) to avoid injury; (5) to learn principles of self-administration of heparin flush solution in the home environment; and (6) to maintain short- and long-term infusion cannulas in the home environment.

Home Care

Appropriate when precautions are adhered to and patient teaching is adequate and accurate.

Administration in Other Clinical Settings

Appropriate when precautions are adhered to and patient teaching is adequate and accurate.

Nursing Interventions

The physician should be notified of all side effects. The drug should be discontinued and appropriate measures instituted. Protamine sulfate is a heparin antagonist specifically indicated to reverse overdosage.

Hetastarch

US: Hespan

Plasma volume expander   pH 5.5

ACTION

Plasma volume expander with properties similar to those found in dextran. Approximates colloidal properties of human albumin. Excreted through the kidneys.

INDICATIONS/USES

Used as adjunctive therapy in treatment of shock resulting from burns, hemorrhage, sepsis, surgery, or trauma. Also used in leukapheresis to improve harvesting of granulocytes.

USUAL DOSE

Shock: Depends on degree of fluid loss and hemoconcentration levels; 500 ml (30 g) is usually given. Total dose should not exceed 1500 ml/24 h or 20 ml/kg body wt.

Leukapheresis: 250–700 ml in continuous centrifuge procedures.

PREPARATION/RECONSTITUTION

Administer as a 6% solution in 500-ml bottle available from manufacturer. *Note: Osmolality is 310 mOsm/L.*

INCOMPATIBILITIES

Unknown at this time.

RATE/MODE OF ADMINISTRATION

IV push: No.

Intermittent: No.

Continuous: Applicable; usually at rate of 20 ml/kg/h by electronic infusion device; rate is reduced in burns or presence of septic shock. Rate in leukapheresis is at constant ratio to venous whole blood, or 1:8.

Filter: Not applicable.

NURSING CONSIDERATIONS

Nursing Diagnoses

1. Potential for alteration in comfort, related to drug side effects.
2. Potential for alteration in nutrition: decreased, related to possible vomiting.

Acute Care

Hetastarch is for IV use only; it is not a substitute for whole blood or plasma proteins. Monitor patient's vital signs and urinary output every 5–15 min for the initial hour of infusion and hourly thereafter. Maintain adequate hydration. Does not interfere with blood typing or crossmatching. Monitor patient's hemoglobin, hematocrit, electrolyte, and serum protein levels during therapy. Monitor leukocyte and platelet counts, leukocyte differential, PT, and PTT during leukapheresis.

Precautions

Use with caution in heart disease, renal insufficiency, congestive heart failure, pulmonary edema, hepatic dysfunction. May reduce the coagulability of circulating blood; patient should be observed for evidence of increased bleeding or circulatory overload.

Contraindications

Severe congestive heart failure, bleeding disorders, renal failure with oliguria or anuria.

Side Effects

Gastrointestinal: Vomiting.
Dermatologic: Urticaria, itching, peripheral edema.
Other: Chills, fever, headache, muscle pains, anaphylaxis.

Patient/Caregiver Teaching

Instruct patient (1) to report all side effects immediately and (2) to provide accurate medical history and drug profile.

Home Care

Not appropriate.

Administration in Other Clinical Settings

Not appropriate.

Nursing Interventions

The physician must be notified of all side effects immediately. Resuscitative equipment should be readily available, including antihistamines, ephedrine, or epinephrine. The drug should be discontinued at first sign of allergic reaction and other means to sustain circulation instituted.

Histamine phosphate

Natural substance   pH 3–6

ACTION

Dilates vessels causing flushing, lowering peripheral resistance, and decreasing blood pressure.

INDICATIONS/USES

Used to establish presumptive diagnosis of pheochromocytoma.

USUAL DOSE

0.01 mg as initial dose; if no response after 5 min, administer 0.05 mg. Sequence is important to ensure validity of test results.

PREPARATION/RECONSTITUTION

Administer undiluted.

INCOMPATIBILITIES

Unavailable; consider incompatible in syringe or solution.

RATE/MODE OF ADMINISTRATION

IV push: Applicable by sideport of infusion of 5% dextrose in water or 0.95% sodium chloride solution.
Intermittent: No.
Continuous: No.
Filter: Not applicable in less than 1-ml dose.

NURSING CONSIDERATIONS

Nursing Diagnoses

1. Potential for alteration in nutrition, related to drug side effects.
2. Potential for ineffective breathing pattern, related to dyspnea and bronchial constriction.
3. Potential for injury, related to drug side effects.

Acute Care

Ensure resting blood pressure of 150/110 or lower prior to administration. Have epinephrine and phentolamine available for hypertensive reaction. Place patient on bed rest and initiate slow infusion of 5% dextrose in water or 0.9% sodium chloride solution prior to administration. Collect 2-hour urine sample for catecholamine assays; upon completion, histamine may be administered by IV Y-site. Repeat urine sample and record blood pressure and pulse every 30 sec for 15 min following injection. Anticipated response includes flushing, headache, decrease in blood pressure followed by increase in blood pressure within 2 min.

Precautions

Minute doses may precipitate asthmatic attack in those with bronchial disease. Withhold antihypertensives, sedatives, narcotics, and sympathomimetic drugs for 24–72 h before the histamine test.

Contraindications

Known hypersensitivity to histamine products, hypo- or hypertension, vasomotor instability, history of bronchial asthma, history of urticaria, and intense renal, pulmonary, or cardiac diseases.

Side Effects

Gastrointestinal: Abdominal cramps, diarrhea, vomiting.
Neurologic: Visual disturbances, syncope, dizziness, faintness, collapse with convulsions, nervousness.
Other: Hyper- or hypotension, metallic taste, palpitations, tachycardia.

Patient/Caregiver Teaching

Instruct patient (1) to report all side effects immediately; (2) to provide accurate medical history and drug profile; and (3) to ensure accuracy of urine samples.

Home Care

Not recommended.

Administration in Other Clinical Settings

Appropriate in a supervised setting.

Nursing Interventions

The physician should be notified of all side effects immediately. In case of accidental overdose, apply tourniquet to obstruct venous flow proximal to IV site and administer epinephrine and antihistamines. Resuscitative equipment should be readily available.

Hydralazine hydrochloride

US: Apresoline

Antihypertensive agent   pH 3.4—4.0

ACTION

Antihypertensive agent that lowers blood pressure by direct relaxation of smooth muscle of arteries and arterioles. Action begins within 2–10 min following injection. Some excretion in the urine.

INDICATIONS/USES

Used in the treatment of severe essential hypertension and for vasodilation in cardiogenic shock.

USUAL DOSE

Adults: 10–40 mg; increase gradually as needed. Maximum dose is 300–400 mg/24 h.
Children: 0.1–0.2 mg/kg body wt every 4–6 h.

PREPARATION/RECONSTITUTION

Administer undiluted.

INCOMPATIBILITIES

Aminophylline, ampicillin, calcium disodium edetate, ethacrynic acid, hydrocortisone, phenobarbital, verapamil, 10% fructose, 10% dextrose in lactated Ringer's injection.

RATE/MODE OF ADMINISTRATION

IV push: Applicable; 10 mg over 1 min.
Intermittent: No.
Continuous: No.
Filter: Not applicable in less than 1-ml dose.

NURSING CONSIDERATIONS

Nursing Diagnoses

1. Potential for alteration in oral mucous membrane, related to drug side effects.
2. Potential for injury, related to drug side effects.
3. Potential for alteration in nutrition: decreased, related to effects of drug.

Acute Care

Monitor blood pressure every 5 min until stable; check every 15 min thereafter during hypertensive crisis. IV use recommended only when oral route is not possible. Patient may develop a tolerance to the drug. Color changes occur in most 10% dextrose solutions.

Precautions

May be used in conjunction with a β-adrenergic-blocking drug; may potentiate effects. Tricyclic antidepressants may be contraindicated. Potentiated by anesthetic agents, ethacrynic acid, MAO inhibitors, triamterene, and other antihypertensive drugs. Inhibits action of epinephrine, levarterenol. Use with caution in those with impaired renal function, cerebrovascular accidents, coronary insufficiency, headache, increased intracranial pressure, congestive heart failure, tachycardia, pregnancy.

Contraindications

Known hypersensitivity, coronary artery disease, mitral valve rheumatic heart disease.

Side Effects

Neurologic: Anxiety, depression, numbness, paresthesias, tingling.
Gastrointestinal: Vomiting, dry mouth, nausea, unpleasant taste.
Other: Tachycardia, postural hypotension, palpitations.
Major: Angina, blood dyscrasias, coronary insufficiency, delirium, dependent edema, ileus, and myocardial ischemia and infarction.

Patient/Caregiver Teaching

Instruct patient (1) to report all side effects immediately and (2) to provide accurate medical history and drug profile.

Home Care

Not recommended.

Administration in Other Clinical Settings

Not recommended.

Nursing Interventions

The physician must be notified of all side effects immediately. Symptomatic treatment reverses most minor side effects. Ganglionic blocking agents may be ordered to control tachycardia. Numbness, tingling, and paresthesias may be controlled by administration of pyridoxine. If major side effects occur, discontinue treatment and notify physician. Resuscitative equipment should be readily available.

Hydrocortisone sodium phosphate

US: Hydrocortone Phosphate

Antiinflammatory agent   pH 7.5–8.5

ACTION

A principal hormone of the adrenal cortex and a potent metabolic antiinflammatory agent. Crosses placental barrier and is secreted in breast milk.

INDICATIONS/USES

Used in the treatment of adrenocortical insufficiency and as supplementary therapy for severe allergic reactions. Used in shock patients who are unresponsive to conventional therapies and in acute exacerbation of disease for those receiving steroid therapy.

USUAL DOSE

Adults: 15–240 mg/day; dosage is usually given at 12-h intervals. Total dose not to exceed 1 g/24 h.
- Acute adrenal insufficiency: 10 mg; repeat every 8 h by infusion.

Children: 2–8 mg/kg body wt/24 h.
- Acute adrenal insufficiency: 1–2 mg/kg IV push; then 150–250 mg/kg in divided doses.

Infants: Total dose not to exceed 150 mg/kg/24 h in divided doses.

PREPARATION/RECONSTITUTION

Administer without further mixing or dilution; use a separate syringe.

INCOMPATIBILITIES

Calcium gluconate, cephalothin, chloramphenicol, erythromycin, heparin sodium, kanamycin, methicillin, nitrofurantoin, phenobarbital, prochlorperazine, promazine, tetracycline, vancomycin, vitamin B complex with C.

RATE/MODE OF ADMINISTRATION

IV push: 25 mg or fraction thereof over 1 min; decrease rate if patient complains of tingling sensation along wall of the vein.

Intermittent: No.

Continuous: Applicable; add medication to appropriate amount of 0.9% sodium chloride solution or 5% dextrose in water and infuse.

Filter: Applicable for infusion purposes; not applicable in less than 1-ml dose.

NURSING CONSIDERATIONS

Nursing Diagnoses

1. Potential for injury, related to weakness.
2. Potential for alteration in fluid volume, related to drug side effects.

Acute Care

Product is heat-sensitive; follow manufacturer's guidelines for storage. May mask signs of infection. May increase patient's blood pressure and cause salt and water retention. Restrictions of salt, potassium, and calcium are needed. May increase insulin needs in diabetics. Monitor serum potassium levels; may potentiate hypokalemia in conjunction with digitalis products, amphotericin B, or potassium-depleting diuretics. Administer prior to 9 am to reduce suppression of patient's own adrenocortical activity.

Precautions

Inhibited by anticonvulsants, some antihistamines, ephedrine, propranolol, and barbiturates. Inhibits action of anticoagulants, aspirin, isoniazid. Potentiates theophyllines and cyclosporine. Dose adjustments may be needed for patients receiving cyclophosphamide. Do not discontinue therapy abruptly; wean patient to avoid rebound elevation of temperature. Maintain on ulcer regime and antacids prophylactically.

Contraindications

Unless a life-threatening emergency exists, the following conditions should be considered absolute contraindications to use: hypersensitivity to any product component, including sulfites, and systemic fungal infections. Other contraindications: active or latent peptic ulcer disease, acute psychoses, chickenpox, congestive heart failure, diabetes mellitus, diverticulitis, hypertension, myasthenia gravis, osteoporosis, pregnancy, fresh intestinal anastomoses, ocular herpes simplex, renal insufficiency, thromboembolic tendency, vaccinia.

Side Effects

Electrolyte disturbances: Calcium imbalance, other electrolyte disorders.
Gastrointestinal: Perforation.
Neurologic: Burning, tingling, weakness, headache, euphoria, psychic disturbances.
Other: Menstrual irregularities, hypersensitivity reactions, masking of infection, Cushing's syndrome, alteration of glucose metabolism.

Patient/Caregiver Teaching

Instruct patient (1) to report all side effects immediately but to realize many are transient and (2) to provide accurate medical history and drug profile.

Home Care

Appropriate for use following initial administration in the inpatient environment and if patient is stable.

Administration in Other Clinical Settings

Appropriate for use following initial administration in the inpatient environment and if patient is stable.

Nursing Interventions

The physician should be notified of all side effects. Resuscitative equipment should be readily available, including epinephrine.

Hydrocortisone sodium succinate

US: A-hydrocort, Lifocort-100, Solu-Cortef

Antiinflammatory agent   pH 7–8

ACTION

Adrenocortical steroid with potent metabolic and antiinflammatory effects. Crosses the placental barrier and is secreted in breast milk.

INDICATIONS/USES

Used in the treatment of acute adrenocortical insufficiency, acute hypersensitivity reactions, aspiration pneumonitis, bilateral adrenalectomy, severe shock, systemic lupus erythematosus relapse, antineoplastic therapy, severe infection with toxicity.

USUAL DOSE

Adults
- Initial: 100–500 mg; may repeat every 1–6 h as needed.
- Severe shock: Up to 2 g or more every 2–4 h; do not use longer than 48–72 h. Never administer more than 8 g/24 h.

Children: 0.16–1.0 mg/kg body wt every 8–12 h, up to maximum single dose of 500 mg.

PREPARATION/RECONSTITUTION

Reconstitute the vial provided by manufacturer, or reconstitute each 250 mg with 2 ml bacteriostatic water for injection. Agitate gently to mix solution.

INCOMPATIBILITIES

Aminophylline, ampicillin, bleomycin, chlorpromazine, colistimethate, dimenhydrinate, diphenhydramine, doxorubicin, ephedrine, heparin sodium, hydralazine, hydroxyzine, kanamycin, lidocaine, meperidine, methicillin, nafcillin, netilmicin, oxytetracycline, phenobarbital, promethazine, tetracycline, vancomycin.

RATE/MODE OF ADMINISTRATION

IV push: 500 mg or fraction thereof over 1 min; usual route of choice.

Intermittent: May be administered over 15 min in 30–50 ml compatible infusate.

Continuous: Only on order of physician and as directed.

Filter: Appropriate only in greater than 1-ml dose; refer to institutional guidelines.

NURSING CONSIDERATIONS

Nursing Diagnoses

1. Potential for injury, related to drug side effects.
2. Potential for alteration in nutrition: decreased, related to aggravation of peptic ulcer.
3. Potential for impaired social interaction, related to psychoses.

Acute Care

Product is sensitive to heat and light; discard unused solution after 3 days. May cause elevated blood pressure and salt and water retention. Salt restriction and potassium and calcium replacement should be considered. May increase insulin needs in diabetics. Administer before 9 am to reduce suppression of adrenocortical activity. Monitor serum potassium levels; may cause hypokalemia with digitalis products, amphotericin B, or potassium-depleting diuretics.

Precautions

May mask signs of infection. Do not stop treatment abruptly; wean patient to avoid rebound elevation of body temperature. Maintain patient on ulcer regime and antacid therapy prophylactically. Inhibited by anticonvulsants, some antihistamines, ephedrine, propranolol, and barbiturates. Dosage adjustment may be required with cyclophosphamide. Inhibits anticoagulants, aspirin, isoniazid. Potentiates action of theophyllines and cyclosporine.

Contraindications

The following are considered absolute contraindications to treatment with hydrocortisone sodium succinate: hypersensitivity to any product component, including sulfites, and systemic fungal infections. Other contraindications include active or latent peptic ulcer disease, acute psychoses, chickenpox, diabetes mellitus, diverticulitis, hypertension, myasthenia gravis, ocular herpes simplex, osteoporosis, pregnancy, renal insufficiency, congestive heart failure, fresh intestinal anastomoses, thromboembolic tendencies, vaccinia.

Side Effects

Neurologic: Weakness, tingling, euphoria.
Other: Menstrual irregularities, perforation and hemorrhage from aggravation of peptic ulcer, headache, sweating, thromboembolism, alteration of glucose metabolism.

Patient/Caregiver Teaching

Instruct patient (1) to report all side effects immediately but to realize many are transient and (2) to provide accurate medical history and drug profile.

Home Care

Appropriate after initial inpatient course of treatment and patient stabilization.

Administration in Other Clinical Settings

Appropriate after initial inpatient course of treatment and patient stabilization.

Nursing Interventions

The physician should be notified of all side effects. Epinephrine should be available for emergency use. Resuscitative equipment should be available.

Hydromorphone hydrochloride
US: Dilaudid

Analgesic   pH 4.0–5.5

ACTION
Provides potent analgesia without hypnotic effects; an opium derivative. Detoxified in the liver and excreted in the urine. Secreted in breast milk.

INDICATIONS/USES
Used in the treatment of moderate to severe, acute or chronic pain.

USUAL DOSE
1–4 mg every 4–6 h.

PREPARATION/RECONSTITUTION
Dilute with 5 ml sterile water or normal saline for injection.

INCOMPATIBILITIES
Alkalies, bromides, iodides, prochlorperazine, sodium bicarbonate.

RATE/MODE OF ADMINISTRATION
IV push: Administer 2 mg over 4–5 min.
Intermittent: No.
Continuous: No.
Filter: Not applicable in less than 1-ml dose.

NURSING CONSIDERATIONS
Nursing Diagnoses
1. Potential for alteration in nutrition: decreased, related to drug side effects.
2. Potential for injury, related to drowsiness.
3. Potential for ineffective breathing pattern, related to action of drug.

Acute Care

Observe patient frequently; monitor vital signs. Keep patient in supine position to avoid orthostatic hypotension and fainting. Administer with caution in the elderly and in those with hepatic or renal dysfunction.

Precautions

Oxygen, controlled respiratory equipment, and naloxone must be readily available at all times. May increase ventricular response rate in presence of supraventricular tachycardias. Cough reflex is suppressed. Potentiated by phenothiazines and other CNS depressants. May cause apnea in the asthmatic patient. Symptoms of abdominal conditions may be masked.

Contraindications

Diarrhea caused by poisoning until the toxic material has been eliminated; known hypersensitivity; premature infants or labor and delivery of premature infants; respiratory depression.

Side Effects

Gastrointestinal: Nausea, vomiting, anorexia, constipation.
Neurologic: Drowsiness, dizziness, respiratory depression, somnolence.
Other: Hypotension, anaphylaxis, urticaria.

Patient/Caregiver Teaching

Instruct patient (1) to report all side effects immediately and (2) to provide accurate medical history and drug profile.

Home Care

Not recommended unless as a component of a specific home pain management program.

Administration in Other Clinical Settings

Not recommended.

Nursing Interventions

The physician must be notified of all side effects immediately. Resuscitative equipment must be readily available.

Imipenem-cilastatin

US: Primaxin

Antibacterial agent   pH 6.5–7.5

ACTION
Broad-spectrum antibacterial agent. Excreted in the urine; may cross the placental barrier.

INDICATIONS/USES
Used to treat serious infections of lower respiratory tract, urinary tract, skin and skin structure, bone, and joint; and gynecologic, intraabdominal, and polymicrobic infections. Also used to treat bacterial septicemia and endocarditis.

USUAL DOSE
250–1000 mg every 6–8 h; not to exceed the lower of 50 mg/kg body wt/24 h or 4 g/24 h. Safety for use in children under age 12 not established.

PREPARATION/RECONSTITUTION
Reconstitute powder in vial in 10-ml compatible infusate from a 100-ml infusion container and shake well to form a suspension; further dilute in 50–100 ml of same infusate; again add 10 ml of this solution to the vial and return to the infusate to ensure complete transfer of vial contents and administer. Available in 120-ml infusion bottles for ease of dilution.

INCOMPATIBILITIES
All aminoglycosides; consider incompatible in syringe or solution with any other bacteriostatic drug.

RATE/MODE OF ADMINISTRATION
IV push: No.
Intermittent: 500 mg over 20–30 min.
Continuous: No.
Filter: Applicable; use consistent with institutional guidelines.

277

NURSING CONSIDERATIONS
Nursing Diagnoses
1. Potential for injury, related to alteration in bleeding parameters.
2. Potential for alteration in nutrition, related to drug side effects.

Acute Care
Sensitivity studies should be performed prior to use to determine susceptibility of the causative organism. Use with caution in those with a history of allergic reactions. Stable for 4 h following preparation at room temperature; refrigerate for 24 h but do not freeze. Rotate infusion sites faithfully to minimize danger of thrombophlebitis.

Precautions
Reduce total daily dose if renal dysfunction present; dose is calculated according to degree of impairment consistent with manufacturer's recommendations. Avoid prolonged use of drug and subsequent possibility of superinfection. Use only if necessary in pregnancy and lactation. Monitor electrolyte balance; drug contains high sodium content (3.2 mEq/g).

Contraindications
Known sensitivity to drug or its components.

Side Effects
Gastrointestinal: Abdominal pain, diarrhea, gastroenteritis, glossitis, heartburn, hemorrhagic colitis, increased salivation, nausea, vomiting, pharyngeal pain.

Neurologic: Tinnitus, transient hearing loss in the hearing impaired, vertigo, seizures, somnolence, paresthesias, headache, myoclonus.

Cardiopulmonary: Dyspnea, hyperventilation, hypotension.

Other: Pseudomembranous colitis; positive direct Coombs' test; presence of WBC, RBC, protein, casts, bilirubin, or urobilinogen in the urine; elevated alkaline phosphatase, SGOT, SGPT, bilirubin, creatinine, BUN, or LDH.

Patient/Caregiver Teaching

Instruct patient (1) to report accurate drug allergy and sensitivity history and (2) to learn principles of home self-administration of this drug.

Home Care

Appropriate following applicable teaching plan.

Administration in Other Clinical Settings

Appropriate following applicable teaching plan.

Nursing Interventions

The physician should be advised of all side effects immediately. Administer anticonvulsants if focal tremors, myoclonus, or seizures occur. If symptoms persist, decrease dose or discontinue the drug and notify the physician. Hemodialysis may reverse overdose and associated toxicities.

Immune globulin intravenous

US: Gamimune, IGIV, Sandoglobulin, Immunoglobulin, IgG, Gammagard

Immune serum   pH 6.4–7.2

ACTION

An immune serum that contains 5% immune globulin; provides immediate antibody levels that last for 3 wk.

INDICATIONS/USES

Used to maintain and treat those unable to produce adequate amounts of IgG antibodies, such as those in need of immediate increase in intravascular immunoglobulin levels, those with small muscle mass or bleeding tendencies in which IM injection is contraindicated, or patients with combined immunodeficiency disease. Sandoglobulin may be used to temporarily increase platelet count in those with idiopathic thrombocytopenic purpura.

USUAL DOSE

Gamimune: 100 mg/kg body wt; may repeat monthly as needed. May increase to 200 mg/kg or lesser dose given at 2-wk intervals if adequate IgG levels or clinical response is not obtained.

Sandoglobulin: 200 mg/kg as single dose infusion; repeat monthly as needed. May increase to 300 mg/kg or lesser dose more frequently if adequate IgG levels or clinical response is not obtained.

* Idiopathic thrombocytopenic purpura: 400 mg/kg for 5 consecutive days.

PREPARATION/RECONSTITUTION

Gamimune: Administer undiluted, or dilute with given amount of 5% dextrose for injection.

Sandoglobulin: Dilute with normal saline diluent provided to make a 3% solution; invert to allow solution to flow into the IV container.

INCOMPATIBILITIES

Considered incompatible with any other drug or solution due to specific use and potential for development of anaphylaxis.

RATE/MODE OF ADMINISTRATION

Gamimune

IV push: No.

Intermittent: No.

Continuous: 0.01–0.02 ml/kg/min over first 30 min; if no discomfort is noted, may increase to 0.02–0.04 ml/kg/min by electronic infusion device.

Filter: Applicable.

Sandoglobulin

IV push: No.

Intermittent: No.

Continuous: 0.5–1 ml/min for 15–30 min; then increase rate to 1.5–2.5 ml/min. Increase rate following initial infusion to

2.0–2.5 ml/min. May increase strength of solution to 6% after first dose beginning at 1.0–1.5 ml/min and increasing to 2.0–2.5 ml/min in 15–30 min. Infuse by electronic infusion device for greatest accuracy.

Filter: Applicable.

NURSING CONSIDERATIONS

Nursing Diagnoses

1. Potential for impaired skin integrity, related to angioedema and urticaria.
2. Potential for alteration in comfort, related to drug side effects.

Acute Care

Use intravenous form of drug only; check label carefully. Do not skin test to avoid localized chemical skin reaction. Monitor vital signs and observe patient continuously during infusion. Do not administer live virus vaccines from 2 wk before to 3 mon after administration of immune globulin IV. Store Gamimune at 2–8° C; discard partially used vials and do not use if turbid or frozen. Store Sandoglubulin below 20° C; discard partially used vials.

Precautions

Emergency equipment and resuscitative supplies must be at bedside. Use with caution in those with isolated IgA deficiency or history of prior systemic allergic reaction. Use with caution in pregnant women.

Contraindications

Known allergic response to gamma globulin or preexisting selective anti-IgA deficiencies.

Side Effects

Circulatory: Angioedema, erythema, fever, urticaria, hypotensive reaction (following too rapid rate of administration).

Patient/Caregiver Teaching

Instruct patient (1) to report all side effects immediately; (2) to provide accurate medical history and drug profile; and (3) to learn principles of home administration.

Home Care
Appropriate; administer initial dose in monitored environment.

Administration in Other Clinical Settings
Appropriate; administer initial dose in monitored environment.

Nursing Interventions
The physician must be notified of all side effects immediately; resume slower infusion if symptoms subside. Epinephrine, diphenhydramine, oxygen, vasopressors, and artificial ventilation are indicated for extreme response to drug.

Indomethacin sodium trihydrate

US: Indocin IV

Nonsteroidal antiinflammatory
agent   pH 6.0–7.5

ACTION
An antiinflammatory, analgesic, and antipyretic agent; exact mechanisms of action are unknown.

INDICATIONS/USES
Used following 48 h of ineffective medical management in the closure of hemodynamically significant patent ductus arteriosis in premature infants weighing 500–1750 g.

USUAL DOSE
Three doses are given at 12–24 h as course of treatment, as follows:

Less than 48 h: 0.2 mg/kg body wt; 0.1 mg/kg; 0.1 mg/kg.
2–7 days: 0.2 mg/kg; 0.2 mg/kg; 0.2 mg/kg.
More than 7 days: 0.2 mg/kg; 0.25 mg/kg; 0.25 mg/kg.

PREPARATION/RECONSTITUTION

Reconstitute solution with 1-2 ml of 0.9% sodium chloride or water for injection. Discard any unused portion.

INCOMPATIBILITIES

Unknown.

RATE/MODE OF ADMINISTRATION

IV push: Applicable; over 5-10 sec; further dilution not recommended.
Intermittent: No.
Continuous: No.
Filter: Not applicable in less than 1-ml dose.

NURSING CONSIDERATIONS

Nursing Diagnoses

1. Potential alteration in breathing patterns, related to toxic effects.
2. Potential sensory-perceptual alteration, related to CNS effects.
3. Potential alteration in comfort, related to drug side effects.

Acute Care

Monitor patient closely during therapy. Arrange for kidney function tests between doses; if severe renal impairment is noted, do not administer next dose.

Precautions

Use with caution in patients with renal dysfunction. Avoid extravasation and resultant local irritation. May increase bleeding. Use with caution in premature infants receiving digitalis (may prolong half-life of digitalis preparations).

Contraindications

Concurrent anticoagulant therapy.

Side Effects

Hematologic: Bleeding, disseminated intravascular coagulation (DIC).
Renal: Oliguria; reduced urine sodium, potassium, and chloride; elevated BUN.
Respiratory: Apnea, pulmonary hemorrhage.

Patient/Caregiver Teaching

Instruct patient (1) to report all side effects immediately; (2) provide accurate drug profile; and (3) to explain disease process and treatment to parents.

Home Care

Not recommended unless patient can be well monitored.

Administration in Other Clinical Settings

Appropriate.

Nursing Interventions

Monitor patient closely throughout therapy. Report all side effects to physician immediately.

Insulin injection (regular)

US: Beef Regular Iletin II, Humulin R, Novolin R, Pork Regular Iletin II, Purified Pork Insulin, Regular Iletin I
CAN: Iletin Regular (Lilly), Insulin-Toronto (Connaught Novo)

Catalyst in carbohydrate metabolism   pH 7.4

ACTION

A catalyst in carbohydrate metabolism in combination with adrenal, anterior pituitary, and thyroid hormones. Reduces liver's capacity to put glucose into the bloodstream; potassium is deposited in the liver. Rapidly absorbed and readily distributed throughout the body; not found in breast milk.

INDICATIONS/USES

Used in the treatment of diabetic coma, ketoacidosis, in combination with glucose to treat hyperkalemia, and to induce insulin shock in psychotherapy.

USUAL DOSE

Varies with clinical condition of patient; ranges from 2–100 U/h.
Low-dose treatment in ketoacidosis or diabetic coma: Loading dose of
    2.4–7.2 U; then 2.4–7.2 U/h.

PREPARATION/RECONSTITUTION

Administer undiluted; may administer as an infusion in 0.9% or 0.45% sodium chloride solution.

INCOMPATIBILITIES

Aminophylline, amobarbital, chlorothiazide, dobutamine, heparin sodium, penicillin G potassium, phenytoin, sodium bicarbonate, thiopental.

RATE/MODE OF ADMINISTRATION

IV push: 50 U or fraction thereof over 1 min.
Intermittent: No.
Continuous: As ordered by physician consistent with patient's clinical needs; administer by electronic infusion device to ensure accuracy.
Filter: Applicable for infusion purposes only; use consistent with institutional guidelines.

NURSING CONSIDERATIONS

Nursing Diagnoses

1. Potential for injury, related to drowsiness and weakness.
2. Potential for alteration in comfort, related to psychic disturbances.
3. Potential for alteration in nutrition, related to drug side effects.

Acute Care

Use regular insulin for IV use only; read label carefully. All insulin is standardized at 100 U/ml; use only if clear solution. Potency may be reduced when in solution; polyvinylchloride IV tubing and bags may present greater risk of reduction of drug potency. The percentage absorbed is inversely proportional to the concentration of insulin (the larger the dose, the less absorption); refer to manufacturer's literature for additional information. Monitor patient carefully to determine appropriateness of response to treatment. Insulin is inactivated at pH greater than 7.5; store in refrigerator or in cool, dark room.

Precautions

In low-dose treatment of diabetic coma or ketoacidosis, initial priming dose of 10 U, followed by 2–12 U/h will achieve normal plasma levels of 100–200 μU/ml of blood. Monitor blood glucose levels as ordered. Hypovolemia is a common side effect of diabetic acidosis; monitor patient's response. In combination with MAO inhibitors or alcohol, death may occur. Inhibited by corticosteroids, thiazide diuretics, dobutamine, epinephrine, furosemide, smoking. Affects serum potassium levels; exercise caution in those taking digitalis products.

Contraindications

None when used as a lifesaving measure.

Side Effects

Circulatory: Ashen color, clammy skin, nervousness, sweating, weakness, drowsiness.
Gastrointestinal: Hunger, nausea.
Others: Tremors, faintness, fatigue.
Advanced: Coma, convulsions, disorientation, hypokalemia, psychic disturbances, unconsciousness, hypersensitivity reaction.

Patient/Caregiver Teaching

Instruct patient (1) to report all side effects immediately and (2) to learn principles of self-glucose monitoring.

Home Care

Appropriate.

Administration in Other Clinical Settings

Appropriate.

Nursing Interventions

The physician should be notified of all side effects immediately. Discontinue drug; glucagon may be ordered to counteract overdose. Oral carbohydrates and 50% IV glucose may be ordered.

Intravenous fat emulsion

US: Intralipid 10% and 20%, Liposyn 10% and 20%, Liposyn II 10% and 20%, Travamulsion 10% and 20%

Nutrient emulsion   pH 6.0–8.9

ACTION

Parenteral nutrient with osmolarity of 280 mOsm/L and containing emulsified fat particles. Total caloric value is 1.1 cal/ml for 10% solution. Metabolized and used as an energy source.

INDICATIONS/USES

Used in the treatment of essential fatty acid deficiency; to provide additional source of caloric intake for those requiring parenteral nutrition.

USUAL DOSE

Adults

- Total parenteral nutrition: 500 ml of 10% or 250 ml of 20% emulsion on first day; increase dose gradually but do not exceed 60% of patient's total caloric intake or 2.5 g/kg body wt.
- Essential fatty acid deficiency: 8%–10% of total caloric intake each 24 h.

Children

- Total parenteral nutrition: Up to 1 g/kg; increase dose gradually but do not exceed 60% of total caloric intake or 4 g/kg.

PREPARATION/RECONSTITUTION

Administer as supplied.

INCOMPATIBILITIES

Do not mix with any electrolyte or other nutrient solution except as a component of total nutrient admixture (triple-mix solution). Do not place medications or additives in container.

RATE/MODE OF ADMINISTRATION

IV push: No.
Intermittent: No.
Continuous

- Adults: Yes, by electronic infusion device; administer 1 ml/min for first 15–30 min (10% solution); then increase to administer 500 ml over 4–6 h. Administer 0.5 ml/min of 20% solution for first 15–30 min; then increase rate to infuse 250 ml over 4–6 h.

- Children: Yes, by electronic infusion device; administer 0.1 ml/min of 10% solution for first 10–15 min; administer 0.05 ml/min of a 20% solution. If no untoward reaction, increase rate to administer 1 g/kg over 4 h; not to exceed rate of 50 ml/h (20%) or 100 ml/h (10%).

Filter: 1.2-μ filter applicable; use consistent with institutional guidelines.

NURSING CONSIDERATIONS

Nursing Diagnoses

1. Potential for injury, related to dizziness.
2. Potential for alteration in comfort: pain, related to drug side effects.
3. Potential for ineffective breathing pattern, related to drug side effects.

Acute Care

Infuse separately or as a component of total nutrient admixture. If administered as a separate infusion, maintain container higher than all other lines; fat emulsion has a low specific gravity and could run back into other solutions. Follow manufacturer's recommendations for storage of emulsion. Do not use if there appears to be an oiling out of the emulsion. Monitor patient's response to treatment.

Precautions

Obtain baseline liver profile, hemogram, coagulation and platelet studies. Exercise caution in administration of lipid emulsion to neonates (intravascular fat accumulation in lungs has occurred). Use with caution in those with jaundice, pulmonary disease, anemia, coagulation defect, or danger of fat embolism.

Contraindications

Pathologic hyperlipemia, lipoid nephrosis, acute pancreatitis with hyperlipemia, severe egg allergies, any condition that disturbs normal fat metabolism.

Side Effects

Gastrointestinal: Nausea, vomiting.
Neurologic: Dizziness, flushing, headache, pressure over eyes, focal seizures.
Other: Hyperlipemia, hypercoagulability, back pain, chest pain, cyanosis, dyspnea, thrombophlebitis.

Patient/Caregiver Teaching

Instruct patient (1) to report all side effects immediately; (2) to provide accurate medical history and drug and allergy profiles; and (3) to practice principles of home self-administration by electronic infusion device.

Home Care

Appropriate.

Administration in Other Clinical Settings

Appropriate.

Nursing Interventions

The physician should be notified of all side effects. In the event of accidental overdose, stop infusion and obtain venous sample for plasma, triglyceride concentration, plasma light-scattering activity by nephelometry.

Iron dextran injection
US: Imferon IV, Proferdex

Iron replacement agent   pH 5.2−6.5

ACTION
Absorbed into the hemoglobin to increase iron stores in the blood.

INDICATIONS/USES
Used in the treatment of iron-deficiency anemia and hemophilia; used when IM therapy is contraindicated.

USUAL DOSE
Adults
- Test dose: 0.5 ml (25 mg); wait 1 h, then increase gradually to 2 ml/24 h and repeat daily. Total calculated dose has been administered as an infusion.

Children: 0.5 ml (25 mg); wait 1 h, then increase gradually to 1 ml/24 h for children from 5−10 kg and repeat daily until desired results are obtained. Refer to product literature for manufacturer's recommendations.

PREPARATION/RECONSTITUTION
Administer undiluted or in 200−1000 ml of 0.9% sodium chloride solution.

INCOMPATIBILITIES
Any other drug in solution or syringe.

RATE/MODE OF ADMINISTRATION
IV push: 1 ml or fraction thereof over 1 min.
Intermittent: No.
Continuous: Applicable after test dose of 25 mg over 5 min; then infuse over 1−2 h by electronic infusion device.
Filter: Not applicable.

NURSING CONSIDERATIONS

Nursing Diagnoses

1. Potential for alteration in comfort, related to drug side effects.
2. Potential for alteration in cardiac output, related to too rapid injection of drug.

Acute Care

Use IV form of drug only; discontinue oral iron before initiating iron dextran IV. Increases joint pain and swelling in those with rheumatoid arthritis. Keep patient in supine position following administration to prevent postural hypotension and possible injury.

Precautions

Inhibited by chloramphenicol; inhibits doxycycline. Monitor serum ferritin assays in prolonged treatment. Use with caution in those with asthma or allergies. Use only if necessary in liver disease, pregnancy, lactation, or childbearing years.

Contraindications

Allergic reaction; any other form of anemia; infants younger than 4 mo.

Side Effects

Gastrointestinal: Nausea.
Neurologic: Dizziness, shivering, headache, transitory paresthesias.
Other: Itching, rash, leukocytosis, arthritic reactivation, chest pain, hypotension, lymphadenopathy, PVCs, tachycardia, shock.

Patient/Caregiver Teaching

Instruct patient (1) to report all side effects immediately and (2) to provide accurate medical history and drug profile.

Home Care

Not routinely recommended.

Administration in Other Clinical Settings

Appropriate only in well-monitored setting.

Nursing Interventions

The physician must be notified of all side effects immediately. Treat allergic symptoms as needed.

Isoproterenol hydrochloride

US: Isuprel hydrochloride

Beta-receptor stimulant   pH 3.5—4.5

ACTION

Exerts positive inotropic and chronotropic actions on the heart, increasing stroke volume, cardiac output, cardiac work, coronary flow, and venous return. Excreted in the urine.

INDICATIONS/USES

Used in the treatment of atrioventricular heart block and cardiac standstill; some ventricular dysrhythmias; and bronchospasm. Used in the management of shock and in cardiac catheterization to simulate exercise.

USUAL DOSE

Adults: Varies according to mode of administration; refer to rate and mode of administration.
- Intracardiac: 0.02 mg of a 1:5000 solution.
- Bronchospasm: 0.01 to 0.02 mg of a 1:50,000 solution; repeat as needed.

Children: One tenth to one half of adult dose; adjust according to patient's response to treatment.

PREPARATION/RECONSTITUTION

Infusion: 2 mg (10 ml) of a 1:5000 solution in 500 ml of 5% dextrose in water (4 μg equals 1 ml).

Bronchospasm or direct IV: Dilute 0.2 mg (1 ml) of 1 : 5000 solution with 10 ml normal saline for injection.
Intracardiac: 1 : 5000 solution undiluted.

INCOMPATIBILITIES

Aminophylline, carbenicillin, diazepam, epinephrine, sodium bicarbonate.

RATE/MODE OF ADMINISTRATION

IV push: 0.02–0.06 mg (1–3 ml of a 1 : 50,000 solution); give over 1 min.
Intermittent: No.
Continuous: Administer 1–5 μg/min of a 1 : 250,000 solution. Give each 1 ml of solution (4 μg) over 1 min; increase dose as needed; use electronic infusion device to ensure accuracy.
Intracardiac: 0.1 ml of a 1 : 5000 solution over 1 sec.

NURSING CONSIDERATIONS

Nursing Diagnoses

1. Potential for alteration in cardiac output: increased, related to drug action.
2. Potential for alteration in comfort: pain, related to drug side effects.
3. Potential for alteration in nutrition, related to drug side effects.

Acute Care

Monitor rate of infusion carefully and decrease as needed according to patient's response to treatment. Do not use if pink or brown or if a precipitate is present. Monitor cardiac status, central venous pressure, blood pressure, and urine flow measurements during therapy.

Precautions

Intracardiac or IV injection in cardiac standstill must be accompanied by cardiac massage to perfuse the drug into the myocardium. May be administered alternately with epinephrine but not concurrently, or else death will result from overstimulation of the myocardium. Use with caution when inhalant anesthetics are being used. Use with caution in those with coronary insufficiency, diabetes mellitus, hyperthyroidism, and known sensitivities. Antagonized by propranolol. Potentiated by tricyclic antidepressants.

Contraindications

Those with tachycardia induced by digitalis intoxication.

Side Effects

Cardiovascular: Angina, cardiac dysrhythmias, flushing, palpitations, sweating, tachycardia, cardiac dilation, marked hypotension, pulmonary edema.

Other: Nausea, nervousness, vomiting.

Patient/Caregiver Teaching

Instruct patient (1) to report all side effects immediately and (2) to provide an accurate medical history and drug profile.

Home Care

Not recommended in IV form.

Administration in Other Clinical Settings

Not recommended in IV form.

Nursing Interventions

The physician must be notified of all side effects immediately. Decrease rate of infusion or discontinue the drug for ventricular rate over 110/min.

Kanamycin sulfate

US: Kantrex, Klebcil

Aminoglycoside antibiotic   pH 4.5

ACTION

An aminoglycoside antibiotic with neuromuscular blocking action; bactericidal against many gram-negative organisms. Usual half-life is 2–3 h; prolonged in infants, postpartum females, fever, hepatic dysfunction and ascites, spinal cord injury, the elderly. Half-life is shortened in the severe burn patient. Excreted in high concentrations through the kidney; secreted in breast milk.

INDICATIONS/USES

Used in the short-term treatment of serious infections caused by susceptible organisms.

USUAL DOSE

Up to 15 mg/kg body wt/24 h in 2–4 equally divided doses based on ideal weight of lean body mass; not to exceed total dose of 1.5 g in 24 h.

PREPARATION/RECONSTITUTION

Dilute each 500 mg in 100 ml of 5% dextrose in water, 5% dextrose in 0.9% sodium chloride solution, or 0.9% sodium chloride solution, or in concentration of not more than 2.5 mg/ml.

INCOMPATIBILITIES

Amphotericin B, ampicillin, carbenicillin, cefoxitin, cephalothin, cephapirin, chlorpheniramine, heparin sodium, hydrocortisone, penicillins.

RATE/MODE OF ADMINISTRATION

IV push: No.
Intermittent: 3–4 ml/min administered over 30–60 min.
Continuous: No.
Filter: Applicable; use consistent with institutional guidelines.

NURSING CONSIDERATIONS

Nursing Diagnoses

1. Potential for injury, related to vertigo and neuromuscular blockade.
2. Potential for sensory-perceptual alteration: auditory, related to drug side effects.

Acute Care

Discard unused vials after 48 h; use extreme caution if treatment is required over 7–10 days. Sensitivity studies should be performed prior to administration to determine susceptibility of the causative organisms. Monitor urine output, BUN, creatinine, and creatinine clearance level. Routine evaluation of hearing function is needed. Monitor peak and trough levels to avoid peak serum concentrations above 30 μg/ml and trough concentrations above 5 μg/ml; the desired level is 8–16 μg/ml. Maintain good hydration.

Precautions

Reduce daily dose in event of renal impairment. Potentiated by anesthetics, other neuromuscular blocking agents, antineoplastics, phenothiazines, and sodium citrate. Ototoxicity may be potentiated by concomitant administration of loop diuretics (not recommended). Digoxin dose may require adjustment. Superinfection may occur as a result of overgrowth.

Contraindications

Known kanamycin or aminoglycoside sensitivity; prior hearing loss.

Side Effects

Neurologic: Vertigo, tinnitus, headache, paresthesias.
Other: Skin rash, thrombophlebitis, apnea, azotemia, elevated BUN, creatinine.

Patient/Caregiver Teaching

Instruct patient (1) to report all side effects immediately; (2) to provide accurate medical history and drug profile; and (3) to learn principles of home self-administration.

Home Care

Appropriate for use following initial treatment in inpatient facility.

Administration in Other Clinical Settings

Appropriate for use following initial treatment in inpatient facility.

Nursing Interventions

The physician should be notified of all side effects. Treatment is symptomatic; reduction in dose may be required. Calcium salts or neostigmine may reverse neuromuscular blockade. Emergency resuscitative equipment should be readily available.

L-Hyoscyamine sulfate

US: Levsin

Anticholinergic   pH 3.0−6.5

ACTION

An anticholinergic and antispasmodic drug that inhibits gastrointestinal motility, reduces gastric secretions, and controls excessive pharyngeal, tracheal, and bronchial secretions. Prompt onset of action lasting 4−6 h. Metabolized in the liver and excreted in the urine; traces may occur in breast milk.

INDICATIONS/USES

Used as adjunctive therapy in peptic ulcer disease, spastic colitis, pylorospasm, dysentery, cystitis, diverticulitis, irritable bowel syndrome, neurogenic bowel disorders. Also used to treat biliary and renal colic and as a diagnostic tool in hypotonic duodenography. Useful as an antidote for overdose of anticholinesterase agents.

USUAL DOSE

Gastrointestinal disorders: 0.25−0.5 mg 3−4 times daily at 4-h intervals.
Reversal of neuromuscular blockade: 0.2 mg for each 1 mg of neostigmine.
Hypotonic duodenography: 0.25−0.5 mg administered 5−10 min prior to initiation of procedure.

PREPARATION/RECONSTITUTION

Administer undiluted.

INCOMPATIBILITIES

Because hyoscyamine is one of the optical isomers containing atropine, physical and chemical compatibility information related to atropine may apply.

RATE/MODE OF ADMINISTRATION

IV push: As a single dose over 1 min.
Intermittent: No.

Continuous: No.
Filter: Not applicable in less than 1-ml dose.

NURSING CONSIDERATIONS

Nursing Diagnoses

1. Potential for sensory-perceptual alteration: visual, related to drug side effects.
2. Potential for injury, related to weakness.
3. Potential for alteration in comfort, related to drug side effects.

Acute Care

Having patient void prior to dose will help to decrease possibility of urinary retention. Use with caution in autonomic neuropathy, cardiac dysrhythmias, congestive heart failure, coronary artery disease, dehydration, hypertension, and hyperthyroidism.

Precautions

Obtain accurate medical profile. Potentiated by alkalizing agents, tricyclic antidepressants, synthetic narcotic analgesics, antihistamines, MAO inhibitors, phenothiazines, and others. Antagonized by histamine products, reserpine. Concomitant administration of digoxin, cholinergics, levodopa, neostigmine, and diphenhydramine may cause adverse effects; exercise caution. Will cause cardiac dysrhythmias with cyclopropane anesthetics.

Contraindications

Glaucoma, hypersensitivity, intestinal atony, myasthenia gravis, obstructive disease of the gastrointestinal system, paralytic ileus, ulcerative colitis, unstable cardiovascular status.

Side Effects

Gastrointestinal: Dry mouth.
Neurologic: Blurred vision, headache, nervousness.
Cardiovascular: Palpitations, tachycardia, weakness.
Genitourinary: Urinary hesitancy, urinary retention.
Other: Heat prostration, increased ocular tension, mydriasis, urticaria, anaphylaxis.

Patient/Caregiver Teaching

Instruct patient (1) to report all side effects immediately; (2) to provide accurate medical history and drug profile; and (3) to void prior to administration of each dose of medication.

Home Care

Not recommended.

Administration in Other Clinical Settings

For ambulatory cases in which full respiratory support is readily available.

Nursing Interventions

The physician must be notified of all side effects immediately. Symptomatic treatment may be advised. Physostigmine 0.5–2.0 mg IV may be used to reverse overdose; monitor side effects carefully. Thiopental sodium 2% may decrease excitement. Cooling measures increase patient comfort level. Mechanical ventilatory equipment must be readily available.

Lidocaine hydrochloride

US: Xylocaine
CAN: Xylocard (Astra)

Anesthetic and antiarrhythmic   pH 5–7

ACTION

A local anesthetic agent and antiarrhythmic. Onset of action 2 min; lasts 10–20 min. Crosses the placental barrier. Metabolized in the liver and excreted in the urine.

INDICATIONS/USES

Used to treat ventricular dysrhythmias such as PVCs or ventricular tachycardias occurring during myocardial infarction.

USUAL DOSE

Adults
- Initial: 1.0–1.5 mg/kg body wt; may repeat in 5 min up to maximum of 300 mg in 1 h. 1 mg/kg; may repeat 0.5 mg/kg every 8–10 min to a total of 3 mg/kg as needed; follow with infusion at rate of 1–4 mg/min.
- Prophylaxis: 75-mg bolus; repeat 50-mg bolus every 5 min if ventricular ectopic activity is present, up to maximum of 275 mg.

Children: 1 mg/kg as a bolus; follow with infusion of 20–50 μg/kg/min.

PREPARATION/RECONSTITUTION

Adults: Administer bolus dose undiluted; dilute 1 g to 250 ml or 500 ml of 5% dextrose in water to yield 2–4 mg/ml of lidocaine solution.

Children: Add 120 mg to 100 ml of 5% dextrose in water; 12.0–2.5 ml/kg/h will deliver 20–50 μg/kg/min.

INCOMPATIBILITIES

Ampicillin, cefazolin, phenytoin; physically incompatible with many drugs.

RATE/MODE OF ADMINISTRATION

IV push: 50 mg over 1 min.
Intermittent: No.
Continuous: Applicable by electronic infusion device as ordered.
Filter: Applicable for infusion purposes; refer to institutional guidelines.

NURSING CONSIDERATIONS

Nursing Diagnoses

1. Potential for sensory-perceptual alteration: visual, related to drug side effects.
2. Potential for alteration in nutrition: decreased, related to possible vomiting.
3. Potential for alteration in cardiac output, related to drug action.

Acute Care

Use IV form of the drug only. Monitor flow rate and patient's ECG continually. Keep a bolus dose available at all times at bedside. Discard diluted solution after 24 h.

Precautions

Therapeutic serum levels range from 1.5–6.0 μg/ml; above 7 μg/ml may be toxic. Discontinue drug when patient's cardiac condition stabilizes or signs of toxicity are evident. Use with caution in severe renal or hepatic dysfunction, hypovolemia, shock, all forms of heart block, untreated bradycardia. Reduce dose in patients with congestive heart failure, reduced cardiac output, digitalis toxicity with AV block. Potentiated by β-adrenergic blockers and cimetidine. May produce cardiac depression with phenytoin. Potentiates neuromuscular blockade of muscle relaxants and aminoglycoside antibiotics.

Contraindications

Known sensitivity; Stokes-Adams syndrome; other severe first-, second-, or third-degree heart block without benefit of artificial pacemaker in place.

Side Effects

Neurologic: Apprehension; blurred vision; dizziness; euphoria; lightheadedness; sensations of heat, cold, and numbness; tinnitus; convulsions; tremors; twitching; unconsciousness.
Gastrointestinal: Vomiting.
Cardiopulmonary: Hypotension, respiratory depression, prolonged PR interval, widened QRS complex, malignant hyperthermia, bradycardia, cardiac arrest or collapse.

Patient/Caregiver Teaching

Instruct patient (1) to report all side effects immediately and (2) to provide accurate medical history and drug profile.

Home Care

As a local anesthetic only; may be administered as an infusion, following bolus dose in select situations only.

Administration in Other Clinical Settings
May be administered as an infusion, following bolus dose in select situations only.

Nursing Interventions
The physician should be notified of all side effects immediately. Epinephrine and corticosteroids may reverse anaphylaxis. Diazepam may relieve CNS stimulation. Vasopressors correct hypotension. Resuscitative equipment should be readily available.

Lincomycin hydrochloride
US: Lincocin
CAN: Lincocin (Astra)

Antibiotic   pH 3.0–5.5

ACTION
Interferes with protein synthesis of bacterial organisms. Actively excreted in bile and urine; crosses the placental barrier and is secreted in breast milk.

INDICATIONS/USES
Used in the treatment of infections caused by life-threatening susceptible gram-positive and anaerobic organisms that do not respond to other less toxic antibiotics; used when patients are allergic to penicillins.

USUAL DOSE
Adults: 600–1000 mg every 8–12 h; total doses of 4–8 g/24 h have been given in some situations.
Children: 10–20 mg/kg body wt/24 h in 2 or 3 divided doses.

PREPARATION/RECONSTITUTION

1 g to a minimum of 100 ml 5% dextrose in water, 0.9% sodium chloride solution, or other compatible solution; larger quantities of drug should be diluted in greater amounts of diluent.

INCOMPATIBILITIES

Ampicillin, carbenicillin, kanamycin, phenytoin; compatible in solution with penicillin for 4 h only.

RATE/MODE OF ADMINISTRATION

IV push: No.
Intermittent: Preferred, not to exceed 1 g/h.
Continuous: No.
Filter: Applicable; use consistent with institutional guidelines.

NURSING CONSIDERATIONS

Nursing Diagnoses

1. Potential for alteration in comfort, related to drug side effects.
2. Potential for injury, related to hematopoietic changes in the blood.

Acute Care

Sensitivity studies must be performed prior to administration of this drug. Keep patient in supine position following injection to prevent hypotension. Avoid prolonged use and subsequent danger of superinfection caused by overgrowth. Monitor blood cell counts and liver function studies. Discard unused solution after 24 h; adhere to minimum rate of administration recommended by manufacturer.

Precautions

May cause severe colitis; observe patient carefully for evidence of diarrhea. May potentiate other neuromuscular blocking agents. Too rapid injection may cause hypotension and cardiac arrest; epinephrine should be readily available for emergency use. Use with caution in the elderly and those with allergic tendencies.

Contraindications

Known sensitivity to this drug; colitis; known monilial infections unless they are being concurrently treated; minor bacterial or viral infections; preexisting hepatic dysfunction.

Side Effects

Hematologic: Agranulocytosis, leukopenia, neutropenia.
Circulatory: Hypotension, anaphylaxis, cardiac arrest.

Other: Jaundice, elevated SGOT, pruritus ani, skin rash, vaginitis, enterocolitis.

Patient/Caregiver Teaching

Instruct patient (1) to report all side effects immediately and (2) to provide accurate medical history and drug profile.

Home Care

Appropriate following teaching in principles of self-administration.

Administration in Other Clinical Settings

Appropriate.

Nursing Interventions

The physician must be notified of all side effects immediately. Treatment is symptomatic. Administration of fluids, antihistamines, corticosteroids, and vasopressors may be indicated. Hemodialysis or CAPD may reverse toxic blood levels.

Lorazepam

US: Ativan

Sedative

ACTION

A benzodiazepine that relieves anxiety and produces sedation. Effective in 15–20 min; lasts up to 16 h. Some amount of drug is slowly excreted in the urine. Crosses the placental barrier and is secreted in breast milk.

INDICATIONS/USES

Used as a preanesthetic medication for adult patients.

USUAL DOSE

2 mg or 0.044 mg/kg body wt 15−20 min prior to procedure; 0.05 mg/kg may be given for greater lack of recall. Patients over age 50 generally receive no more than 2 mg.

PREPARATION/RECONSTITUTION

Dilute with equal volume of sterile water, 5% dextrose in water, or 0.9% sodium chloride solution.

INCOMPATIBILITIES

Undetermined.

RATE/MODE OF ADMINISTRATION

IV push: 2 mg over 1 min.
Intermittent: No.
Continuous: No.
Filter: Not applicable in less than 1-ml dose.

NURSING CONSIDERATIONS

Nursing Diagnoses

1. Potential for ineffective breathing pattern, related to drug side effects.
2. Potential for injury, related to delirium and restlessness.
3. Potential for alteration in sensory-conceptual pattern: visual, related to drug side effects.

Acute Care

Patient should remain on bed rest for 3 h following injection; assistance may be required for up to 8 h following dosage. Avoid extravasation; select appropriate vessel to ensure patency and adequate hemodilution. Maintain patency of airway. Usually administered IM; rarely given IV. Refrigerate and use only freshly prepared solutions.

Precautions

Potentiates narcotics, phenothiazines, antihistamines, barbiturates, MAO inhibitors, and tricyclic antidepressants. Potentiated by alcohol and other CNS depressants. Scopolamine increases level of sedation, hallucinations, and irrational behavior.

Contraindications

Known hypersensitivity to benzodiazepines; acute narrow-angle glaucoma; psychoses; pregnancy, labor, delivery, lactation; children.

Side Effects

Respiratory: Apnea, airway obstruction.
Neurologic: Confusion, crying, delirium, depression, drowsiness, hallucinations, restlessness.

Patient/Caregiver Teaching

Instruct patient (1) to report all side effects immediately; (2) to provide accurate medical history and drug profile; and (3) to be careful to remain in supine position.

Home Care

Not recommended.

Administration in Other Clinical Settings

Not recommended.

Nursing Interventions

The physician must be notified of all side effects immediately. Resuscitative equipment must be readily available, including full respiratory support. Promote excretion of drug through fluid and electrolyte administration and osmotic diuretics. Anticholinergic overdose may be reversed by administration of physostigmine 0.5–4.0 mg at 1 mg/min (may cause seizures).

Lymphocyte immune globulin

US: Antithymocyte globulin, Atgam

Immunosuppressant   pH 6.8

ACTION

Lymphocyte selective immunosuppressant that reduces the number of thymus-dependent lymphocytes and contains low concentrations of antibodies against other elements in the bloodstream. Serum half-life is 5–8 days.

INDICATIONS/USES

Used in management of allograft rejection in renal transplant patients; adjunct to other immunosuppressive therapy to delay initial rejection episodes.

USUAL DOSE

Adults: Range is 10–30 mg/kg body wt/24 h; given concomitantly with other immunosuppressive therapy; skin test is required.
- Delay onset of renal allograft rejection: 15 mg/kg/24 h for 14 days; then every other day for 7 doses (administer initial dose 24 h before or after transplant).
- Treat allograft rejection: 10–15 mg/kg/24 h for 14 days; then every other day for 7 more doses (administer initial dose when rejection episode is diagnosed).

Children: 5–25 mg/kg/24 h for 14 days; then every other day for total of 21 doses in 28 days.

PREPARATION/RECONSTITUTION

In solution; further dilute total daily dose with 0.45% or 0.9% sodium chloride solution; invert saline container while injecting drug so contact is not made with air in container. Dilute at rate of 1 mg/ml IV fluid.

INCOMPATIBILITIES

Considered incompatible in syringe or solution with any other drug or solution besides 0.45% or 0.9% sodium chloride solution; precipitates with dextrose solution. Avoid polyvinylchloride IV containers.

RATE/MODE OF ADMINISTRATION

IV push: No.

Intermittent: Administer in equally divided doses over a minimum of 4 h.

Continuous: No.

Filter: Applicable to 0.2–1-μ range; use consistent with institutional guidelines.

NURSING CONSIDERATIONS

Nursing Diagnoses

1. Potential for alteration in comfort: pain, related to drug side effects.
2. Potential for alteration in nutrition: decreased, related to effects of drug.
3. Potential for injury, related to hematopoietic properties of drug.

Acute Care

Administer under the direction of a highly trained and specialized physician in an acute care environment only. Intradermal skin test is required prior to administration. Use 0.1 ml of a 1 : 1000 dilution in normal saline and a saline control. Do not administer if a systemic reaction occurs. If a limited reaction (10-mm wheal) occurs, proceed with caution. Causes chemical phlebitis in peripheral veins; do not use peripheral venous system. Keep refrigerated before and following dilution; discard diluted solution after 12 h.

Precautions

Anaphylaxis may occur even with negative skin test; exercise caution. Monitor patient for signs of leukopenia, thrombocytopenia, infection. Notify physician promptly of any side effects. Resuscitative equipment must be readily available at patient's bedside. Use caution in repeat courses of therapy. *Note: Administer through vascular shunt, arteriovenous fistula, or high-flow central vein.*

Contraindications

Systemic hypersensitivity reaction to previous injection.

Side Effects

Hematologic: Leukopenia, thrombocytopenia, clotted arteriovenous fistula.

Gastrointestinal: Diarrhea, nausea, stomatitis.

Other: Infusion site pain, chest pain, chills, arthralgia, urticaria, wheal, flare, hypotension.

Patient/Caregiver Teaching

Instruct patient (1) to report all side effects immediately; (2) to report accurate medical history and drug profile; and (3) to report itching or rash.

Home Care

Not recommended.

Administration in Other Clinical Settings

Not recommended.

Nursing Interventions

The physician should be notified of all side effects immediately. Discontinue if anaphylaxis, severe thrombocytopenia, or severe leukopenia occur. Hemolysis of any clinical significance may require erythrocyte transfusion, IV mannitol, furosemide, sodium bicarbonate, and adequate fluids. Treat anaphylaxis immediately with epinephrine, diphenhydramine, oxygen, vasopressors, corticosteroids, and artificial ventilation. Resuscitative equipment must be readily available.

Magnesium sulfate

CAN: Magnesium
(Abbott, NovoPharm)

CNS depressant   pH 5.5–7.0

ACTION

A CNS depressant and depressant of smooth, skeletal, and cardiac muscle. Mild diuretic effect. Immediate onset of action that lasts about 30 min. Excreted in the urine and crosses the placental barrier.

INDICATIONS/USES

Used in the treatment of convulsive states, severe hypomagnesemia, nutritional supplementation in total parenteral nutrition, cerebral edema, uterine tetany.

USUAL DOSE

Convulsive states: 1–4 g of a 10% solution; repeat as needed but not to exceed 30–40 g/24 h.
Hyperalimentation
- Adults: 8–24 mEq/24 h.
- Infants: 2–10 mEq/24 h.
Hypomagnesemia: 5 g to 1000 ml 5% dextrose in water or 0.9% sodium chloride solution.

PREPARATION/RECONSTITUTION

Administer undiluted or add to IV for a minimum 20% solution.

INCOMPATIBILITIES

Alcohol, alkalies, calcium gluconate, calcium gluceptate, clindamycin, dobutamine, hydrocortisone, IV fat emulsion 10%, phosphates, sodium bicarbonate, tobramycin, vitamin B complex.

RATE/MODE OF ADMINISTRATION

IV push: 1.5 ml of a 10% solution over 1 min.
Intermittent: No.

Continuous: Over 3 h; not to exceed 3 ml/min. Administer by electronic infusion device to ensure accuracy.

Filter: Not applicable in less than 1-ml dose; appropriate for use with infusion consistent with institutional guidelines.

NURSING CONSIDERATIONS

Nursing Diagnoses

1. Potential for injury, related to flaccid paralysis.
2. Potential for alteration in cardiac output: decreased, related to drug side effects.
3. Potential for alteration in comfort: temperature, related to drug actions.

Acute Care

Discontinue IV administration when desired therapeutic effect has been obtained. Test knee jerk prior to each subsequent dose of medication; if absent, do not give additional magnesium sulfate. Respiratory emergency equipment must be readily available at all times. Observe patient constantly.

Precautions

Do not administer during the 2 h preceding delivery of a toxemic patient; may cause magnesium toxicity in the newborn requiring ventilatory assistance. Maintain minimum of 100 ml of urine output every 4 h. Each gram contains 8.12 mEq of magnesium (normal body contains 20–30 g of magnesium). Potentiates neuromuscular blocking agents.

Contraindications

Heart block or myocardial damage.

Side Effects

Neurologic: Absence of knee jerk reflex, flaccid paralysis.
Respiratory: Respiratory depression and failure.
Cardiovascular: Cardiac arrest, circulatory collapse, flushing, hypotension, hypothermia, increased PR interval, prolonged ST interval, increased QRS complex, sweating.

Patient/Caregiver Teaching

Instruct patient (1) to report all side effects immediately and (2) to provide accurate medical history and drug profile.

Home Care

Appropriate for use as a component of total parenteral nutrition formula.

Administration in Other Clinical Settings

Appropriate for use as a component of total parenteral nutrition formula.

Nursing Interventions

The physician must be notified of all side effects immediately. Calcium gluconate and calcium gluceptate are specific antidotes; 5–10 mEq reverses respiratory depression and heart block associated with overdose. Dopamine reverses symptoms of hypotension. Resuscitate patient as needed.

Mannitol

US: Osmitrol

Osmotic diuretic   pH 4.5–7.0

ACTION

Sugar alcohol and effective osmotic diuretic; excreted in the urine along with water.

INDICATIONS/USES

Used as prophylaxis of acute renal failure; to reduce intracranial pressure and brain mass before and following surgery; and to reduce high intraocular pressure. Promotes excretion of toxic substances from sedative overdose. Used in the oliguric phase of acute renal failure.

USUAL DOSE

Adults: 1–2 g/kg body wt or 50–200 g/24 h; 1 g equals approximately 5.5 mOsm. The following solutions are available: 25%, 20%, 15%, 10%, 5%.

- Reduction of intracranial pressure and brain mass: 1.5–2.0 g/kg as a 15%–25% solution.
- Oliguria: 300–400 mg/kg of a 20% or 25% solution; up to 100 g of a 15% or 20% solution.
- Prevention of acute renal failure: 50–100 g as a 5%–25% solution.
- Reduction of intraocular pressure: 1.5–2 g/kg as a 15%, 20%, or 25% solution; may be used 60–90 min prior to surgery.

Children: 1–2 g/kg or 30–60 g/m^2 as a 15% or 20% solution.

PREPARATION/RECONSTITUTION

Administer undiluted; dissolve all crystals prior to administration. Warm ampule or bottle in hot water and shake vigorously; cool to body temperature prior to using.

INCOMPATIBILITIES

Potassium chloride, sodium chloride, whole blood.

RATE/MODE OF ADMINISTRATION

IV push: No.
Intermittent: Over 30–90 min; administer test dose over 3–5 min.

- Glomerular filtration: 100 ml of a 20% solution in 180 ml 0.9% sodium chloride solution at 20 ml/min.

Continuous: Follow guidelines for intermittent method.
Filter: Applicable consistent with institutional guidelines.

NURSING CONSIDERATIONS

Nursing Diagnoses

1. Potential for sensory-perceptual alteration: visual, related to drug side effects.
2. Potential for alteration in nutrition, related to side effects.
3. Potential for alteration in cardiac output: related to effects of drug.

Acute Care

Use only freshly prepared solutions; discard any unused portions. Administer test dose in those with marked oliguria or impaired renal function. Administration of 200 mg/kg over 3–5 min produces urine output of 40 ml in 1 h. Urine output should then exceed 30–50 ml/h; monitor carefully. Monitor IV site carefully to avoid infiltration and other complications. Maintain hydration.

Precautions

Calcium disodium edetate increases the amount of mannitol absorbed. Evaluate cardiac status. May cause deafness when administered with kanamycin. Monitor electrolytes faithfully. Insert Foley catheter as needed to monitor urinary output.

Contraindications

Anuria, fluid and electrolyte depletion, pregnancy, congestive heart failure, severe dehydration, severe renal insufficiency, edema associated with capillary fragility.

Side Effects

Neurologic: Convulsions, blurred vision, dizziness, headache.
Genitourinary: Urinary retention, polyuria followed by oliguria.
Cardiovascular: Chills, chest pain, diuresis, edema, fever, congestive heart failure, hyperosmolality, hyper- or hypotension, pulmonary edema, thrombophlebitis.

Patient/Caregiver Teaching

Instruct patient (1) to report all side effects immediately and (2) to provide accurate medical history and drug profile.

Home Care

Appropriate with physician specialist supervision and with highly qualified home IV program.

Administration in Other Clinical Settings

Appropriate with physician specialist supervision.

Nursing Interventions

The physician must be notified of all side effects immediately. If urine output is less than 30–50 ml/h, discontinue drug and notify physician. Hemodialysis may be indicated to clear mannitol, reduce serum osmolality, and reverse physical condition.

Mechlorethamine hydrochloride

US: Mustargen, Nitrogen mustard, HN2

Alkylating agent   pH 3–5

ACTION
A cell-cycle-phase nonspecific alkylating agent with antitumor activity. Absorbed and metabolized immediately; excreted in the urine changed.

INDICATIONS/USES
Used to suppress or retard neoplastic growth with good response in Hodgkin's disease, lymphosarcoma, chronic myelocytic or lymphocytic leukemia, bronchogenic carcinoma, polycythemia vera, mycosis fungoides, metastatic effusions.

USUAL DOSE
0.4 mg/kg body wt as a single dose; may divide into 2–4 doses and administer daily for 2–4 days. Usually allow 3–6 wk between courses of therapy.

PREPARATION/RECONSTITUTION
Reconstitute 10-mg vial with 10 ml sterile water or sodium chloride for injection for a concentration of 1 mg/ml; do not remove needle and syringe. Hold securely and shake to dissolve completely; withdraw desired amount. Follow precautions as detailed in Appendix 14 to avoid exposure to drug and components.

INCOMPATIBILITIES
Any other drug in solution or syringe.

RATE/MODE OF ADMINISTRATION

IV push: Total daily dose equally distributed over 3–5 min by sideport of a freely flowing infusion.

Intermittent: No.

Continuous: No.

Filter: Not applicable in less than 1-ml dose; use nonaerosolization needle to prepare drug.

NURSING CONSIDERATIONS

Nursing Diagnoses

1. Potential for disturbance of self-concept, related to drug side effects.
2. Potential for injury, related to immunosuppression.
3. Potential for alteration in nutrition: decreased, related to effects of drug.

Acute Care

Follow precautions for handling of cytotoxic waste as described in Appendix 14. Must be administered under the direction of a physician specialist. Highly toxic; do not inhale. Avoid contact with mucous membranes and skin. Treat accidental exposure with copious irrigation with water for 15 min; follow with 2% sodium thiosulfate rinse. Mix solution immediately prior to use due to instability of admixed solution. Neutralize unused portion with equal volume of sodium thiosulfate–sodium bicarbonate and allow to stand for 45 min, then discard. Do not use if discolored. Discontinue breast-feeding. Do not allow drug to extravasate; will cause sloughing and necrosis. Maintain adequate hydration.

Precautions

Observe closely for signs of infection. Narrow margin of safety requires frequent monitoring of blood parameters. Use with caution in those receiving radiation therapy, other antineoplastic agents, or in the immunocompromised patient. May interact with amphotericin B. Do not use in the presence of severe suppurative inflammation.

Contraindications

Terminal stages of malignancy; leukemia with infectious granuloma.

Side Effects

Gastrointestinal: Anorexia, nausea, vomiting, diarrhea.
Hematologic: Bleeding, bone marrow depression, leukopenia, petechiae, hemolytic anemia.
Neurologic: Vertigo, cerebrovascular accidents, weakness, depression.
Other: Alopecia, thrombophlebitis, hyperuricemia, jaundice, death.

Patient/Caregiver Teaching

Instruct patient (1) to report all side effects immediately; (2) to provide accurate medical history and drug profile; and (3) to avoid contact between skin and drug.

Home Care

Appropriate when treated as biohazardous waste products. Precautions for handling and disposal must be considered in planning patient care.

Administration in Other Clinical Settings

Appropriate when treated as biohazardous waste product. Precautions for handling and disposal must be considered in planning patient care.

Nursing Interventions

The physician must be advised of all side effects immediately. Use 2% sodium thiosulfate solution for external contact and cleaning purposes. Inject isotonic sodium thiosulfate with a fine hypodermic needle into indurated area of extravasation. Administration of chlorpromazine may control nausea.

Meperidine hydrochloride
US: Demerol

Narcotic analgesic   pH 3.5–6.0

ACTION
A synthetic narcotic analgesic with onset of action in 5 min, lasting up to 2 h. Elevates pain threshold. Crosses placental barrier. Metabolized in the liver, excreted in the urine, and secreted in breast milk.

INDICATIONS/USES
Used to provide relief of moderate to severe pain, as a preoperative medication, to support anesthesia, and to provide obstetric analgesia.

USUAL DOSE
Adults: 10–50 mg; repeat every 3–4 h as needed.
Children: Not recommended in IV form.

PREPARATION/RECONSTITUTION
Add 5 ml sterile water or normal saline for injection or other IV solution to dilute; prefilled cartridge is commercially available.

INCOMPATIBILITIES
Aminophylline, furosemide, heparin sodium, hydrocortisone sodium succinate, methicillin, morphine, phenytoin, sodium bicarbonate, sodium iodide, thiopental.

RATE/MODE OF ADMINISTRATION
IV push: As a single dose over 4–5 min.
Intermittent: No.
Continuous: Diluted to 1 mg/ml and administered as patient-controlled analgesia solution consistent with physician's orders.
Filter: Not applicable in less than 1-ml dose. Applicable for continuous infusion; use consistent with institutional guidelines.

NURSING CONSIDERATIONS

Nursing Diagnoses

1. Potential for ineffective breathing pattern: related to drug side effects.
2. Potential for injury, related to dizziness and postural hypotension.
3. Potential for alteration in cardiac output, related to action of drug.

Acute Care

Emergency resuscitative equipment should be readily available. Observe patient frequently; monitor vital signs regularly. Keep patient supine to avoid orthostatic hypotension and fainting. Cough reflex is suppressed.

Precautions

Dependence may occur. Use with caution in glaucoma, head injuries, increased intracranial pressure, asthmas, chronic obstructive pulmonary disease, convulsions, hepatic or renal dysfunction, respiratory depression. Potentiated by anticholinergics, cimetidine, tricyclic antidepressants, MAO inhibitors, neuromuscular blocking agents, phenothiazines, general anesthetics, other narcotics, CNS depressants, alcohol.

Contraindications

Known hypersensitivity to meperidine; diarrhea resulting from poisoning unless toxic material has been eliminated; pregnancy before labor; lactation; premature infants.

Side Effects

Gastrointestinal: Nausea, vomiting.
Neurologic: Dizziness, flushing, lightheadedness, restlessness, syncope, convulsions, tremors, dilated pupils.
Cardiovascular: Cardiovascular collapse, cold and clammy skin, shock, postural hypotension.
Other: Respiratory depression.

Patient/Caregiver Teaching

Instruct patient (1) to report all side effects immediately; (2) to provide accurate medical history and drug profile; and (3) to learn principles of patient-controlled analgesia, including use of infusion equipment.

Home Care

Appropriate when administered as a component of a patient-controlled analgesia program by a qualified home care agency.

Administration in Other Clinical Settings

Appropriate.

Nursing Interventions

The physician should be notified of all side effects immediately. Narcan reverses symptoms of respiratory depression. Symptomatic relief including oxygen and artificial respiration may be used.

Mephentermine sulfate
US: Wyamine

Vasopressor   pH 4.0–6.5

ACTION

A vasopressor, effective within 1–2 min for a period of 1–2 h. Excreted in the urine.

INDICATIONS/USES

Used in the treatment of hypotensive states not associated with hemorrhage, such as myocardial infarction. Used to enhance surgical, postoperative, obstetric, and spinal anesthesia.

USUAL DOSE

15–45 mg initially; follow by repeat doses of 15–45 mg as needed. Continuous infusion may be used.

PREPARATION/RECONSTITUTION

Administer undiluted or add to 5% dextrose in water (600 mg to 500 ml delivers 1 mg/ml).

INCOMPATIBILITIES
Epinephrine, hydralazine.

RATE/MODE OF ADMINISTRATION
IV push: Applicable.
Intermittent: No.
Continuous: Applicable; administer 0.5–1.0 mg/kg body wt by continuous infusion by electronic infusion device.
Filter: Applicable for continuous infusion; use consistent with institutional guidelines.

NURSING CONSIDERATIONS
Nursing Diagnoses
1. Potential for alteration in nutrition: decreased, related to drug side effects.
2. Potential for anxiety, related to drug side effects.

Acute Care
Monitor blood pressure every 2 min until stable; then every 5 min thereafter. Discontinue medication temporarily after condition has stabilized; restart as needed.

Precautions
Potentiated or inhibited by Rauwolfia alkaloids and others. Potentiated by MAO inhibitors; hypertensive crisis may result. May cause hypotension and bradycardia with hydantoins. Diluted infusion may be needed to maintain blood pressure in hemorrhagic shock until whole blood replacement is available.

Contraindications
Known sensitivity. Overdosage of phenothiazines: further hypotension results, possibly followed by irreversible shock.

Side Effects
Gastrointestinal: Anorexia.
Neurologic: Anxiety, nervousness.
Other: Hypertension, cardiac dysrhythmias.

Patient/Caregiver Teaching
Instruct patient (1) to report all side effects immediately and (2) to provide accurate medical history and drug profile.

Home Care
Appropriate in highly monitored setting.

Administration in Other Clinical Settings
Appropriate in highly monitored setting.

Nursing Interventions
The physician should be notified of all side effects immediately. If hypertension occurs, discontinue drug and notify physician.

Metaraminol bitartrate
US: Aramine

Vasopressor   pH 3.5–4.5

ACTION
A potent vasopressor that constricts blood vessels, increases peripheral resistance, and elevates systolic and diastolic pressures. Inactivated in the body and excreted in the urine. Effective within 1–2 min; maximum effect up to 1 h.

INDICATIONS/USES
Used in the treatment of acute hypotensive states from anesthesia, hemorrhage, medication reaction, cardiogenic shock, trauma, septicemia, surgical complications.

USUAL DOSE
Adults: 0.5–5.0 mg in emergency situation; otherwise, infuse 15–100 mg in 500 ml.
Children: 0.01 mg/kg body wt as single dose or 1 mg/25 ml dextrose or saline for infusion.

PREPARATION/RECONSTITUTION
Single dose up to 5 mg undiluted; dilute for infusion in 500 ml 5% dextrose in water or 0.9% sodium chloride solution.

INCOMPATIBILITIES

Amphotericin B, ampicillin, cephalothin, dexamethasone, erythromycin, heparin sodium, hydrocortisone phosphate, hydrocortisone, invert sugar, lactated Ringer's injection, methicillin, methylprednisolone, oxacillin, penicillin G potassium or sodium, phenytoin, prednisolone, sodium bicarbonate, sodium lactate, thiopental.

RATE/MODE OF ADMINISTRATION

IV push: 5 mg over 1 min.

Intermittent: No.

Continuous: Applicable by electronic infusion device to regulate flow.

Filter: Applicable for infusion purposes only.

NURSING CONSIDERATIONS

Nursing Diagnoses

1. Potential for injury, related to dizziness.
2. Potential for alteration in cardiac output: related to action of drug.

Acute Care

Monitor blood pressure every 5 min until desired effect is obtained; then every 15 min thereafter. Discontinue IV administration if infiltration occurs; may result in tissue necrosis and sloughing (see Appendix 13).

Precautions

Hypertension may remain even when drug is discontinued. Potentiated by MAO inhibitors and tricyclic antidepressants. Use with caution in hepatic, cardiac, and thyroid disease and in hypertension and diabetes. May cause dysrhythmias with digitalis.

Contraindications

Do not use with cyclopropane or halothane anesthetic agents.

Side Effects

Neurologic: Dizziness, nervousness.

Cardiovascular: Cardiac arrest, cardiac dysrhythmias, hypertension, tachycardia.

Patient/Caregiver Teaching

Instruct patient (1) to report all side effects immediately and (2) that side effects may occur with minimal dosing.

Home Care

Not recommended.

Administration in Other Clinical Settings

Not recommended.

Nursing Interventions

The physician must be notified of all side effects immediately. Most treatment is symptomatic. Resuscitative equipment should be readily available, including nitroprusside or phentolamine. Extravasation may be reversed by injection of 5–10 mg phentolamine diluted in 10–15 ml normal saline throughout tissue in the involved area.

Methicillin sodium

US: Staphcillin

Bactericidal antibiotic   pH 7–8

ACTION

A semisynthetic penicillin used for bactericidal action against gram-positive organisms, especially pencillinase-producing staphylococci. Excreted in the urine and secreted in breast milk.

INDICATIONS/USES

Used in treatment of serious infections caused by penicillinase-producing staphylococci.

USUAL DOSE

Adults: 4–12 g/24 h every 4–6 h in divided doses; do not exceed 2 g/12 h if creatinine clearance is less than 10 ml/min.

Children: 100–300 mg/kg body wt/24 h every 4–6 h in divided
   doses.

Neonates
   - Under 2 kg and up to 7 days: 50 mg/kg/24 h in divided doses
     every 12 h.
     Meningitis: 100 mg/kg/24 h.
   - Under 2 kg and over 7 days: 75 mg/kg/24 h in divided doses
     every 8 h.
     Meningitis: 150 mg/kg/24 h.
   - Over 2 kg and up to 7 days: 75 mg/kg/24 h in divided doses
     every 8 h.
     Meningitis: 150 mg/kg/24 h.
   - Over 2 kg and over 7 days: 100 mg/kg/24 h in divided doses
     every 6 h.
     Meningitis: 150–200 mg/kg/24 h.

PREPARATION/RECONSTITUTION

Reconstitute each 1-g vial with 1.5 ml sterile water for injection to
produce 500 mg/ml. Dilute further as directed by the manufacturer.

INCOMPATIBILITIES

Do not mix with any other drug. Incompatible with aminophylline,
ascorbic acid, cephalothin, chloramphenicol, codeine, hydrocortisone sodium succinate, lincomycin, metaraminol, methadone,
morphine, promethazine, sodium bicarbonate, vancomycin, vitamin B complex.

RATE/MODE OF ADMINISTRATION

IV push: 10 ml properly diluted over 1 min or longer (no faster than
   200 mg/min).
Intermittent: Divided doses over 30 min each.
Continuous: May administer individual dose up to 8 h if needed.
Filter: Applicable; use consistent with institutional guidelines.

NURSING CONSIDERATIONS

Nursing Diagnoses

1. Potential for injury, related to alteration in clotting parameters.
2. Potential for alteration in patterns of urinary elimination, related
   to drug side effects.

Acute Care

Sensitivity studies are needed to determine susceptibility of causative organism to this drug. Monitor patient carefully for signs of allergic reaction. Avoid superinfection caused by overgrowth following prolonged use. Initial solution stable for 24 h at room temperature and 4 days if refrigerated. Inactivates aminoglycosides; do not mix in same IV container.

Precautions

Use caution in infant dosing. Abnormal blood levels may occur because of underdeveloped renal function. Inhibited by chloramphenicol, erythromycin, tetracyclines. Rapid injection will lead to thrombophlebitis; inject slowly. Concomitant administration of β-adrenergic blockers may increase risk of anaphylaxis. Potentiates action of anticoagulants.

Contraindications

Known hypersensitivity to penicillin or cephalothin; pregnancy.

Side Effects

Hematologic: Anemia, eosinophilia, neutropenia.
Gastrointestinal: Stomatitis, glossitis, oral *Candida.*
Other: Skin rash, serum sickness, nephrotoxicity, anaphylaxis.

Patient/Caregiver Teaching

Instruct patient (1) to report all side effects immediately; (2) to provide accurate medical history and drug profile; and (3) to learn principles of home self-administration.

Home Care

Appropriate for use following initial dosing in inpatient environment.

Administration in Other Clinical Settings

Appropriate for use following initial dosing in inpatient environment.

Nursing Interventions

The physician should be notified of all side effects immediately. Hemodialysis or peritoneal dialysis may be used to counteract overdose.

Methocarbamol

US: Robaxin

Skeletal muscle depressant   pH 4—5

ACTION
A skeletal muscle depressant acting on interneural blocking agent. Metabolized in the liver and excreted in the urine.

INDICATIONS/USES
Used in the treatment of acute neuromusculoskeletal injury; acute exacerbation of chronic musculoskeletal disorders; convulsive states associated with strychnine poisoning, tetanus, black widow spider bite, lead poisoning, acute alcoholism, opiate withdrawal.

USUAL DOSE
Adults: 1 g every 8 h for 3 days; dosage may be as high as 3 g every 6 h for treatment of tetanus given as 1—2 g IV push followed by infusion of balance.
Children
- Tetanus: 15 mg/kg body wt initially; repeat every 6 h as needed.

PREPARATION/RECONSTITUTION
Administer undiluted or dilute single dose in no more than 250 ml isotonic sodium chloride or 5% dextrose in water.

INCOMPATIBILITIES
Unknown at this time.

RATE/MODE OF ADMINISTRATION
IV push: 300 mg over 2 min.
Intermittent: No.
Continuous: Applicable as single dose in 250-ml solution.
Filter: Applicable; use consistent with institutional guidelines.

NURSING CONSIDERATIONS

Nursing Diagnoses

1. Potential for injury, related to irritating nature of drug.
2. Potential for sensory-perceptual alteration: vision, related to drug side effects.
3. Potential for alteration in nutrition: decreased, related to drug side effects.

Acute Care

Observe injection site carefully to avoid danger of extravasation. Blood aspirated back into the syringe does not mix with methocarbamol. Keep patient in recumbent position for 15 min after injection to prevent postural hypotension. Store drug at room temperature following dilution; do not refrigerate.

Precautions

May interfere with several laboratory tests, including 5-HIAA, VMA. Potentiated by alcohol, CNS depressants, MAO inhibitors, and phenothiazines. Exercise caution in pregnancy and lactation.

Contraindications

Known hypersensitivity; renal pathology. Do not use with propoxyphene (Darvon).

Side Effects

Neurologic: Diplopia, dizziness, drowsiness, fainting, flushing, headache, lightheadedness, metallic taste, lack of muscular coordination, nystagmus, vertigo, convulsions, syncope, blurred vision.
Other: Pain at injection site, sloughing of tissue, thrombophlebitis, anaphylaxis, bradycardia.

Patient/Caregiver Teaching

Instruct patient (1) to report all side effects immediately; (2) to provide accurate medical history and drug profile; (3) to avoid use of alcohol; and (4) to learn principles of home self-administration.

Home Care

Appropriate after initial dosing in monitored inpatient environment.

Administration in Other Clinical Settings
Appropriate.

Nursing Interventions
The physician should be notified of all side effects immediately. Epinephrine, steroids, and antihistamines should be available to counteract symptoms.

Methotrexate

US. Mexate, Amethopterin, MTX

Antimetabolite, folic acid
antagonist   pH 8.5

ACTION
Cell cycle specific for the S phase; interrupts mitotic process during nucleic acid synthesis. Excreted unchanged in the urine within 6 h; does not cross blood–brain barrier.

INDICATIONS/USES
Used to suppress or retard gestational choriocarcinoma; mycosis fungoides, meningeal leukemia; palliation for acute lymphocytic leukemia; cancers of the breast, lung, head, and neck; lymphosarcoma; adjuvant for osteosarcoma.

USUAL DOSE
Choriocarcinoma: 15–30 mg/24 h for 5 days; repeat after 7–12 days if no evidence of toxicity.

Leukemia: 3.3 mg/m² daily with prednisone 50 mg/m²; administer 3–6 times weekly as tolerated for up to 8 wk. Leucovorin rescue requires highly individualized increased dosing regimens.

- Maintenance: 2.5 mg/kg body wt every 24 days.

Psoriasis: 10–25 mg wk; not to exceed 50 mg.

PREPARATION/RECONSTITUTION

Refer to Appendix 14 for information on handling of cytotoxic agents; special handling and precautions required in dealing with this drug. Add 5 mg of drug to 2 ml sterile water for injection; each ml equals 2.5 mg of methotrexate.

INCOMPATIBILITIES

Bleomycin, fluorouracil, metoclopramide, prednisolone.

RATE/MODE OF ADMINISTRATION

IV push: 10 mg over 1 min.
Intermittent: No.
Continuous: No.
Filter: Not indicated in less than 1-ml dose.

NURSING CONSIDERATIONS

Nursing Diagnoses

1. Potential for alteration in nutrition: decreased, related to drug side effects.
2. Potential for impairment of skin integrity: actual, related to drug side effects.

Acute Care

Person administering this drug must be thoroughly familiar with leucovorin rescue process. Protect from light; may be frozen. Use as soon as possible following reconstitution; with preservatives, use within 24 h. Use preservative-free solution for intrathecal use. Refer to Appendix 14 for guidelines on handling cytotoxic drugs. Must be administered under the direction of a physician specialist. Maintain adequate hydration.

Precautions

Monitor CBC counts, bone marrow biopsies, chest radiograph; renal and liver function tests before, during, and after therapy. Observe patient carefully for signs of infection. Concomitant administration of the following drugs may produce toxicity: alcohol, antibacterials, salicylates, hepatotoxic drugs, sulfonamides, tranquilizers, phenylbutazone, phenytoin, pyrimethamine. Discontinue breast-feeding (has caused fetal death and congenital anomalies). Prophylactic administration of antiemetics reduces nausea and vomiting.

Contraindications

Not recommended during pregnancy; not recommended in hepatic, renal, or bone marrow damage.

Side Effects

Gastrointestinal: Diarrhea, enteritis, GI ulceration, gingivitis, nausea, oral ulcerations, pharyngitis, stomatitis, vomiting, hepatotoxicity.

Genitourinary: Cystitis, menstrual dysfunction.

Other: Pruritus, rash, hemorrhage from any site, acne, alopecia, chills, depigmentation, edema.

Patient/Caregiver Teaching

Instruct patient (1) that some side effects are transient, but to report all side effects immediately and (2) to avoid injury.

Home Care

Appropriate after initial dosing in an inpatient environment and with monitoring by highly qualified home IV program.

Administration in Other Clinical Settings

Appropriate after initial dosing in an inpatient environment.

Nursing Interventions

The physician must be notified of all side effects immediately. To counteract inadvertent overdosage, administer Citrovorum factor, folinic acid (leucovorin) promptly. Dose needed may equal that of methotrexate. Administer within 1 h and repeat every 4–6 h times 4 doses.

Methoxamine hydrochloride

US: Vasoxyl

Vasopressor   pH 3–5

ACTION
Vasopressor with immediate onset of action lasting about 1 h. Excreted in the urine.

INDICATIONS/USES
Used in prevention and treatment of hypotension during anesthesia; shock resulting from traumatic, surgical, or medical conditions; and termination of episodes of paroxysmal supraventricular tachycardia.

USUAL DOSE
3–5 mg; may repeat after 15 min; follow with continuous drip infusion.

PREPARATION/RECONSTITUTION
Administer undiluted or add 40 mg to 250 ml of 5% dextrose in water.

INCOMPATIBILITIES
Alkaline compounds.

RATE/MODE OF ADMINISTRATION
IV push: 5 mg over 2 min.
Intermittent: No.
Continuous: Applicable at rate of 5 ml/min by electronic infusion device.
Filter: Applicable for continuous infusion; use consistent with institutional guidelines.

NURSING CONSIDERATIONS

Nursing Diagnoses

1. Potential for alteration in nutrition: decreased, related to drug side effects.
2. Potential for alteration in urinary elimination: related to drug side effects.

Acute Care

Discontinue IV infusion if infiltration occurs; avoid tissue necrosis and sloughing. IV administration is for acute emergencies only (systolic blood pressure is 60 mmHg or less). Check blood pressure every 2 min until stabilized; then every 5 min.

Precautions

May cause severe hypertension after administration of ergot alkaloids. Potentiated by MAO inhibitors, thyroid preparation, tricyclic antidepressants, and others. Replace blood, plasma, fluids, and electrolyte needs in hypovolemia.

Contraindications

Do not use in combination with local anesthetics.

Side Effects

Cardiovascular: Bradycardia, hypertension.
Other: Projectile vomiting, urinary urgency.

Patient/Caregiver Teaching

Instruct patient (1) to report all side effects promptly and (2) to provide accurate medical history and drug profile.

Home Care

Not recommended.

Administration in Other Clinical Settings

Not recommended.

Nursing Interventions

The physician must be notified of all side effects immediately. Atropine may be used to reverse effects of bradycardia. Treat extravasation with liberal injection of 5–10 mg phentolamine diluted in 10–15 ml normal saline.

Methyldopate hydrochloride

US: Aldomet, Methyldopa

Antihypertensive   pH 3.5–4.2

ACTION

An antihypertensive that permeates brain tissue without affecting cardiac output. Maximum action occurs in 2–3 h and lasts 10 h. Excreted through the urine in small amounts. Crosses the placental barrier and is secreted in breast milk.

INDICATIONS/USES

Used in the treatment of hypertensive crisis in patients with renal or cardiac insufficiencies.

USUAL DOSE

Adults: 250–500 mg every 6 h; a maximum of 1 g every 6 h may be given.
Children: 20–40 mg/kg body wt/24 h every 6 h in divided doses; maximum dose is the lesser of 65 mg/kg or 3 g.

PREPARATION/RECONSTITUTION

Dilute single dose in 100–200 ml of 5% dextrose in water.

INCOMPATIBILITIES

Amphotericin B, tetracycline.

RATE/MODE OF ADMINISTRATION

IV push: No.
Intermittent: Applicable over 30–60 min.
Continuous: No.
Filter: Applicable; use consistent with institutional guidelines.

NURSING CONSIDERATIONS

Nursing Diagnoses

1. Potential for injury, related to anemia.

2. Potential for sensory-perceptual alteration, related to drug side effects.

3. Potential for alteration in comfort, related to edema.

Acute Care

Monitor patient's blood pressure every 30 min until stabilized. Obtain baseline liver function tests and CBC count. Monitor urinary output to ensure adequacy. Drug is more effective when given concomitantly with diuretics.

Precautions

Use with caution in those with hepatic or renal disease, lactation, pregnancy. Potentiated by MAO inhibitors, CNS depressants, and verapamil; when given in combination, death may occur. Potentiates oral anticoagulants, oral antidiabetics, levarterenol, all hypertensive drugs, and levodopa. Inhibited by tricyclic antidepressants. Monitor patient's response carefully; drug reaction may occur with adrenergics, amphetamines, antidepressants, sympathomimetics.

Contraindications

Known hypersensitivity; hepatic dysfunction.

Side Effects

Neurologic: Depression, dizziness, dry mouth, nightmares, sedation.
Circulatory: Mild postural hypotension, paradoxical hypertension, fever.
Other: Apprehension, hemolytic anemia, nasal congestion.

Patient/Caregiver Teaching

Instruct patient (1) to report all side effects immediately; (2) to provide accurate medical history and drug profile; and (3) to monitor intake and output.

Home Care

Not recommended.

Administration in Other Clinical Settings

Not recommended.

Nursing Interventions

The physician should be notified of all side effects immediately. Administration of dopamine or levarterenol counteracts effect of hypotension from overdose. Acute overdose may be reversed by hemodialysis.

Methylprednisolone sodium succinate

US: Solu-Medrol

Steroid   pH 7−8

ACTION

An antiinflammatory and adrenocortical steroid agent with less tendency to cause excessive potassium and calcium excretion and sodium and water retention. Primarily excreted in the feces and urine; 75% is excreted within 24 h. Crosses the placental barrier and appears in breast milk.

INDICATIONS/USES

Used in the treatment of hypersensitivity reactions and dermatologic conditions; used as adjunctive treatment following administration of epinephrine in allergic reactions. Also used in severe shock, ulcerative colitis, extreme infections, esophageal burns, chemotherapy.

Usual Dose

Adults: 10−40 mg; repeat every 2−6 h as needed.
- High-dose therapy: 30 mg/kg body wt may be administered.
- Shock: 1000 mg or more every 4 h as needed.

Children: No less than 0.5 mg/kg/24 h.

DILUTION

Available as a Mix-O-Vial; dilute only with the diluent provided by the manufacturer.

INCOMPATIBILITIES

Aminophylline, calcium gluconate, cephalothin, chlorpromazine, cytarabine, 5% dextrose in 0.45% sodium chloride solution, diphenhydramine, insulin, meperidine, metaraminol, nafcillin, penicillin G sodium and potassium, promethazine, tetracycline, thiopental, vitamin B complex and vitamin B complex with C. When doses greater than 80 mg are given, incompatibilities may occur with specific IV solutions; refer to manufacturer's recommendations for use.

RATE/MODE OF ADMINISTRATION

IV push: 500 mg over 1 min or more.
Intermittent: Not preferred, but may be given over 10–20 min.
Continuous: Not preferred route.
Filter: Applicable in doses greater than 1 ml.

NURSING CONSIDERATIONS

Nursing Diagnoses

1. Potential for alteration in comfort, related to drug side effects.
2. Potential for alteration in tissue perfusion, related to drug action.

Acute Care

Monitor patient's blood pressure carefully; may cause hypertension and salt and water retention. May be necessary to restrict salt and potassium; may need to replace calcium intake. Do not stop treatment abruptly; wean patient from medication to avoid adrenocortical insufficiency. Those on long-term therapy may be monitored following withdrawal for 24 mo. May increase insulin needs in diabetics. Discard unused solutions after 8 h.

Precautions

Maintain on ulcer regimen and provide prophylactic antacids as needed. Inhibited by anticonvulsants, antihistamines, ephedrine, propanolol. Inhibits anticoagulants and salicylates. Potentiates theophyllines and cyclosporine. May cause hypokalemia when used in conjunction with digitalis products, amphotericin B, or potassium-depleting diuretics. Use with caution after renal transplantation.

Contraindications

Absolute (unless life-threatening condition): Hypersensitivity; newborns; systemic fungal infection.

Relative: Acute psychoses, chickenpox, congestive heart failure, peptic ulcer, diabetes mellitus, diverticulitis, hypertension, osteoporosis, pregnancy, renal insufficiency, septic shock, thromboembolic disease, vaccinia.

Side Effects

Circulatory: Hypertension, hypersensitivity reaction, sweating, weakness.

Other: Electrolyte disorders, calcium imbalances, euphoria, glycosuria, menstrual irregularities, increased intracranial pressure, peptic ulcer perforation, transitory burning/tingling.

Patient/Caregiver Teaching

Instruct patient (1) to report all side effects immediately and (2) to provide accurate medical history and drug profile.

Home Care

Appropriate following inpatient course of treatment; patient must be monitored carefully, and emergency medications must be readily available.

Administration in Other Clinical Settings

Appropriate following inpatient course of treatment; patient must be monitored carefully, and emergency medications must be readily available.

Nursing Interventions

The physician should be notified of all side effects immediately. Epinephrine should be readily available.

Metoclopramide hydrochloride

US: Reglan

Dopamine antagonist   pH 3–5

ACTION

Stimulates tone of gastric contractions and increases peristalsis of duodenum and jejunum. Relaxes lower esophageal and pyloric sphincters. Onset of action within 1–3 min and lasting 1–2 h.

INDICATIONS/USES

Used to facilitate small bowel intubation; to stimulate gastric and intestinal emptying of barium in radiologic imaging; and to prevent nausea and vomiting associated with administration of antineoplastic therapies.

USUAL DOSE

Adults
- Small bowel intubation: 10 mg as a single dose.
- Antiemetic: 2 mg/kg body wt 30 min prior to administration of antineoplastic therapy; may repeat every 2 h for 2 doses, then every 3 h for 3 doses.

Children
- Small bowel intubation: 6–14 yr, 2.5–5.0 mg; under age 6, 0.1 mg/kg.

DILUTION

Administer undiluted if not in excess of 10 mg; otherwise, dilute in 50 ml of 5% dextrose in water, Ringer's injection, lactated Ringer's injection, or 0.9% sodium chloride solution.

INCOMPATIBILITIES

Calcium gluconate, cephalothin, chloramphenicol, cisplatin, erythromycin, methotrexate, penicillin G potassium, tetracycline, sodium bicarbonate.

RATE/MODE OF ADMINISTRATION
IV push: Applicable, 10 mg over 2 min.
Intermittent: Applicable over 15 min.
Continuous: No.
Filter: Applicable; use consistent with institutional guidelines.

NURSING CONSIDERATIONS
Nursing Diagnoses
1. Potential for injury, related to dizziness.
2. Potential for alteration in comfort, related to drug side effects.

Acute Care
Use with caution in pregnancy and lactation; may increase milk production. Too rapid injection by IV route causes anxiety, restlessness, drowsiness.

Precautions
Single dose usually does not produce side effects. Insulin reactions may occur from gastric stasis; adjust insulin dose accordingly. May potentiate extrapyramidal effects with concomitant use of phenothiazines and antipsychotic drugs.

Contraindications
Those cases in which gastric motility is not advised including obstruction, perforation, GI hemorrhage; known hypersensitivity; epilepsy; pheochromocytoma.

Side Effects
Gastrointestinal: Bowel disorders, nausea.
Neurologic: Insomnia, headache, drowsiness, dizziness, restlessness, disorientation.
Other: Methemoglobinemia in neonates.

Patient/Caregiver Teaching
Instruct patient (1) to report all side effects immediately; (2) to provide accurate medical history and drug profile; and (3) to avoid injury.

Home Care
Appropriate if monitored carefully.

Administration in Other Clinical Settings
Appropriate if monitored carefully.

Nursing Interventions
The physician should be notified of all side effects. Overdose may be reversed by administration of diphenhydramine. Resuscitative equipment should be available as needed.

Metoprolol tartrate
US: Lopressor

Adrenergic blocking agent pKa 9.68 (ionizable)

ACTION
Adrenergic blocking agent that reduces the size of the infarct and incidence of fatal dysrhythmias. Works within 1–2 min and lasts 3–4 h. Excreted as metabolites in the urine.

INDICATIONS/USES
Used to reduce cardiac mortality in hemodynamically stable persons with suspected or defined myocardial infarct.

USUAL DOSE
5 mg; repeat at 2-min intervals for 2 additional doses. If well tolerated, switch to oral medication.

PREPARATION/RECONSTITUTION
Administer undiluted.

INCOMPATIBILITIES
All other drugs in syringe.

RATE/MODE OF ADMINISTRATION
IV push: Single dose of 5 mg over 1 min.
Intermittent: No.

Continuous: No.
Filter: No.

NURSING CONSIDERATIONS
Nursing Diagnoses
1. Potential for alteration in cardiac output, related to possible side effects.
2. Potential for alteration in tissue perfusion, related to action of drug.

Acute Care
Monitor ECG and blood pressure continuously; discontinue drug if adverse symptoms (including bradycardia less than 45 beats/min and heart block greater than first degree) occur. No adjustment in dose is required for those with renal disease. Use caution in the presence of digitalis-induced heart failure.

Precautions
May antagonize antihistamines, antiinflammatory agents, ritodrine. Potentiated by anesthetics, cimetidine, furosemide, phenothiazines, phenytoin. Potentiates antidiabetics, insulin, lidocaine, narcotics, muscle relaxants, theophyllines, thyroid agents. Do not use concomitantly with verapamil; may result in severe myocardial depression and AV conduction. Reduce dose gradually to avoid rebound angina, myocardial infarction, ventricular dysrhythmias.

Contraindications
Second- or third-degree heart block, first-degree heart block with PR interval greater than 0.24 sec, systolic blood pressure less than 100 mmHg, moderate or severe cardiac failure, heart rate less than 45 beats/min.

Side Effects
Cardiovascular: Bradycardia; cardiac failure; first-, second- or third-degree heart block.
Neurologic: Syncope, tiredness, visual disturbances, vertigo, headache, dizziness, confusion.
Respiratory: Dyspnea, respiratory distress.
Other: Headache, rash.

Patient/Caregiver Teaching

Instruct patient (1) to report all side effects immediately; (2) to provide accurate medical history and drug profile; and (3) to avoid injury precipitated by side effects of drug.

Home Care

Not recommended.

Administration in Other Clinical Settings

Not recommended.

Nursing Interventions

The physician should be notified of all side effects immediately. Discontinue the drug and treat side effects consistent with patient's needs. Atropine reverses bradycardia; isoproterenol may be used with caution if atropine is not effective. Transvenous cardiac pacing may be indicated. Hypotension is best treated with IV fluids or vasopressors but use with extreme caution. Cardiac failure may be treated with digitalis, diuretics, dobutamine, isoproterenol, or glucagon as needed. Resuscitative equipment should be readily available.

Metronidazole hydrochloride

US: Flagyl IV, Flagyl IV RTU CAN: Flagyl (Rhone-Poulenc), Neo-Metric (Neolab)

Bactericidal antibiotic   pH 5–7

ACTION

Bactericidal with cytotoxic effects active against specific protozoa and anaerobes. Prompt onset of action with duration of 8 h. Excreted in urine; some in feces. Crosses placental and blood–brain barriers; secreted in breast milk.

INDICATIONS/USES

Used in treatment of serious infections of skin, skin structure, gynecologic system, bone and joint, CNS, respiratory tract, intraabdominal wall. Used in perioperative prophylaxis and hepatic encephalopathy, and as a radiosensitizer to enhance susceptibility of tumors resistant to radiation therapy.

USUAL DOSE

Loading: 15 mg/kg body wt; follow with 7.5 mg/kg in 6 h and every 5 h thereafter for 7–10 days as needed. Do not exceed 4 g/24 h.
Perioperative: 15 mg/kg 60 min before surgery for 30–60 min; follow with 7.5 mg/kg in 6 h and repeat in 12 h.

PREPARATION/RECONSTITUTION

Solutions are prediluted and ready to use except Flagyl IV. Reconstitute Flagyl IV with 4.4 ml sterile water or 0.9% sodium chloride for injection for a concentration of 100 mg/ml. Further dilute to 8 mg/ml with 0.9% sodium chloride, 5% dextrose in water, or lactated Ringer's solution for infusion. Then neutralize prior to use with 5 mEq sodium bicarbonate per 500 mg of drug.

RATE/MODE OF ADMINISTRATION

IV push: No.
Intermittent: Applicable as a slow infusion over 60 min; discontinue primary IV during use. Do not use plastic containers in a series connection because of risk of air embolism. Avoid contact with aluminum in needles and syringes.
Continuous: Applicable.
Filter: Applicable; use consistent with institutional guidelines.

NURSING CONSIDERATIONS

Nursing Diagnoses

1. Potential for alteration in comfort, related to drug side effects.
2. Potential for sensory-perceptual alteration: taste, related to drug side effects.

Acute Care

Follow directions for dilution carefully. Carbon dioxide gas may be generated as a result of dilution of Flagyl IV and subsequent neutralization with sodium bicarbonate; may require venting. Rate should be ordered by physician. Sensitivity studies are required to ensure susceptibility of the causative organism to this drug. Avoid prolonged use and subsequent superinfection caused by overgrowth. Discard diluted and neutralized solutions in 24 h. Store at room temperature before and after dilution; do not refrigerate. Protect from light during storage.

Precautions

An anaerobic/aerobic infection requires use of additional antibiotics. May cause decreased SGOT level. Avoid alcohol and disulfiram. Inhibited by barbiturates, cimetidine, phenytoin. Potentiates oral anticoagulants. Reduce and adjust dose in those with hepatic dysfunction; observe for toxicities. Use with caution in those with edema, those taking corticosteroids, or those with impaired cardiac function, CNS disease, or blood dyscrasias.

Contraindications

Known hypersensitivity, first trimester of pregnancy.

Side Effects

Gastrointestinal: Abdominal pain, diarrhea, vomiting, nausea.
Hematologic: Neutropenia.
Neurologic: Convulsions, dizziness, headache, metallic taste, peripheral neuropathy, syncope.
Other: Thrombophlebitis, pruritus.

Home Care

Appropriate.

Administration in Other Clinical Settings

Appropriate.

Nursing Interventions

The physician should be notified of all side effects. Onset of convulsions or peripheral neuropathy requires reassessment of benefit/risk of treatment. Hemodialysis or peritoneal dialysis reverses overdose. Resuscitate as needed.

Mezlocillin sodium

US: Mezlin

Antibiotic   pH 4.5–8.0

ACTION

Extended spectrum penicillin; bactericidal against many gram-positive and gram-negative bacteria including aerobic and anaerobic strains. Effective against *Klebsiella* and *Pseudomonas*. Prompt onset of action; excreted in the urine. Crosses the placental barrier and is secreted in breast milk.

INDICATIONS/USES

Used in treatment of serious infections of respiratory system, urinary tract, gynecologic and skin structures, septicemia, intraabdominal infections. Used as perioperative prophylaxis in contaminated cases.

USUAL DOSE

Adults: 200–300 mg/kg body wt/24 h in 4–6 divided doses; do not exceed 24 g/24 h.
  • Perioperative: Single dose 30–90 min before procedure.
Children 1 mo to 12 yr: 50 mg/kg every 4 h.
  • Perioperative: Single dose 30–90 min prior to procedure.
Neonates
  • Less than 7 days: 75 mg/kg every 12 h.
  • Over 7 days and less than 2 kg: 75 mg/kg every 8 h.
  • Over 7 days and more than 2 kg: 75 mg/kg every 6 h.
  • Perioperative: Single dose 30–90 min prior to procedure.

PREPARATION/RECONSTITUTION

Dilute each gram with 10 ml sterile water, 5% dextrose, or 0.9% sodium chloride for injection; shake vigorously. Dilute to minimum 10% concentration for direct IV administration. May further dilute in desired volume of 50–100 ml of compatible infusate for alternate use; refer to manufacturer's recommendations.

INCOMPATIBILITIES
Aminoglycosides, amphotericin B, chloramphenicol, lincomycin, polymyxin B, promethazine, tetracycline, vitamin B with C.

RATE/MODE OF ADMINISTRATION
IV push: Applicable over 3–5 min.
Intermittent: Applicable over 30 min; discontinue primary infusion during administration. Use full 30 min for pediatric dose.
Continuous: No.
Filter: Applicable; use consistent with institutional guidelines.

NURSING CONSIDERATIONS
Nursing Diagnoses
1. Potential for alteration in nutrition: decreased, related to drug side effects.
2. Potential for injury, related to alteration in bleeding parameters.
3. Potential for injury, related to drug side effects.

Acute Care
Sensitivity studies should be performed prior to use of this drug. Monitor patient for early signs of allergic reaction. Avoid prolonged use and subsequent superinfection caused by overgrowth. Monitor electrolyte and blood levels. Confirm patency of vein and avoid extravasation or intraarterial injection. Drug is stable at room temperature for 72 h; warm to 37°C in water bath for 20 min if precipitation occurs after refrigeration. Shake vigorously; change in color does not affect potency.

Precautions
May be used concurrently with other drugs such as gentamicin; administer in separate infusions. Continue drug for minimum of 2 days after cessation of symptoms of infection. Reduction of dose appropriate only for renal impairment with creatinine clearance below 30 ml/min. Risk of bleeding potentiated with concomitant anticoagulant therapy. Concomitant use of β-adrenergic blockers may increase risk of anaphylaxis. Neuromuscular excitability or convulsions may result from higher than normal doses of drug.

Contraindications
Known sensitivity to penicillin or multiple allergens.

Side Effects

Gastrointestinal: Nausea, diarrhea, vomiting.

Neurologic: Convulsions, neuromuscular excitability, taste sensation.

Hematologic: Thrombocytopenia, neutropenia, leukopenia, eosinophilia, decreased hemoglobin or hematocrit, bleeding abnormalities.

Other: Elevated SGOT, SGPT, BUN; fever; interstitial nephritis; skin rash; urticaria; thrombophlebitis.

Patient/Caregiver Teaching

Instruct patient (1) to report all side effects immediately; (2) to provide accurate medical history and drug profile; and (3) to avoid injury.

Home Care

Appropriate.

Administration in Other Clinical Settings

Appropriate.

Nursing Interventions

The physician must be notified of all side effects. Severe symptoms require medication to be discontinued. Allergic reactions may be reversed by administration of appropriate antihistamines. Hemodialysis or peritoneal dialysis reverses overdose.

Miconazole

US: Monistat IV

Antifungal agent   pH 3.7–5.7

ACTION

Antifungal agent, metabolized in the liver with some excretion in the urine.

INDICATIONS/USES

Used in treatment of serious systemic fungal infections, including coccidioidomycosis, candidiasis, cryptococcosis.

USUAL DOSE

Adults: 200 mg initial dose, then 600–3600 mg/24 h in 3 equally divided doses every 8 h.

Children: 20–40 mg/kg body wt in 3 equally divided doses; do not exceed 15 mg/kg per infusion.

PREPARATION/RECONSTITUTION

Dilute single dose in 200 ml 0.9% sodium chloride or 5% dextrose in water.

INCOMPATIBILITIES

Unknown; do not mix with other drugs in syringe or solution.

RATE/MODE OF ADMINISTRATION

IV push: No.
Intermittent: Applicable over 30–60 min.
Continuous: No.
Filter: Applicable.

NURSING CONSIDERATIONS

Nursing Diagnoses

1. Potential for injury, related to drug side effects.
2. Potential for alteration in cardiac output, related to action of drug.

Acute Care

Patient should be hospitalized while initiating treatment. Monitor blood counts, lipids, electrolytes before and during treatment. Avoid rapid injection; may cause tachycardia or dysrhythmias. Monitor plasma levels of both drugs when administering with phenytoin. Administration of antiemetics prior to dose minimizes nausea and vomiting. Discard darkened solution.

Precautions

Potentiates coumarin drugs; monitor bleeding parameters and adjust anticoagulant dose accordingly. May antagonize amphotericin B. Use with caution in pregnancy. Pruritus is a common occurrence.

Contraindications
Known sensitivity; children under 1 yr.

Side Effects
Gastrointestinal: Diarrhea, nausea, vomiting, anorexia.
Cardiovascular: Phlebitis, tachycardia, flushing, fever, dysrhythmia, anaphylaxis.
Other: Pruritus, rash.

Patient/Caregiver Teaching
Instruct patient (1) to report all side effects immediately; (2) to report accurate medical history and drug profile; and (3) to realize that pruritus is a common side effect.

Home Care
Appropriate after course of hospitalized therapy.

Administration in Other Clinical Settings
Appropriate after course of hospitalized therapy.

Nursing Interventions
The physician should be notified of all side effects; infusion rate may need to be decreased to allay side effects.

Midazolam hydrochloride
US: Versed

CNS depressant   pH 3

ACTION
CNS depressant with half-life range from 1.2 to 12.3 h. Metabolized and excreted in the urine. Crosses placental barrier.

INDICATIONS/USES
Used to produce sedation, relieve anxiety, and impair memory of perioperative events. Also used as preinduction anesthesia.

USUAL DOSE

Conscious sedation for procedure in healthy adults under age 60: 1.0–2.5 mg immediately before procedure. Monitor patient's response and adjust dose accordingly. Reduce by 30% in presence of narcotic premedication or other CNS depressants.

Conscious sedation for procedure in healthy adults over age 60: 0.5–1.5 mg immediately before procedure. Monitor patient's response and titrate dose accordingly. Reduce by 50% in presence of narcotic premedication or other CNS depressants.

Induction of anesthesia: 0.15–0.35 mg/kg body wt depending on age, condition, premedication. Allow 2 min to monitor effect.

PREPARATION/RECONSTITUTION

Dilute with normal saline or 5% dextrose in water in sufficient quantity to permit slow titration, such as 1 mg in 4 ml.

INCOMPATIBILITIES

Unknown.

RATE/MODE OF ADMINISTRATION

IV push: Single dose over 2 min for conscious sedation: single dose over 20–30 sec for induction anesthesia. Rapid injection may cause respiratory depression. Physician should be present when medication is administered.

Intermittent: No.

Continuous: No.

Filter: No.

NURSING CONSIDERATIONS

Nursing Diagnoses

1. Potential for ineffective breathing pattern, related to drug side effects.
2. Potential for alteration in cardiac output, related to action of drug.
3. Potential for injury, related to neurologic side effects.

Acute Care

Increased cough reflex and laryngospasm may occur; therefore, use topical anesthetic agent with this drug during perioral endoscopy and premedication with a narcotic for bronchoscopy. Monitor respiratory and cardiac function. Resuscitative equipment should be readily available. Compatible in syringe with morphine, meperidine, atropine, or scopalamine. Maintain bed rest for 3 h after IV injection.

Precautions

Maintain patent airway and support adequate ventilation. Avoid extravasation or arterial injection. Potentiated by narcotics, alcohol, barbiturates, other CNS depressants, antihistamines, tricyclic antidepressants. Potentiates halothane, inhalation anesthetics, thiopental.

Contraindications

Known hypersensitivity, acute angle-closure glaucoma, open-angle glaucoma unless being treated, pregnancy, childbirth, lactation, shock, coma, infants and children under age 18, acute alcohol intoxication with depressed vital signs.

Side Effects

Respiratory: Apnea, airway obstruction, bronchospasm, depressed respiration, hyperventilation, laryngospasm, shallow respirations, tachypnea.

Cardiovascular: Bradycardia, cardiac arrest, cardiac dysrhythmias, fluctuation in vital signs, hypotension, vasovagal episode.

Neurologic: Vertigo, dizziness, headache, hyperexcitation, slurred speech, syncope, ataxia, blurred vision.

Other: Nightmares, redness and phlebitis at injection site.

Patient/Caregiver Teaching

Instruct patient (1) to report all side effects immediately and (2) to provide accurate medical history and drug profile.

Home Care

Not recommended.

Administration in Other Clinical Settings

Not recommended unless continuous monitoring of respiratory and cardiac function is possible.

Nursing Interventions

The physician should be notified of all side effects immediately. Promote excretion through fluid and electrolyte replacement with osmotic diuretics. Dopamine, levaterenol, metaraminol may reverse hypotension. Resuscitate as needed.

Minocycline hydrochloride

US: Minocin

Antibiotic   pH 2.0–2.8

ACTION

Broad-spectrum antibiotic that is bacteriostatic against many gram-negative and gram-positive organisms. Crosses placental barrier and is secreted in breast milk.

INDICATIONS/USES

Used to treat serious infections caused by susceptible organisms and as a substitute for contraindicated penicillin or sulfonamide therapy.

USUAL DOSE

Adults: 200 mg; then 100 mg every 12 h. Do not exceed 400 mg/24 h in presence of normal renal function.
Children over age 8: 4 mg/kg body wt followed by 2 mg/kg every 12 h.

PREPARATION/RECONSTITUTION

Reconstitute 100 mg with 5 ml sterile water for injection for a concentration of 20 mg/ml; may further dilute as needed in 500–1000 ml of compatible solution.

INCOMPATIBILITIES

Unknown. Forms precipitate with calcium.

RATE/MODE OF ADMINISTRATION

IV push: No.
Intermittent: Applicable in appropriate dilution.
Continuous: No.
Filter: Applicable.

NURSING CONSIDERATIONS

Nursing Diagnoses

1. Potential for alteration in nutrition, related to side effects.
2. Potential for injury, related to vertigo.

Acute Care

Stable at room temperature for 24 h. Sensitivity studies are needed to determine appropriateness of therapy prior to treatment with minocycline. Ensure patency of vein and avoid extravasation. Thrombophlebitis may occur. Check expiration date of product and discard expired drugs; may cause nephrotoxicity.

Precautions

Use with extreme caution in renal or hepatic dysfunction; monitor parameters carefully. May cause skeletal retardation in fetus and infants and permanent tooth discoloration in children under age 8. Potentiates digoxin and anticoagulants. Inhibited by alkalizing agents, barbiturates, calcium, cimetidine, phenytoin, iron and magnesium salts, sodium bicarbonate.

Contraindications

Known hypersensitivity to tetracyclines.

Side Effects

Gastrointestinal: Nausea, vomiting, diarrhea, dysphagia, entero-
    colitis.
Other: Blood dyscrasias, anogenital lesions, dizziness, vertigo, rash.

Patient/Caregiver Teaching

Instruct patient (1) to report all side effects immediately; (2) to be aware that photosensitivity may occur; and (3) to provide accurate medical history and drug profile.

Home Care
Appropriate.

Administration in Other Clinical Settings
Appropriate.

Nursing Interventions
The physician should be notified of all side effects. Treat symptomatically and discontinue drug.

Mitomycin
US: Mitomycin-C, Mutamycin

Antibiotic antineoplastic agent   pH 6–8

ACTION
A toxic antibiotic antineoplastic that is cell-cycle-phase nonspecific; most useful in G and S phases. Metabolized in the liver with some excretion in the urine.

INDICATIONS/USES
Used as palliative treatment as an adjunct to surgery, radiation, or for those whose carcinomas are resistant to other antineoplastic agents. Helpful in treatment of gastric, pancreatic, cervical, breast, bronchogenic, head, and neck carcinomas and malignant melanoma.

USUAL DOSE
20 mg/m^2 as single dose or 2 mg/m^2 daily for 5 days. Wait 2 days, then repeat 2 mg/m^2 daily for additional 5 days to reach total dose of 20 mg/m^2. Schedule may be repeated in 6–8 wk.

PREPARATION/RECONSTITUTION
Follow precautions as defined in Appendix 14 for handling cytotoxic drugs and biohazardous waste. Reconstitute 5 mg with 10 ml

sterile water for injection for a concentration of 500 μg/ml; allow to stand at room temperature until completely in solution.

INCOMPATIBILITIES
Bleomycin sulfate.

RATE/MODE OF ADMINISTRATION
IV push: Single dose over 5–10 min.
Intermittent: No.
Continuous: As ordered, potent in 5% dextrose in water for 3 h.
Filter: No.

NURSING CONSIDERATIONS
Nursing Diagnoses
1. Potential for alteration in nutrition: decreased, related to side effects.
2. Potential for injury, related to immunosuppression.

Acute Care
See Appendix 14 for handling and precautions. Ensure patency of vein and avoid extravasation and resultant cellulitis and tissue necrosis. Monitor bleeding parameters before, during, and 7–10 wk following treatment. Stable at room temperature for 7 days; up to 14 days if refrigerated. Prophylactic administration of antiemetics allays nausea and vomiting.

Precautions
Assess patient for signs of bone marrow depression or infection. Used with other antineoplastics and radiation in reduced doses to achieve tumor remission. Discontinue treatment if no response after 2 courses of this drug. Dosage is based on average weight in presence of edema. Use with caution in those with renal dysfunction.

Contraindications
Known hypersensitivity; thrombocytopenia; coagulation disorders; WBC count below 4000; platelet count below 150,000; serum creatinine above 1.7 mg; serious infections.

Side Effects
Gastrointestinal: Anorexia, nausea, vomiting, mouth ulcers, stomatitis.

Respiratory: Dyspnea, pneumonia.
Cardiovascular: Anaphylaxis, hypertension.
Hematologic: Thrombocytopenia, leukopenia, microangiopathic hemolytic anemia, bleeding.
Other: Thrombophlebitis, skin toxicity, paresthesias, elevated BUN, confusion, anaphylaxis, alopecia (related to total dose).

Patient/Caregiver Teaching

Instruct patient (1) to report all side effects immediately; (2) to recognize hair loss as a side effect; (3) to provide accurate medical history and drug profile; and (4) to avoid injury.

Home Care

Appropriate if administered by qualified IV nurse.

Administration in Other Clinical Settings

Appropriate if administered by qualified IV nurse.

Nursing Interventions

The physician should be notified of all side effects immediately. Discontinue drug if dyspnea, nonproductive cough, pulmonary infiltrates occur. Extravasation may be minimized by treatment with LA dexamethasone injected into indurated area with fine hypodermic needle. Hematologic effects require discontinuation of drug.

Morphine sulfate
CAN: Epimorph (Robins), Morphine H.P. (Sabex)

Narcotic analgesic   pH 3–6

ACTION

A narcotic analgesic and respiratory depressant. Detoxified in the liver and excreted in the urine. Crosses the placental barrier and is secreted in breast milk.

INDICATIONS/USES

Used to relieve severe pain and apprehension from coronary occlusion, malignancy, traumatic injury, renal or biliary colic, burns, pulmonary edema. Provides postoperative relief of pain.

USUAL DOSE

2.5–15.0 mg; repeat every 2–4 h as needed or administer protocol for patient-controlled analgesia with appropriate lockout interval as ordered. *Note: Daily amounts in excess of 1 g may be needed in severe pain management.*

PREPARATION/RECONSTITUTION

Dilute with 5 ml sterile water or normal saline for injection; use compatible infusate for PCA infusion.

INCOMPATIBILITIES

Aminophylline, heparin sodium, meperidine, methicillin, phenobarbital, phenytoin, sodium bicarbonate, sodium iodide, thiopental.

RATE/MODE OF ADMINISTRATION

IV push: Applicable over 4–5 min.
Intermittent: No.
Continuous: Applicable as PCA infusion.
Filter: Appropriate for infusion purposes.

NURSING CONSIDERATIONS

Nursing Diagnoses

1. Potential for ineffective breathing pattern, related to respiratory decompression.
2. Potential for hypothermia, related to drug side effects.
3. Potential for alteration in nutrition: decreased, related to side effects.
4. Potential for alteration in elimination, related to side effects.

Acute Care

Physical dependence may result. Resuscitative equipment, including oxygen and naloxone, should be available prior to use. Monitor vital signs carefully. Maintain patient in supine position to avoid orthostatic hypotension and fainting.

Precautions

Tolerance may occur; withhold drug for 1–2 wk to restore effectiveness of medication. Use with extreme caution in head injury, increased intracranial pressure, craniotomy. Symptoms of acute abdominal condition may be masked. Potentiated by phenothiazines, CNS depressants, MAO inhibitors, neuromuscular blocking agents, and adrenergic blocking agents.

Contraindications

Acute alcoholism, benign prostatic hypertrophy, diarrhea caused by poisoning until toxin has been eliminated, hypersensitivity to opiates, respiratory depression, biliary tract surgery, patients taking MAO inhibitors, premature infants, or labor and delivery of premature infants.

Side Effects

Respiratory: Respiratory depression, Cheyne-Stokes respiration.
Neurologic: Pinpoint pupils, excitation, coma.
Cardiovascular: Tachycardia, anaphylaxis, hypotension.
Other: Constipation, neonatal apnea, hypothermia, death.

Patient/Caregiver Teaching

Instruct patient (1) to report all side effects immediately; (2) to learn principles of PCA administration; and (3) to provide accurate medical history and drug profile.

Home Care

Appropriate as a component of a home pain management program administered by qualified personnel.

Administration in Other Clinical Settings

Appropriate in monitored environments.

Nursing Interventions

The physician should be notified of all side effects immediately. Naloxone reverses respiratory depression. Patent airway, oxygen, artificial ventilation must be used as needed.

Moxalactam disodium

US: Moxam

Third-generation cephalosporin

ACTION

Third-generation cephalosporin bactericidal to many gram-positive, gram-negative, and anaerobic organisms. Excreted in the urine. Crosses the placental barrier and is secreted in breast milk.

INDICATIONS/USES

Used in treatment of serious infections of lower respiratory system, urinary tract, intraabdominal, skin and skin structure, bone and joint, CNS, and bacterial septicemia.

USUAL DOSE

Adults: 2–12 g/24 h in equally divided doses every 8–12 h for 5–10 days. May administer 250 mg every 12 h up to 4 g every 8 h as needed.

Children

- Birth to 1 wk: 50 mg/kg body wt every 12 h. *Note: Buildup of cephalosporins in neonates may increase half-life of drugs, resulting in less frequent dosing for young infants.*
- 1–4 wk: 50 mg/kg every 8 h.
- Infants: 50 mg/kg every 6 h.
- Others: 50 mg/kg every 8 h; up to 200 mg/kg may be needed; loading dose of 100 mg/kg may be given in gram-negative meningitis.

PREPARATION/RECONSTITUTION

Reconstitute each gram with 10 ml sterile water, 5% dextrose in water, or 0.9% sodium chloride solution.

INCOMPATIBILITIES

Aminoglycosides. Do not mix with other drugs in syringe or solution.

RATE/MODE OF ADMINISTRATION

IV push: Single dose over 3–5 min; may be given sideport by infusion.

Intermittent: Preferred; further dilute to at least 20 ml/g with compatible infusate and administer over 30 min.

Continuous: Applicable if added to 500–1000 ml compatible infusate and administered over 6–24 h.

Filter: Applicable.

NURSING CONSIDERATIONS

Nursing Diagnoses

1. Potential for decreased urinary elimination, related to nephrotoxicity.
2. Potential for injury, related to hematologic side effects.

Acute Care

Sensitivity studies should be obtained prior to use of this drug. Administer within 24 h of preparation; selected solutions may be preserved for 96 h with refrigeration. Use with caution in the penicillin-sensitive patient because of the potential for cross sensitivity. Avoid concurrent administration of bacteriostatic agents. Rotate infusion sites and monitor carefully to avoid thrombophlebitis.

Precautions

Will produce symptoms of acute alcohol intolerance with alcohol. May be used concomitantly with aminoglycosides in severe infections; do not mix drugs. Use with caution in those with renal and hepatic dysfunction. Adverse reaction may occur with promethazine, procainamide, muscle relaxants, potent diuretics, aminoglycosides. *Pseudomonas* infections require higher doses. Contains 3.8 mEq sodium per gram. Causes hypoprothrombinemia; recommend 10 mg/wk prophylactic vitamin K. Use of vitamin K and limiting dose to 4 g/24 h will avoid platelet dysfunction.

Contraindications

Known hypersensitivity to cephalosporins or penicillins.

Side Effects

Hematologic: Bleeding; decreased hemoglobin, hematocrit, PT, and platelet count; leukopenia; platelet dysfunction; thrombocytopenia; transient neutropenia; eosinophilia.

Gastrointestinal: Vomiting, pseudomembranous colitis, diarrhea.

Other: Vaginitis; elevated SGOT, SGPT, total bilirubin, alkaline phosphatase, LDH, and BUN; false-positive reaction for urine glucose except with Tes-Tape or Keto-Diastix.

Patient/Caregiver Teaching

Instruct patient (1) to report all side effects immediately; (2) to provide accurate medical history and drug profile; and (3) to learn principles of home self-administration.

Home Care

Appropriate if administered by qualified professionals.

Administration in Other Clinical Settings

Appropriate if administered by qualified professionals.

Nursing Interventions

The physician should be notified of all side effects immediately. Hemodialysis may be helpful in overdose. Bleeding tendencies may be reversed by administration of vitamin K, fresh frozen plasma, packed RBC, platelet concentrates. Bleeding from platelet dysfunction should be treated by discontinuing moxalactam and treating with cefamandole or cefoperzone.

Nafcillin sodium

US: Nafcil, Unipen

Bactericidal antibiotic   pH 6.0–6.5

ACTION

Bactericidal against penicillin G–sensitive and –resistant strains of

Staphylococcus aureus and other gram-positive organisms. Small quantities excreted in the urine; secreted in breast milk.

INDICATIONS/USES

Used in treatment of infection caused by penicillinase-producing staphylococci.

USUAL DOSE

Adults: 500–1000 mg every 4 h.

Children over 1 mo: 50–100 mg/24 h every 6 h in divided doses for moderate infection; 100–200 mg/kg body wt/24 h every 4–6 h in divided doses for more serious infection.

PREPARATION/RECONSTITUTION

Reconstitute each 500-mg vial with 1.7 ml sterile water for injection; each ml equals 250 mg. Further dilute each 500 mg with 15–30 ml of 5% dextrose in water or other compatible infusate.

INCOMPATIBILITIES

Aminoglycosides, aminophylline, ascorbic acid, bleomycin, methylprednisolone, hydrocortisone sodium succinate, oxytetracycline, solutions with a pH below 5 or above 8.

RATE/MODE OF ADMINISTRATION

IV push: 500 mg over 5 min.

Intermittent: Applicable in concentration of 2–40 mg/ml over 30–60 min.

Continuous: Applicable.

Filter: Applicable.

NURSING CONSIDERATIONS

Nursing Diagnoses

1. Potential for alteration in comfort, related to drug side effects.

2. Potential for alteration in nutrition: decreased, related to side effects.

3. Potential for injury, related to hematologic side effects.

Acute Care

Stable in solutions at concentrations of 2–40 mg/ml for 24 h at room temperature and 96 h if refrigerated. Refrigerate unused medication after initial preparation/reconstitution and discard after 7 days. Sensitivity studies to determine susceptibility of causative organisms should be done before administration. Determine allergy history.

Precautions

Prolonged use of drug may cause superinfection. Monitor renal, hepatic, and hematopoietic functions during long-term treatment. Inactivated by chloramphenicol, erythromycin, tetracyclines. Potentiated by probenecid. Rapid injection may cause thrombophlebitis. Inhibits aminoglycosides; do not mix in same container. Risk of bleeding increased with anticoagulant therapy.

Contraindications

Known hypersensitivity to penicillin; infants less than 1 mo old.

Side Effects

Hematologic: Bleeding.
Gastrointestinal: Nausea, diarrhea, vomiting.
Integumentary: Skin rash, urticaria, pruritus.
Other: Anaphylaxis.

Patient/Caregiver Teaching

Instruct patient (1) to report all side effects immediately; (2) to provide accurate medical history and drug profile; and (3) to learn principles of home self-administration.

Home Care

Appropriate.

Administration in Other Clinical Settings

Appropriate.

Nursing Interventions

The physician should be notified of all side effects. Discontinue drug if severe symptoms occur and treat symptomatically with antihistamines, epinephrine, corticosteroids. Hemodialysis or peritoneal dialysis may reverse overdose.

Nalbuphine hydrochloride

US: Nubain

Narcotic agonist-antagonist   pH 3.5

ACTION
Narcotic agonist-antagonist analgesic producing relief of pain in 2–3 min and lasting about 3–5 h. Some excretion in the urine. Crosses the placental barrier and is secreted in breast milk.

INDICATIONS/USES
Used to provide relief of moderate to severe pain, as a preoperative analgesic and supplement to surgical anesthesia, and for obstetric analgesia in labor.

USUAL DOSE
10 mg; repeat every 3–6 h as needed. Maximum daily dose is 160 mg.

PREPARATION/RECONSTITUTION
Administer undiluted.

INCOMPATIBILITIES
Diazepam, pentobarbital.

RATE/MODE OF ADMINISTRATION
IV push: 10 mg over 3–5 min; titrate according to response.
Intermittent: No.
Continuous: No.
Filter: Not recommended.

NURSING CONSIDERATIONS
Nursing Diagnoses
1. Potential for sensory-perceptual defect: visual, related to drug side effects.

2. Potential for ineffective breathing pattern, related to respiratory depression.
3. Potential for injury, related to neurologic side effects.

Acute Care

Sudden withdrawal may precipitate symptoms; wean patient from drug. Oxygen and respiratory resuscitative equipment should be readily available. Physical dependence may develop with abuse.

Precautions

Potentiated by phenothiazines, CNS depressants, psychotropic agents, sedatives. May need to reduce doses of both drugs; reduce to one quarter if previous medication was a narcotic. Use with care in asthma, respiratory depression, renal or hepatic dysfunction, and myocardial infarction.

Contraindications

Hypersensitivity, head injury, pregnancy and lactation, children under age 18, biliary surgery.

Side Effects

Cardiovascular: Bradycardia, hyper- or hypotension, tachycardia.
Neurologic: Vertigo, blurred vision, dry mouth, dizziness, sedation.
Other: Vomiting, urinary urgency, nausea, anaphylaxis.

Patient/Caregiver Teaching

Instruct patient (1) to report all side effects immediately and (2) to provide accurate medical history and drug profile.

Home Care

Not recommended.

Administration in Other Clinical Settings

Appropriate in ambulatory surgery setting when administered under direction of licensed physician.

Nursing Interventions

The physician should be notified of all side effects immediately. Naloxone hydrochloride may reverse respiratory depression. Complete respiratory resuscitative equipment should be available.

Naloxone hydrochloride
US: Narcan

Narcotic antagonist   pH 3.0–4.5

ACTION
Narcotic antagonist with prompt onset of action and duration of 1–4 h. Excreted in the urine.

INDICATIONS/USES
Used to reverse narcotic depression, as an antidote for natural and synthetic narcotics, and to diagnose acute opiate overdose.

USUAL DOSE
Adults
- Narcotic overdose: 0.4–2.0 mg; repeat in 2–3 min for 3 doses as needed.
- Postoperative narcotic depression: 0.1–0.2 mg at 2- to 3-min intervals until desired response is obtained; titrate to avoid excessive reduction of analgesia.

Children
Note: Use ampules containing 0.02 mg/ml.
- Narcotic overdose: 0.01 mg/kg body wt; repeat as for adults.
- Postoperative narcotic depression: 0.005–0.01 mg at 2- to 3-min intervals.

Neonates: 0.01 mg/kg into umbilical vein.

PREPARATION/RECONSTITUTION
Administer undiluted or dilute with sterile water for injection; may add to 5% dextrose in water or 0.9% sodium chloride solution for infusion.

INCOMPATIBILITIES
Preparations containing sulfites, alkaline pH, long-chain or high-molecular-weight anions.

RATE/MODE OF ADMINISTRATION

IV push: Each 0.4 mg over 15 sec.
Intermittent: No.
Continuous: 2 mg/500 ml equals concentration of 0.004 mg/ml.
Filter: Applicable for infusion only.

NURSING CONSIDERATIONS

Nursing Diagnoses

1. Potential for altered cardiac output; related to drug side effects.
2. Potential for alteration in nutrition, related to GI side effects.

Acute Care

Observe patient constantly. Discard infusion after 24 h.

Precautions

Does not produce respiratory depression with nonnarcotic drug overdose. Oxygen and artificial respiratory equipment should be readily available. Precipitates acute withdrawal symptoms in narcotic addicts; use caution. Safety for use in lactation and pregnancy not yet established. Exercise caution in those with cardiac disease or who are receiving cardiotoxic drugs.

Contraindications

Known hypersensitivity, pregnancy (except during labor).

Side Effects

Gastrointestinal: Nausea, vomiting.
Cardiovascular: Tachycardia, fibrillation, pulmonary edema, hypo- or hypertension.
Other: Elevated PTT, irritability and crying in the newborn.

Patient/Caregiver Teaching

Instruct patient (1) to report all side effects immediately and (2) to provide accurate medical history and drug profile.

Home Care

Not recommended.

Administration in Other Clinical Settings

Under the supervision of a licensed physician only.

Nursing Interventions

The physician should be notified of all side effects immediately. Resuscitate as needed.

Neostigmine methylsulfate
US: Prostigmin

Anticholinesterase   pH 5.9

ACTION

Anticholinesterase and antagonist of skeletal muscle relaxants that restores normal transmission of nerve impulses.

INDICATIONS/USES

Used as an antidote for tubocurarine, atropine, and hyoscine and to treat myasthenia gravis.

USUAL DOSE

Adults: 0.5–2.0 mg as antidote for tubocurarine; repeat as needed, not to exceed 5 mg.
  • Myasthenia gravis: 0.5 mg/titrate.
Children: 40 μg/kg with 20 μg/kg body wt of atropine as antidote for tubocurarine.

PREPARATION/RECONSTITUTION

Administer undiluted.

INCOMPATIBILITIES

Do not mix with any other drug.

RATE/MODE OF ADMINISTRATION

IV push: 0.5 mg over 1 min.
Intermittent: No.
Continuous: No.
Filter: No.

NURSING CONSIDERATIONS

Nursing Diagnoses

1. Potential for decreased cardiac output, related to drug action.
2. Potential for alteration in comfort, related to side effects.

Acute Care

The physician should be present when neostigmine is administered IV. Ensure appropriateness of drug for IV use; check label carefully. Effectiveness may be monitored by use of a peripheral nerve stimulator device.

Precautions

Administer atropine sulfate 0.5–1.2 mg before IV neostigmine when using this drug to reverse tubocurarine; atropine may mask symptoms of neostigmine overdose. Have epinephrine readily available for emergency use. Patient should be hyperventilated. Drug action may be inhibited by corticosteroids and magnesium. May induce premature labor in near-term pregnancy.

Contraindications

High concentrations of inhalant anesthesia; known sensitivity to bromides and neostigmine; mechanical intestinal/urinary obstruction; peritonitis.

Side Effects

Cardiovascular: Bradycardia, hypotension, cardiac dysrhythmias, pulmonary edema.
Gastrointestinal: Nausea, vomiting, abdominal cramps, anorexia, diarrhea.
Other: Muscle weakness, increased salivation, increased bronchial secretions, anxiety, convulsions, paralysis.

Patient/Caregiver Teaching

Instruct patient (1) to report all side effects immediately and (2) to provide accurate medical history and drug profile.

Home Care

Not recommended.

Administration in Other Clinical Settings
Not recommended.

Nursing Interventions
The physician should be notified of all side effects immediately. Atropine sulfate is an antidote for neostigmine and is given in doses of 0.6 mg IV. Endotracheal intubation or tracheostomy may be needed. Artificial ventilation, oxygen, and monitoring should be instituted as needed. Ephinephrine will reverse allergic reactions. Paralysis may be relieved by administration of 2 g pralidoxime chloride/IV; follow with 250 mg every 5 min until desired effect is obtained.

Netilmicin

US: Netromycin

Aminoglycoside antibiotic   pH 3.5–6.0

ACTION
Aminoglycoside antibiotic with neuromuscular blocking action that is bactericidal against specific gram-negative and gram-positive bacilli. Usual half-life is 2–3 h and is prolonged in infants, postpartum females, the elderly, and those with fever. Shorter half-life found in burn patients. Crosses the placental barrier and is secreted in breast milk. Excreted through the kidneys.

INDICATIONS/USES
Used in the short-term management of serious infections; also used when penicillin and other antibiotics are ineffective or contraindicated.

USUAL DOSE
Adults: 1.5–3.25 mg/kg body wt every 12 h; 1.3–2.2 mg/kg may be given every 8 hours for treatment of serious infections. Dosage is based on ideal weight of lean body mass. Patient must have normal kidney function.

Children 6 wk to 12 yr: 1.8–2.7 mg/kg every 8 h or 2.7–4.0 mg/kg every 12 h.

Neonates: 2.0–3.25 mg/kg every 12 h; neonates have immature kidney function.

PREPARATION/RECONSTITUTION

100 mg/ml concentration for adults; 25 mg/ml for pediatrics; and 10 mg/ml for neonates. Further dilute each dose in 50–200 ml of 0.9% sodium chloride solution, 5% dextrose in water, or other compatible infusate.

INCOMPATIBILITIES

Inactivated in solution by carbenicillin, other penicillins, most cephalosporins, dopamine, furosemide, heparin sodium.

RATE/MODE OF ADMINISTRATION

IV push: No.
Intermittent: Applicable over 30 min to 2 h.
Continuous: No.
Filter: Applicable.

NURSING CONSIDERATIONS

Nursing Diagnoses

1. Potential for injury, related to dizziness.
2. Potential for sensory-perceptual alteration, related to drug side effects.

Acute Care

Monitor peak and trough concentrations to avoid peak serums above 16 µg/ml and troughs above 4 µg/ml; desired range is peak 6–10 µg/mL and trough 0.5–2.0 µg/ml. A narrow range exists between toxic and therapeutic levels. Use caution if needed longer than 7–10 days; drug has ototoxic and nephrotoxic properties. Maintain good hydration. Stable for 72 h. Evaluate hearing routinely.

Precautions

Sensitivity studies should be performed to determine susceptibility of causative organisms. Reduce daily dose commensurate with degree of renal impairment; increase intervals between injections.

Monitor BUN, urine output, serum creatinine. Potentiated by anesthetics, citrate-anticoagulated blood, other neuromuscular blocking antibiotics, antineoplastics, muscle relaxants, phenothiazines, sodium citrate; apnea can occur. Potentiated by other ototoxic drugs. Avoid superinfection caused by overgrowth.

Contraindications

Known netilmicin or aminoglycoside sensitivity; renal failure.

Side Effects

Neurologic: Dizziness, headache, lethargy, muscle twitching, numbness, roaring in ears, tingling, tinnitus, convulsions, neuromuscular blockade.

Gastrointestinal: Weight loss, vomiting, nausea.

Cardiovascular: Fever, hyper- or hypotension.

Other: Urticaria, rash, burning at injection site.

Patient/Caregiver Teaching

Instruct patient (1) to report all side effects immediately; (2) to provide accurate medical history and drug profile; and (3) to learn principles of home self-administration.

Home Care

Appropriate.

Administration in Other Clinical Settings

Appropriate.

Nursing Interventions

The physician should be notified of all side effects. Minor side effects should be treated symptomatically. Hemodialysis may reverse overdose. Calcium salts or neostigmine may reverse neuromuscular blockade. Resuscitative equipment may be needed.

Nitroglycerin IV

US: Nitro-Bid IV, Nitrol IV, Nitrostat IV, Tridil

Vaosdilator   pH 5.1

ACTION

Smooth muscle relaxant and vasodilator with onset of action in 1–2 min with duration of 3–5 min. Some excretion in the urine.

INDICATIONS/USES

Used to control blood pressure in perioperative hypertension, congestive heart failure in presence of acute myocardial infarction, controlled hypotension during surgical procedures; treatment of angina in patients unresponsive to therapeutic doses of organic nitrates or beta-blockers.

USUAL DOSE

5 μg/min initially; increase by 5 μg/min increments every 3–5 min until response is noted. If no response at 20 μg/min, then 10 μg/min increases should be used. Refer to manufacturer's recommendations concerning optimum dosing.

PREPARATION/RECONSTITUTION

Dilute and administer as an infusion using only glass bottles and drug-specific infusion tubing. Follow manufacturer's guidelines for dilution and percent solution; may be used in dilutions ranging from 25–500 μg/ml.

INCOMPATIBILITIES

Do not mix with any other drug in syringe or solution.

RATE/MODE OF ADMINISTRATION

IV push: No.
Intermittent: No.
Continuous: Applicable by electronic infusion device.
Filter: Not recommended by manufacturer.

NURSING CONSIDERATIONS

Nursing Diagnoses

1. Potential for alteration in comfort, related to drug side effects.
2. Potential for alteration in cardiac output, related to drug action.

Acute Care

Follow manufacturer's recommendations for use of drug-specific tubing to avoid leeching of plasticizers from polyvinylchloride IV tubing. If changing preparations from 0.8 to 5.0 mg/ml, use new administration set or clear existing set with minimum of 15 ml; adjust dose carefully. Protect medication from light; solution stable for up to 48 h.

Precautions

Maintain adequate systemic blood pressure and coronary perfusion pressure. Monitor heart rate, blood pressure, pulmonary wedge pressure if possible. Observe for tachycardia and fall in pulmonary wedge pressure (precedes shock). Potentiated by alcohol, antihypertensives, β-adrenergic blockers, tricyclic antidepressants. Potentiates nondepolarizing muscle relaxants. Inhibited by sympathomimetics. Use with caution in those with renal/hepatic dysfunction, pericarditis, or postural hypotension. May cause orthostatic hypotension with calcium channel blockers.

Contraindications

Known hypersensitivity to nitrates, hypotension, uncorrected hypovolemia, head trauma, increased intracranial pressure, constrictive pericarditis, cerebral hemorrhage, pericardial tamponade.

Side Effects

Gastrointestinal: Abdominal pain, nausea, vomiting.
Cardiovascular: Angina, hypotension, palpitations, postural hypotension, restlessness, tachycardia, shock, constrictive pericarditis, pericardial tamponade, decreased organ perfusion, death.
Neurologic: Apprehension, dizziness, headache, muscle twitching.
Other: Methemoglobinemia.

Patient/Caregiver Teaching

Instruct patient (1) to report all side effects immediately and (2) to provide accurate medical history and drug profile.

Home Care
Not recommended.

Administration in Other Clinical Settings
Not recommended.

Nursing Interventions
The physician should be notified of all side effects immediately. Resuscitative equipment should be readily available. Reduction of rate and Trendelenburg position may alleviate hypotension and reflex tachycardia. Administer IV fluids. Methemoglobinemia is treated with methylene blue 0.2 ml/kg body wt IV and high flow oxygen.

Norepinephrine
US: Levarterenol bitartrate, Levophed

Vasoconstriction   pH 3.0—4.5

ACTION
Vasoconstrictor that greatly increases blood flow to all vital organs without increasing workload or output of the heart. Rapidly inactivated in the body and excreted in changed form in the urine.

INDICATIONS/USES
Used in all hypotensive states, including anesthesia, drug reactions, hemorrhage, myocardial infarction, pheochromocytomectomy, septicemia, trauma, surgery, sympathectomy, blood reactions.

USUAL DOSE
0.25–0.5 ml/10 kg body wt; average dose is 4 mg to each 1000 ml diluent.

PREPARATION/RECONSTITUTION
Must be diluted in 500–1000 ml of 5% dextrose in water or 5% dextrose in 0.9% sodium chloride solution and administered by infusion.

INCOMPATIBILITIES

Aminophylline, amobarbital, ampicillin, cephalothin, cephapirin, diazepam, heparin sodium, metaraminol, methicillin, oxytocin, pentobarbital, phenobarbital, phenytoin, sodium bicarbonate, sodium iodide, streptomycin, tetracycline, thiopental, whole blood.

RATE/MODE OF ADMINISTRATION

IV push: No.
Intermittent: No.
Continuous: Applicable by electronic infusion device; titrate to patient's needs.
Filter: Applicable.

NURSING CONSIDERATIONS

Nursing Diagnoses

1. Potential for discomfort, related to drug side effects.
2. Potential for alteration in tissue perfusion, related to drug action.

Acute Care

Monitor blood pressure every 2 min until stable, and every 5 min thereafter. Monitor IV flow rate and injection site carefully; avoid extravasation (treat with 5–10 mg phentolamine or 10 mg heparin sodium).

Precautions

Observe patient for development of hypovolemia and replace fluids immediately. Potentiated by amphetamines, antihistamines, tricyclic antidepressants, MAO inhibitors, methylphenidate. May cause hypertension with ergot alkaloids. Causes hypotension and bradycardia when administered with hydantoins.

Contraindications

Mesenteric or peripheral vascular thrombosis; cyclopropane or halothane anesthesias.

Side Effects

Cardiovascular: Bradycardia, chest pain.
Other: Vomiting, photophobia, pallor, necrosis induced by extravasation, headache, ischemia.

Patient/Caregiver Teaching

Instruct patient (1) to report all side effects immediately and (2) to provide accurate medical history and drug profile.

Home Care

Not recommended.

Administration in Other Clinical Settings

Outpatient surgery under care of licensed physician as emergency intervention only.

Nursing Interventions

The physician must be notified of all side effects immediately. Inject 5–10 mg phentolamine diluted in 10–15 ml 0.9% sodium chloride throughout the tissue of extravasated areas. Bradycardia may be reversed with administration of atropine.

Normal serum albumin (human)

US: Albuminar-5 and -25, Buminate 5% and 25%

Plasma protein derivative   pH 6.4–7.4

ACTION

Natural plasma protein used to expand the blood volume. Low sodium content helps maintain electrolyte balance and promote diuresis in presence of edema (contains 130–160 mEq sodium/L).

INDICATIONS/USES

Used in range of 5% or 25% solution for the following conditions: shock, burns, hepatic cirrhosis, cerebral edema. Used as 25% solution in nephrosis, adult respiratory distress syndrome, cardiopulmonary bypass, hyperbilirubinemia, or erythroblastosis fetalis as adjunct to exchange transfusion.

USUAL DOSE

Adults: Depends on hemoglobin and hematocrit and amount of pulmonary/venous congestion present; range is from 5–75 g/24 h. Available as 5% solution in 50-ml, 250-ml, 500-ml, and 1000-ml vials. Do not exceed 250 g/48 h. Available as 25% solution in 50 ml and 100 ml.

- Hypoproteinemia: 1 ml/lb/24 h of 25% solution; maximum dose is 75 g.
- Burns: Maintain albumin level from 2.5 g to just below 4 g/100 ml.

Children: 5–25 g/24 h; 25% solution is usually selected.

- Erythroblastosis fetalis: 1 g/kg body wt 1–2 h before transfusion or with exchange.
- Hypoproteinemia: 3–4 ml/lb (350 mg/kg of 25% solution).

PREPARATION/RECONSTITUTION

May administer undiluted or further diluted with normal saline or 5% dextrose in water.

INCOMPATIBILITIES

Ionosol D-CM, Ionosol G with dextrose 10%.

RATE/MODE OF ADMINISTRATION

IV push: No.

Intermittent: No.

Continuous: Applicable by electronic infusion device and consistent with patient's clinical condition: normal blood volume, 1–2 ml/min; deficient blood volume, 25–50 g as tolerated and repeat 25 g in 15–30 min; shock, 1 ml/min if blood volume normal. Reduce rate of infusion for children and infants to one quarter to one half of adult dose.

Filter: Applicable.

NURSING CONSIDERATIONS

Nursing Diagnoses

1. Potential for alteration in nutrition: decreased, related to drug side effects.
2. Potential for alteration in fluid volume, related to drug action.

Acute Care

Use only clear solution. Store at room temperature below 37 °C and use immediately after opening container. Monitor blood pressure carefully. Evaluate hemoglobin, hematocrit, electrolytes, and serum protein during treatment. Observe patient for signs of bleeding.

Precautions

5% solution is isotonic and osmotically approximates human plasma. 25% solution is hypertonic and the osmotic equivalent of 2 units of fresh frozen plasma. Maintain hydration; provide additional fluids as needed. Obtain central venous pressure readings.

Contraindications

Anemia, cardiac failure, known hypersensitivity, normal or increased intravascular volume.

Side Effects

Gastrointestinal: Nausea, salivation, vomiting.
Other: Circulatory failure, dyspnea, elevation in central venous pressure, hypotension, pulmonary edema.

Patient/Caregiver Teaching

Instruct patient (1) to report all side effects immediately and (2) to provide accurate medical history and drug profile.

Home Care

Not generally given in the home.

Administration in Other Clinical Settings

Appropriate in monitored situations.

Nursing Interventions

The physician should be notified of all side effects immediately. Treat minor side effects symptomatically. Discontinue albumin and treat symptomatically all cases of major side effects. Resuscitate patient as needed.

Oxacillin sodium
US: Bactocill, Prostaphlin

Penicillin antibiotic   pH 8

ACTION

Semisynthetic penicillin bactericidal against penicillinase-producing organisms. Excreted in the urine. Crosses the placental barrier and is secreted in breast milk.

INDICATIONS/USES

Used to treat infection caused by penicillinase-producing staphylococci.

USUAL DOSE

Adults: Over 40 kg: 250–1000 mg every 4–6 h; maximum dose is 12 g/24 h. Under 40 kg: 50–100 mg/kg body wt 24 h in 4 divided doses every 6 h; maximum 200 mg/kg/24 h.

Premature and full-term neonates: 25 mg/kg/24 h every 6 h in 4 equally divided doses.

PREPARATION/RECONSTITUTION

Dilute 500 mg powder in 5 ml sterile water or sodium chloride for injection; may further dilute in 5% dextrose in water or saline, 0.9% sodium chloride, or other compatible infusate.

INCOMPATIBILITIES

Amikacin, levarterenol, metaraminol, oxytetracycline, tetracycline.

RATE/MODE OF ADMINISTRATION

IV push: No.
Intermittent: 1 g (10 ml) over 10 min or in small volume parenteral with concentration of 2 mg/ml.
Continuous: No.
Filter: Applicable.

NURSING CONSIDERATIONS

Nursing Diagnoses

1. Potential for alteration in nutrition: decreased, related to drug side effects.
2. Potential for impairment of skin integrity, related to drug side effects.

Acute Care

Sensitivity studies should be done to determine susceptibility of the organisms. Diluted solution is stable for no more than 6 h. May be used concurrently with aminoglycosides; administer as separate infusions. Rotate IV site frequently to avoid venous irritation.

Precautions

Avoid superinfection caused by overgrowth. Elimination rate is markedly reduced in neonates; use with caution. Inactivated by chloramphenicol, tetracyclines, erythromycins. Potentiated by probenecid. May potentiate heparin sodium. Possible increased risk of anaphylaxis when administered concomitantly with β-adrenergic blockers. Higher than normal doses may lead to neuromuscular excitability or convulsions.

Contraindications

Known sensitivity to penicillin or cephalothin.

Side Effects

Gastrointestinal: Diarrhea, vomiting, nausea.
Other: Pruritus, skin rash, urticaria, thrombophlebitis, hypersensitivity, elevated SGOT.

Patient/Caregiver Teaching

Instruct patient (1) to report all side effects immediately; (2) to provide accurate medical history and drug profile; and (3) to learn principles of home self-administration.

Home Care

Appropriate.

Administration in Other Clinical Settings

Appropriate.

Nursing Interventions

The physician should be notified of all side effects immediately. Treat allergic reaction with antihistamines, epinephrine, and corticosteroids and resuscitate as needed. Overdose may be reversed by hemodialysis or peritoneal dialysis.

Oxymorphone hydrochloride

US: Numorphan

CNS depressant   pH 2.7–4.5

ACTION

CNS depressant related to morphine, but 10 times more potent milligram for milligram. Prompt onset of action lasting 3–4 h. Excreted in the urine. Crosses the placental barrier and is secreted in breast milk.

INDICATIONS/USES

Used to provide relief of moderate to severe pain; obstetric analgesia; relief of anxiety in dyspnea associated with pulmonary edema; anesthesia support.

USUAL DOSE

0.5 mg initial dose; may repeat every 2–4 h as needed, up to 1.5 mg.

PREPARATION/RECONSTITUTION

Dilute with 5 ml sterile water or normal saline for injection.

INCOMPATIBILITIES

Unknown.

RATE/MODE OF ADMINISTRATION

IV push: Applicable, over 4–5 min.
Intermittent: No.

Continuous: No.
Filter: Not applicable in less than 1-ml dose.

NURSING CONSIDERATIONS
Nursing Diagnoses
1. Potential for alteration in nutrition: decreased, related to drug side effects.
2. Potential for ineffective breathing pattern, related to effect of drug.
3. Potential for injury, related to neurologic side effects of drug.

Acute Care
Emergency resuscitative equipment, including full respiratory support, should be readily available. Monitor vital signs and observe patient at frequent intervals. Maintain patient in supine position to avoid orthostatic hypotension and fainting. Physical dependence may result.

Precautions
Use with caution in the following: the elderly, hepatic/renal dysfunction, emphysema, head injury, increased intracranial pressure, respiratory depression, craniotomy. May cause apnea in the asthmatic patient. Symptoms of acute abdominal conditions may be masked. Potentiated by phenothiazines and other CNS depressants. Cough reflex is suppressed. Marked increase in dose may precipitate seizures in presence of history of convulsive disorders.

Contraindications
Diarrhea caused by poisoning until toxin has been eliminated; known hypersensitivity; premature infants; labor and delivery of premature infants; children under age 12 yr.

Side effects
Gastrointestinal: Nausea, vomiting, anorexia, constipation.
Respiratory: Respiratory depression.
Neurologic: Somnolence, dizziness, drowsiness.
Other: Skin rash, urinary retention, anaphylaxis.

Patient/Caregiver Teaching

Instruct patient (1) to report all side effects immediately; (2) to remain in supine position; and (3) to provide accurate medical history and drug profile.

Home Care

Not recommended.

Administration in Other Clinical Settings

In ambulatory surgery, under direction of a licensed physician who is in attendance.

Nursing Interventions

The physician should be notified of all side effects immediately. Minor side effects are treated symptomatically. If severity increases, discontinue drug and notify physician. Naloxone counteracts serious respiratory depression. Resuscitate as needed.

Oxytetracycline hydrochloride IV

US: Terramycin IV

Antibiotic   pH 1.8–2.8

ACTION

Bacteriostatic against many gram-negative and gram-positive organisms. Excreted through the bile to urine and feces. Crosses the placental barrier and is secreted in breast milk.

INDICATIONS/USES

Used in treatment of infections caused by susceptible strains or organisms, including rickettsiae, viruses, spirochetal agents; used in place of sulfonamides and penicillin; administered as an adjunct to amebicides in acute intestinal amebiasis.

USUAL DOSE

Adults: 250–500 mg every 6–12 h; maximum 500 mg every 6 h for 24 hours in presence of normal renal function.

Children over 8 yr: 12 mg/kg body wt/24 h in 2 divided doses; range may be 10–20 mg/kg/24 h.

PREPARATION/RECONSTITUTION

Reconstitute each 500 mg with 10 ml sterile water for injection. Further dilute each 500 mg or fraction thereof with 100 ml 5% dextrose in water or 0.9% sodium chloride solution or other compatible infusate.

INCOMPATIBILITIES

All solutions with a pH greater than 6; amikacin, aminophylline, amobarbital, amphotericin B, ampicillin, carbenicillin, cefazolin, cephalothin, cephapirin, calcium gluconate and gluceptate, cloxacillin, erythromycin, heparin sodium, hydrocortisone phosphate, hydrocortisone sodium succinate, iron dextran, metaraminol, methicillin, methohexital, nafcillin, oxacillin, potassium and sodium penicillin G, phenytoin, polymyxin B, prochlorperazine, sodium bicarbonate, sodium lactate, succinylcholine, tetracycline, vancomycin, vitamin B complex with C, warfarin, lactated Ringer's injection with 5% dextrose, lactated Ringer's injection.

RATE/MODE OF ADMINISTRATION

IV push: 100 mg over minimum of 5 min; do not increase rate.
Intermittent: Applicable.
Continuous: No.
Filter: Applicable.

NURSING CONSIDERATIONS

Nursing Diagnoses

1. Potential for alteration in nutrition, related to dysphagia and other symptoms.
2. Potential for impairment of skin integrity, related to drug side effects.

Acute Care

Store away from heat and light; check expiration date. Store reconstituted drug at 2–8°C and use within 48 h. Ascorbic acid is used as a buffer. Sensitivity studies to determine susceptibility of causative organisms should be done. Ensure patency of IV line and avoid extravasation. Monitor for development of thrombophlebitis.

Precautions

May cause skeletal retardation in the fetus and infants and permanent tooth discoloration in those under age 8. Inhibits bactericidal action of penicillin, ampicillin, oxacillin, and methicillin. May be toxic with sulfonamides. Potentiated by alcohol, barbiturates, cimetidine, phenytoin, other hepatotoxic drugs. May potentiate digoxin and anticoagulants. Inhibited by alkalizing agents; sodium bicarbonate. In presence of syphilis, perform dark-field examination before treatment.

Contraindications

Known hypersensitivity.

Side Effects

Gastrointestinal: Nausea, anorexia, dysphagia, diarrhea, enterocolitis, vomiting.
Other: Skin rash, blood dyscrasias, anogenital lesions, photosensitivity, systemic moniliasis, thrombophlebitis.

Patient/Caregiver Teaching

Instruct patient (1) to report all side effects immediately; (2) to realize the possibility of photosensitivity reaction; (3) to report accurate medical history and drug profile; and (4) to learn principles of home self-administration and monitoring.

Home Care

Appropriate.

Administration in Other Clinical Settings

Appropriate.

Nursing Interventions

The physician should be notified of all side effects immediately. Treatment is symptomatic.

Oxytocin injection

US: Pitocin, Syntocinon

Uterine stimulant   pH 2.5—4.5

ACTION

Posterior pituitary derivative that produces rhythmic contraction of uterine smooth muscle. Rapid action with half-life of 1–6 min. Excreted in the urine; has a mild antidiuretic effect.

INDICATIONS/USES

Used to induce or stimulate labor at term or before; control of postpartum bleeding; treatment of incomplete or inevitable abortion.

USUAL DOSE

Consistent with intended use, dilution, rate of administration.

PREPARATION/RECONSTITUTION

Induction of labor: Dilute 1 ml (10 U) in 1 L 0.9% sodium chloride solution or 5% dextrose in 0.9% sodium chloride solution (10 mU/ml).

Control of postpartum bleeding: Dilute 1–4 ml in 1 L of above infusates (10 to 40 mU/ml).

Incomplete or inevitable abortion: Dilute 1 ml in 500 ml of above infusates (20 mU/ml).

INCOMPATIBILITIES

Levarterenol, prochlorperazine, warfarin.

RATE/MODE OF ADMINISTRATION

IV push: No.

Intermittent: No.

Continuous: Applicable by electronic infusion device using minimal effective rate of infusion and monitoring patient constantly.

- Induction of labor: 1–2 mU/min; increase in equal incre-

ments at 15- to 30-min intervals until contractions simulate
normal labor.

- Control of postpartum bleeding: Aimed at control of uterine
atony; 10–20 mU/min; increase or decrease as needed.
- Incomplete or inevitable abortion: 10 to 20 mU/min.

NURSING CONSIDERATIONS

Nursing Diagnoses

1. Potential for alteration in cardiac output, related to drug side
effects.
2. Potential for injury, related to hemorrhage.
3. Potential for alteration in comfort, related to drug side effects.

Acute Care

Maintain infusion of 0.9% sodium chloride solution without additives at bedside for emergency situation. Should be administered in
the inpatient environment with availability of a physician at all
times. Monitor blood pressure, fetal heart tones, timing and
strength of contractions, resting uterine tone every 15 min or as
needed. Monitor oral intake and observe for evidence of fluid retention (water intoxication has caused maternal death). Do not combine IV and oral routes; use one route of administration only.
Refrigerate drug to store for extended periods. Secreted in breast
milk; nursing may be postponed until 24 h after drug is discontinued. Oxytocin should be given by sideport to allow it to be
discontinued abruptly and to maintain an open IV line.

Precautions

Severe hypertension may result in presence of local anesthesia,
regional anesthesia, and with dopamine, ephedrine, epinephrine,
methoxamine, other vasopressors. Chlorpromazine reverses the
hypertension. Oxytocin-Challenge test is an antepartum test of
uteroplacental insufficiency performed in the high-risk patient by a
physician only. Infuse properly diluted oxytocin (10 mU/ml) at rate
of 0.5 mU/min. Increase rate gradually until contractions are timed
at 3–4 min apart. Monitor fetal heart rate constantly. Monitor for
signs of fetal distress with contractions (evidence of inadequate
placental reserve). Stop infusion.

Contraindications

Abruptio placentae, cephalopelvic disproportion, cesarean section, uterine surgery, dead fetus, fetal distress, fetal malpresentation, known hypersensitivity, hypertonic uterine contractions, medical or obstetric conditions (past or present) of a serious nature, toxemia of pregnancy.

Side Effects

Cardiovascular: Anaphylaxis, cardiac dysrhythmias, fetal bradycardia, fetal death, fluid retention, hypertension.
Other: Afibrinogenemia, subarachnoid hemorrhage, uterine rupture or spasm, postpartum hemorrhage, pelvic hematoma.

Patient/Caregiver Teaching

Instruct patient (1) to report all side effects immediately; (2) to expect some nausea and vomiting; and (3) to provide accurate drug/allergy profile.

Home Care

Not recommended.

Administration in Other Clinical Settings

Not recommended.

Nursing Interventions

The physician should be notified of all side effects immediately. Nausea and vomiting are treated symptomatically. Discontinue drug immediately for uterine hyperactivity or fetal distress and administer oxygen to the mother. Side effects may occur during labor and delivery and into the postpartum period.

Pancuronium bromide

US: Pavulon

Skeletal muscle relaxant   pH 5

ACTION
Skeletal muscle relaxant five times more potent than tubocurarine. Onset of action dose dependent; may begin in 30 sec and last 25 min. Excreted in the urine.

INDICATIONS/USES
Used as an adjunct to general anesthesia and to facilitate endotracheal intubation; also used to manage patients using mechanical ventilation.

USUAL DOSE
Adults: Individualized according to patient's clinical condition and degree and length of muscle relaxation required. 0.04 to 0.1 mg/kg body wt is initial dose; 0.01 mg/kg doses as needed to maintain muscle relaxation at 25–60-minute intervals.
- Endotracheal intubation: 0.06–0.1 mg/kg.

Neonates: Test dose of 0.02 mg/kg required; determine patient's response before proceeding.

PREPARATION/RECONSTITUTION
Administer undiluted.

INCOMPATIBILITIES
Not available.

RATE/MODE OF ADMINISTRATION
IV push: Single dose over 60–90 sec.
Intermittent: No.
Continuous: No.
Filter: No.

NURSING CONSIDERATIONS

Nursing Diagnoses

1. Potential for ineffective breathing pattern, related to drug action.
2. Potential for ineffective airway clearance, related to drug side effects.
3. Potential for alteration in tissue perfusion, related to drug side effects.

Acute Care

Store in refrigerator; maintains potency at room temperature for up to 6 mo. Administer only under the direction of an anesthesiologist; produces apnea. Artificial ventilation with oxygen should be continuous and constantly supervised. Maintain patent airway. Drug action altered by dehydration, electrolyte imbalance, body temperature, acid-base imbalance.

Precautions

Have emergency resuscitative equipment available at all times. Use peripheral nerve stimulator to monitor patient's response to drug. Use with caution in those with hepatic/renal dysfunction. Potentiated by hypokalemia, some carcinomas, inhalant anesthetics, neuromuscular blocking antibiotics, diazepam, calcium salts, carbon dioxide, diuretics, other muscle relaxants, digitalis, magnesium sulfate, MAO inhibitors, quinidine, morphine, lidocaine, meperidine, propranolol, succinylcholine. Antagonized by acetylcholine, anticholinesterases, aminophylline, potassium. Hyperkalemia may result in cardiac dysrhythmias and increased paralysis.

Contraindications

Known hypersensitivity.

Side Effects

Respiratory: Respiratory insufficiency, apnea, airway closure.
Cardiovascular: Shock, hypotension, histamine release, anaphylaxis, hypersensitivity.

Patient/Caregiver Teaching

Instruct patient (1) to report side effects if able to do so and (2) to provide accurate medical history and drug profile.

Home Care
Inappropriate.

Administration in Other Clinical Settings
Not recommended.

Nursing Interventions
The physician must be readily available; all side effects are considered emergencies. Controlled artificial ventilation is mandatory. To reverse muscle relaxation, administer pyridostigmine or neostigmine. Resuscitate as needed.

Penicillin G potassium and Penicillin G sodium

US: Penicillin G, Pfizerpen
CAN: Ayercillin (Ayerst)

Penicillin antibiotic   pH 6–7

ACTION
Bactericidal against penicillin-sensitive microorganisms. Crosses the placental barrier and is secreted in breast milk. Excreted in the urine.

INDICATIONS/USES
Used to treat severe infections caused by penicillin G–sensitive gram-positive, gram-negative, and anaerobic microorganisms; pneumococcal, Vincent's gingivitis, spirochetal infections; meningitis; endocarditis. Also used as prophylaxis against bacterial endocarditis.

USUAL DOSE
Adults: 1,000,000–20,000,000 U/24 h in equally divided doses; doses up to 80,000,000 U/24 h have been given.

Children: 50,000–300,000 U/kg body wt/24 h in equally divided doses every 4–6 h.

Neonates
- Under 2 kg and up to 7 days old:
  50,000 U/kg/24 h in equally divided doses every 12 h;
  for meningitis, administer 100,000 U.
- Under 2 kg and over 7 days old:
  75,000 U/kg/24 h in equally divided doses every 8 h;
  for meningitis, administer 150,000 U.
- Over 2 kg and up to 7 days old:
  50,000 U/kg/24 h in equally divided doses every 8 h;
  for meningitis, administer 150,000 U.
- Over 2 kg and over 7 days old:
  100,000 U/kg/24 h in equally divided doses every 6 h;
  for meningitis, administer 200,000 U.

PREPARATION/RECONSTITUTION

Dilute with sterile water for injection; direct flow of water against the sides of the vial while rotating it; shake vigorously. May be added to 0.9% sodium chloride or dextrose solutions.

INCOMPATIBILITIES

Do not mix with other drugs in solution. Incompatible with acid media, alcohol 5% in dextrose, alkaline media, amikacin, aminophylline, amphotericin B, ascorbic acid, cephalothin, chlorpromazine, dextran, dopamine, heparin sodium, lincomycin, metaraminol, oxytetracycline, phenytoin, prochlorperazine, promazine, promethazine, sodium bicarbonate, tetracycline, thiopental, vancomycin, vitamin B complex with C.

RATE/MODE OF ADMINISTRATION

IV push: No.
Intermittent: Applicable; dilute to at least 100,000 U/ml and administer over 20–60 min.
Continuous: Applicable; use electronic flow control device if available.
Filter: Applicable.

NURSING CONSIDERATIONS

Nursing Diagnoses

1. Potential for alteration in body temperature, related to drug side effects.
2. Potential for alteration in comfort, related to action of drug.
3. Potential for fluid volume excess, related to drug side effects.

Acute Care

Stable at room temperature for at least 24 h; contains 1.7 mEq of the salt in 1,000,000 U. Sensitivity studies should be performed to determine susceptibility of causative organisms. Monitor IV site for evidence of impending phlebitis; rotate site carefully to avoid.

Precautions

Adjust dosage downward for those with impaired kidney function. Evaluate renal and hematopoietic systems periodically. Monitor for signs of electrolyte imbalance caused by potassium or sodium content. Avoid prolonged use and subsequent superinfection caused by overgrowth. Optimal pH range is 6–7. Risk of bleeding with anticoagulants is increased. Inactivates aminoglycosides; administer separately.

Contraindications

Known sensitivity to a penicillin.

Side Effects

Neuromuscular: Arthralgia, prostration, convulsions, hyperreflexia.
Cardiovascular: Sodium-induced congestive heart failure, chills, edema, fever, potassium poisoning with coma.
Other: Urticaria, anaphylaxis.

Patient/Caregiver Teaching

Instruct patient (1) to report all side effects immediately; (2) to provide accurate history and drug profile; and (3) to learn principles of home self-administration.

Home Care

Appropriate.

Administration in Other Clinical Settings
Appropriate.

Nursing Interventions
The physician should be notified of all side effects. Discontinue drug and treat symptomatically. Resuscitate as needed.

Pentamidine isethionate
US: Pentam 300

Antiprotozoal agent   pH 5.4

ACTION
Antiprotozoal agent specifically helpful in dealing with *Pneumocystis carinii*. Excreted in the urine; accumulates in renal failure.

INDICATIONS/USES
Used in treatment of *P. carinii* pneumonia. Used investigationally for treatment of trypanosomiasis and visceral leishmaniasis.

USUAL DOSE
4 mg/kg body wt once daily for 14 days.

PREPARATION/RECONSTITUTION
Dilute each 300 mg in 3–5 ml sterile water or 5% dextrose in water for injection. Single dose may be further diluted in 50–250 ml of 5% dextrose in water for infusion purposes.

INCOMPATIBILITIES
Unavailable. Do not mix with any other drug in solution or syringe.

RATE/MODE OF ADMINISTRATION
IV push: No.
Intermittent: Single dose over 60 min.
Continuous: No.
Filter: Applicable.

NURSING CONSIDERATIONS

Nursing Diagnoses

1. Potential for alteration in urinary elimination, related to side effects.
2. Potential for alteration in tissue perfusion, related to side effects.
3. Potential for alteration in cardiac output, related to action of drug.
4. Potential for alteration in nutrition and comfort, related to GI side effects of drug.

Acute Care

Side effects occur in more than half of patients and may be life-threatening. Keep patient in supine position and observe continuously for sign of adverse reaction. Monitor blood pressure continuously during and after infusion. Emergency resuscitative equipment, including full ventilatory support, must be readily available. Monitor blood glucose levels during treatment and several times following completion of same; may cause pancreatic necrosis and high plasma insulin levels. Obtain base line and periodic BUN, CBC, platelet count, alkaline phosphatase, bilirubin, SGOT, SGPT, serum calcium, and ECG. Stable at room temperature for 24 h; discard unused portion of drug.

Precautions

May cause hyperglycemia and diabetes mellitus. Use with caution in those with hyper- or hypotension, hypo- or hyperglycemia, hypocalcemia, leukopenia, thrombocytopenia, anemia, or hepatic or renal dysfunction. Use only if clearly indicated in pregnancy and lactation.

Contraindications

None if diagnosis of *P. carinii* pneumonia is confirmed.

Side Effects

Some side effects occur after treatment has been completed.

Hematologic: Anemia, leukopenia, thrombocytopenia.
Gastrointestinal: Nausea, anorexia, bad taste in mouth.
Cardiovascular: Cardiac dysrhythmias, hyperkalemia, hypocalcemia, hypoglycemia, hypotension.

Other: Rash, phlebitis, neuralgia, fever, elevated serum creatinine and liver function tests, acute renal failure.

Patient/Caregiver Teaching

Instruct patient (1) to report all side effects immediately; (2) to provide accurate medical history and drug profile; and (3) to avoid injury.

Home Care

Not recommended in IV form.

Administration in Other Clinical Settings

Only if emergency equipment for full resuscitation is available.

Nursing Interventions

The physician should be notified of all side effects. Discontinue drug and resuscitate as necessary.

Pentazocine (lactate)

US: Talwin

Narcotic agonist-antagonist   pH 4–5

ACTION

Potent analgesic with onset of action in 2–3 min, lasting about 2 h. Excreted in the urine. Crosses the placental barrier and is secreted in breast milk.

INDICATIONS/USES

Used as relief for moderate to severe pain; preoperative medication; aid in anesthesia; and obstetric analgesia.

USUAL DOSE

5–30 mg; may repeat every 3–4 h as needed; may decrease to 5–15 mg and repeat every 2 h. 360 mg is maximum dose in 24-h period.

PREPARATION/RECONSTITUTION

Administer undiluted; may also dilute each 5 mg with 1 ml sterile water for injection.

INCOMPATIBILITIES

All barbiturates, aminophylline, glycopyrrolate, sodium bicarbonate.

RATE/MODE OF ADMINISTRATION

IV push: 5 mg over 1 min.
Intermittent: No.
Continuous: No.
Filter: Not applicable in less than 1-ml dose.

NURSING CONSIDERATIONS

Nursing Diagnoses

1. Potential for sensory-perceptual alteration: visual, related to drug side effects.
2. Potential for alteration in comfort, related to effect of drug.
3. Potential for activity intolerance, related to sedation.

Acute Care

Monitor patient during injection and thereafter. Emergency resuscitative equipment should be readily available, including oxygen. May provide less effective analgesia in heavy smokers.

Precautions

Use with caution in bronchial asthma, relief of biliary pain, history of drug abuse, myocardial infarction, during delivery of premature infants, renal or hepatic dysfunction, respiratory depression, history of seizures. Use with caution with CNS depressants.

Contraindications

Head injury, hypersensitivity, pathologic brain conditions, increased intracranial pressure, children under 12 yr.

Side Effects

Neurologic: Blurred vision, apprehension, confusion, depression, disorientation, double vision, dreams, floating feeling, hallucinations, insomnia, muscle tremor, nervousness, nystagmus, paresthesias, sedation, seizures, taste alteration.

Cardiovascular: Circulatory depression, facial edema, flushing, hypertension, shock, tachycardia.

Other: Uterine contraction depression, urinary retention, allergic reaction, perspiration, pruritus, respiratory depression.

Patient/Caregiver Teaching

Instruct patient (1) to report all side effects immediately and (2) to provide accurate medical history and drug profile.

Home Care

Not recommended.

Administration in Other Clinical Settings

Only if physician supervision is provided.

Nursing Interventions

The physician should be notified of all side effects. Discontinue the drug and treat side effects symptomatically. Naloxone may reverse respiratory depression or overdose.

Pentobarbital sodium

US: Nembutal sodium

Sedative   pH 9.0–10.5

ACTION

Sedative, hypnotic barbiturate of short duration and CNS depressant. Onset of action is prompt, lasting 3–4 h. Excreted in the urine in changed form. Crosses the placental barrier and is secreted in breast milk.

INDICATIONS/USES

Used to provide preanesthetic sedation; dental and minor surgical sedation; control of convulsive states; sedation in psychoses.

USUAL DOSE
Adults: 100-mg initial dose; after one full minute administer increments of 25–50 mg; maximum dose ranges from 200–500 mg.
Children: Initial dose is 50 mg.

PREPARATION/RECONSTITUTION
Administer undiluted or dilute in sterile water, sodium chloride for injection, or Ringer's injection. Addition of 9 ml diluent to 1 ml pentobarbital provides 5 mg/ml.

INCOMPATIBILITIES
Atropine, benzquinamide, butorphanol, cefazolin, cephalothin, chlordiazepoxide, chlorpheniramine, chlorpromazine, cimetidine, clindamycin, codeine, dimenhydrinate, diphenhydramine, ephedrine, erythromycin, fructose solutions, hydrocortisone sodium succinate, hydroxyzine, insulin, kanamycin, levarterenol, levorphanol, meperidine, methadone, morphine, nalbuphine, opium alkaloids, oxytetracycline, penicillins, pentazocine, phenytoin, prochlorperazine, sodium bicarbonate, streptomycin, succinylcholine, tetracycline, vancomycin.

RATE/MODE OF ADMINISTRATION
IV push: 50 mg over 1 min; titrate to obtain desired effect.
Intermittent: No.
Continuous: No.
Filter: No.

NURSING CONSIDERATIONS
Nursing Diagnoses
1. Potential for ineffective breathing pattern, related to drug side effects.
2. Potential for alteration in comfort, related to drug side effects.

Acute Care
Use only clear solutions. Record blood pressure, pulse, and respirations every 3–5 min. Maintain patent airway. Rapid injection may cause symptoms of overdose. Ensure patency of vein and avoid extravasation and intraarterial injection resulting in gangrene.

Precautions

Treat the cause of a convulsion. Status epilepticus may occur from rapid withdrawal. Use with caution in status asthmaticus, shock, uremia, depressive state following convulsion, severe hepatic disease. Use with caution in presence of other CNS depressants. Inhibits effectiveness of propranolol, corticosteroids, doxycycline, oral anticoagulants, oral contraceptives, theophylline. May increase orthostatic hypotension with furosemide. Monitor phenytoin and barbiturate levels when given concurrently.

Contraindications

History of porphyria, known hypersensitivity, impaired liver function, pregnancy, premature delivery, severe respiratory depression, and delivery (when maximum effect would be at time of delivery only).

Side Effects

Respiratory: Asthma, bronchospasm, neonatal apnea, respiratory depression, cough reflex depression, laryngospasm.
Neurologic: Sluggish or absent reflexes.
Cardiovascular: Facial edema, fever, hypotension, lowered body temperature, pulmonary edema.
Other: Renal shutdown, thrombocytopenic purpura, pain at or below injection site.

Patient/Caregiver Teaching

Instruct patient (1) to report all side effects immediately; (2) to provide accurate medical history and drug profile; and (3) to avoid injury.

Home Care

Not recommended.

Administration in Other Clinical Settings

Only under medical supervision.

Nursing Interventions

The physician should be notified of all side effects immediately. Discontinue drug for pain at or below injection site. Maintain adequate airway with artificial ventilatory support. Maintain body temperature. Administer IV volume expanders and fluids to maintain circulatory status. Hemodialysis or administration of diuretics will promote elimination of the drug. Use vasopressors to maintain blood pressure.

Perphenazine
US: Trilafon

Phenothiazine antiemetic   pH 4.2–5.6

ACTION
Six times more potent than chlorpromazine. Decreases anxiety and tension, relaxes muscle, sedates and tranquilizes. Onset of action is immediate; slowly excreted through the kidneys.

INDICATIONS/USES
Used to control severe vomiting, intractable hiccups, and acute symptoms such as violent retching associated with surgery.

USUAL DOSE
1 mg; repeat as often as needed, allowing 2–3 min between doses; do not exceed 5 mg.

PREPARATION/RECONSTITUTION
Dilute each 5 mg (1 ml) with 9 ml normal saline for injection; 1 ml will equal 0.5 mg. May be further diluted and administered by infusion.

INCOMPATIBILITIES
Aminophylline, opium alkaloids, oxytocin, pentobarbital, secobarbital, thiopental, vitamin B complex.

RATE/MODE OF ADMINISTRATION
IV push: Applicable over 1 min.
Intermittent: Applicable; refer to further dilution guidelines and administer under direction of physician anesthesiologist.

Continuous: No.
Filter: No.

NURSING CONSIDERATIONS
Nursing Diagnoses
1. Potential for injury, related to neurologic side effects.
2. Potential for alteration in comfort, related to side effects.

Acute Care
Administer IV when absolutely necessary only. Use single-dose, 5-mg ampules only. Handle drug with care to avoid contact dermatitis. Keep patient in supine position and monitor blood pressure during and between doses.

Precautions
Drug intolerance is indicated by temperature without etiology. Potentiates CNS depressants. Reduce dosage of any medication potentiated by phenothiazines by a fourth to a half. Use with caution in coronary disease, severe hyper- or hypotension, and epilepsy.

Contraindications
Not recommended for use in children under age 12. Contraindicated with quinidine, epinephrine, and thiazide diuretics.

Side Effects
Neurologic: Blurred vision, dizziness, dysphagia, extrapyramidal symptoms, excitement, slurred speech, spastic movements.
Circulatory: Tachycardia, elevated blood pressure, hypotension, hypersensitivity reaction, cardiac arrest, anaphylaxis.

Patient/Caregiver Teaching
Instruct patient (1) to report all side effects immediately; (2) to remain in supine position; (3) to provide accurate medical history and drug profile.

Home Care
Not applicable.

Administration in Other Clinical Settings
Not applicable.

Nursing Interventions

Discontinue the drug at onset of side effect and notify physician immediately. Hypotension may be counteracted with IV fluids, dopamine, or levarterenol. Epinephrine is contraindicated for hypotension; further hypotension will develop. Phenytoin may help to control ventricular dysrhythmias. Resuscitate as needed.

Phenobarbital sodium

US: Luminal sodium

Sedative   pH 9.2–10.2

ACTION

Sedative, hypnotic barbiturate with potent anticonvulsant effects; CNS depressant. Prompt onset of action; effects last 6–10 h. Excreted in alkaline urine. Crosses the placental barrier and is secreted in breast milk.

INDICATIONS/USES

Used for prolonged sedation and as an anticonvulsant.

USUAL DOSE

Adults: 100–300 mg; may repeat in 6 h. Not to exceed maximum daily dose of 600 mg.

Children: As an anticonvulsant, 20 mg/kg body wt; then 6 mg/kg every 20 min as needed. Not to exceed 40 mg/kg/24 h.

PREPARATION/RECONSTITUTION

Dilute sterile powder with a minimum of 10 ml sterile water for injection. Available as a sterile premixed solution; further dilute up to 10 ml with sterile water for injection.

INCOMPATIBILITIES

Acidic solutions, alcohol 5% in dextrose, aminophylline, benzquinamide, calcium chloride, cephalothin, chlorpromazine, cimetidine, clindamycin, codeine, diphenhydramine, ephedrine, erythromycin, hydralazine, hydrocortisone sodium succinate, hydroxyzine, insulin, kanamycin, levarterenol, levorphanol, meperidine, magnesium sulfate, methadone, morphine, oxytetracycline, pancuronium bromide, penicillin G potassium, pentazocine, phenytoin, prochlorperazine, promazine, sodium bicarbonate, streptomycin, succinylcholine, tetracycline, thiamine, vancomycin, warfarin.

RATE/MODE OF ADMINISTRATION

IV push: 1 gr (65 mg) over 1 min.
Intermittent: No.
Continuous: No.
Filter: No.

NURSING CONSIDERATIONS

Nursing Diagnoses

1. Potential for ineffective breathing pattern, related to drug side effects.
2. Potential for injury, related to delirium and other neurologic side effects.

Acute Care

Solutions prepared from powder must be made fresh. Use only clear solutions. Discard powder or solution exposed to air for 30 min. Rapid injection may cause symptoms of overdose; inject slowly and monitor patient. Use IV only if IM route is not feasible. Monitor patient continuously. Resuscitative equipment should be readily available. Avoid extravasation and resultant thrombosis.

Precautions

Record vital signs hourly or more often if indicated. Maintain patent airway. Treat cause of a convulsion. Use with caution if other CNS depressants have been given. Inhibits effectiveness of propranolol, corticosteroids, doxycycline, oral anticoagulants, oral contraceptives, theophylline. May increase orthostatic hypotension with furosemide. Monitor phenytoin and barbiturate levels when given concurrently.

Contraindications
Impaired renal function, known hypersensitivity, previous addiction, severe respiratory depression, obstruction, cor pulmonale, history of porphyria.

Side Effects
Respiratory: Asthma, bronchospasm, apnea including neonatal apnea, respiratory depression, cough reflex depression, laryngospasm.
Neurologic: Depression, vertigo, coma, delirium, sluggish or absent reflexes, stupor, flat EEG.
Cardiovascular: Facial edema, hypotension, pulmonary edema, lowered body temperature, renal shutdown.
Other: Fever, dermatitis, nausea, thrombocytopenic purpura.

Patient/Caregiver Teaching
Instruct patient (1) to report all side effects immediately and (2) to provide accurate medical history and drug profile.

Home Care
Not recommended.

Administration in Other Clinical Settings
Not recommended.

Nursing Interventions
The physician should be notified of all side effects immediately. Symptomatic and supportive treatment is indicated. Maintain adequacy of airway with artificial means. Keep patient warm. Administer IV volume expanders and fluid to maintain adequate circulation. Hemodialysis or diuretics promote elimination of the drug. Use vasopressors to maintain blood pressure.

Phentolamine mesylate
US: Regitine

Vasodilator   pH 4.5–6.5

ACTION
A vasodilator and α-blocking agent.

INDICATIONS/USES
Used to prevent and treat hypertensive episodes of pheo-chromocytoma preoperatively and throughout surgery. Used for prevention and treatment of necrosis and sloughing associated with extravasation of dopamine and norepinephrine.

USUAL DOSE
Adults: 5 mg 1–2 h preoperatively; may repeat as needed. To prevent necrosis caused by levarterenol, add 10 mg of phentol-amine to each 1000 ml IV solution containing levarterenol.
• Test dose for pheochromocytoma: 2.5–5.0 mg.
Children: 1 mg.

PREPARATION/RECONSTITUTION
Dilute each 5 mg with 1 ml sterile water for injection; may further dilute with 5–10 ml sterile water for injection.

INCOMPATIBILITIES
Iron salts.

RATE/MODE OF ADMINISTRATION
IV push: 5 mg over 1 min; inject test dose rapidly after pressor response to venipuncture has subsided.
Intermittent: No.
Continuous: No.
Filter: No.

NURSING CONSIDERATIONS

Nursing Diagnoses

1. Potential for alteration in nutrition, related to drug side effects.
2. Potential for injury, related to dizziness.

Acute Care

Use only freshly prepared solutions. Ideally, urinary test for VMA should be performed to diagnose pheochromocytoma. Monitor vital signs every 2 min.

Precautions

Use care in presence of dysrhythmia; patient should ideally have normal sinus rhythm. May be used concomitantly with propranolol. Antagonizes effects of epinephrine and ephedrine.

Contraindications

Coronary insufficiency, coronary artery disease, hypersensitivity, myocardial infarction.

Side Effects

Gastrointestinal: Diarrhea, vomiting, nausea.
Cardiovascular: Tachycardia, cerebrovascular occlusion or spasm, tingling of skin, weakness, cardiac dysrhythmias, hypotension, myocardial infarction, shock.
Other: Nasal stuffiness, dizziness.

Patient/Caregiver Teaching

Instruct patient (1) to report all side effects immediately and (2) to provide accurate medical history and drug profile.

Home Care

Not recommended.

Administration in Other Clinical Settings

Not recommended.

Nursing Interventions

The physician should be notified of all side effects. Treat minor effects symptomatically. If side effects increase in severity, discontinue drug and notify physician. Shock caused by hypotension may be reversed with administration of dopamine. Do not use epinephrine. If tachycardia or cardiac dysrhythmias occur, defer use of digitalis preparations until normal sinus rhythm returns if possible.

Phenylephrine hydrochloride

US: Neo-Synephrine

Vasoconstrictor   pH 3.0—5.5

ACTION

A potent, long-lasting vasoconstrictor. Effective within seconds and lasts about 15 min.

INDICATIONS/USES

Used to maintain adequate blood pressure in inhalation and spinal anesthesia, shocklike states, drug-induced hypotension, hypersensitivity reactions. Also used to treat paroxysmal supraventricular tachycardia, to prolong anesthesia, and as an antidote for chlorpromazine-induced hypotension.

USUAL DOSE

0.2 mg; from 0.1—0.5 mg may be used. May repeat every 10—15 min as needed; never exceed 0.5 mg in a single dose.

PREPARATION/RECONSTITUTION

Varies with mode of administration. For direct IV use, dilute each 1 ml with 9 ml sterile water for injection. For infusion, dilute 10 mg in 500 ml dextrose or sodium chloride solution for a 1 : 50,000 solution.

INCOMPATIBILITIES

Alkaline solutions, iron salts, phenytoin.

RATE/MODE OF ADMINISTRATION

IV push: Applicable over 20–30 sec for paroxysmal supraventricular tachycardia; over 60 sec for other clinical situations.
Intermittent: No.
Continuous: Applicable by electronic infusion device.
Filter: Appropriate for continuous infusion.

NURSING CONSIDERATIONS
Nursing Diagnoses

1. Potential for alteration in cardiac output, related to drug action and side effects.
2. Potential for injury, related to vertigo.

Acute Care

Monitor blood pressure every 2 min until stable. Begin with small dose and increase gradually until desired effect is obtained. Discontinue IV administration if infiltration or thrombosis occurs; can cause sloughing and tissue necrosis.

Precautions

May be administered concurrently with blood volume replacement or volume expanders. Use with caution in the elderly, those with partial heart block, hyperthyroidism, bradycardia, myocardial disease, severe arteriosclerosis. Potentiated by halothane anesthetics, tricyclic antidepressants, MAO inhibitors, other vasopressors; hypertensive crisis and death may result. Use with caution with digitalis. Causes bradycardia when used with hydantoins.

Contraindications

Anesthesia with inhalant anesthetics; hypertension; ventricular tachycardia.

Side Effects

Cardiovascular: Bradycardia, hypertension, ventricular extrasystoles, ventricular tachycardia.
Neurologic: Vertigo, fullness of head, tingling of extremities, tremulousness.
Other: Headache.

Patient/Caregiver Teaching
Instruct patient (1) to report all side effects immediately; (2) to provide accurate medical history and drug profile; and (3) to avoid injury.

Home Care
Not recommended.

Administration in Other Clinical Settings
Under medical supervision only.

Nursing Interventions
The physician should be notified of all side effects immediately. To prevent sloughing and necrosis in extravasated areas, inject 5–10 mg phentolamine diluted in 10–15 ml of normal saline with a fine hypodermic needle throughout the extravasated tissue. Hypertension may be reversed with administration of phentolamine. Treat cardiac dysrhythmias symptomatically and resuscitate as needed.

Phenytoin sodium
US: Dilantin sodium
CAN: Dilantin (P.D., (NovoPharm/ LyphoMed)

Anticonvulsant   pH 12

ACTION
An anticonvulsant; metabolized in the liver and excreted in changed form in the urine. Crosses the placental barrier and is secreted in breast milk.

INDICATIONS/USES
Used in control of grand mal and psychomotor seizures; treatment of choice in status epilepticus. Also used to control seizures in

neurosurgery, treatment of supraventricular and ventricular dysrhythmias.

USUAL DOSE

Adults

- Anticonvulsant: 100–250 mg initially; repeat with 100–150 mg in 30 min as needed. Repeat initial dose every 4 h. Or, loading dose of 600–1000 mg in divided doses over 8–12 h; not to exceed total dose of 20 mg/kg body wt.
- Antiarrhythmic: 50–100 mg every 10–15 min; not to exceed total dose of 15 mg/kg.

Children: 250 mg/m² or 10–15 mg/kg in divided doses of 5–10 mg/kg.

Neonates: 15–20 mg/kg in divided doses of 5–10 mg/kg.

PREPARATION/RECONSTITUTION

Use only the diluent provided by manufacturer; add 2.2 ml to 100-mg vial and 5.2 ml to 250-mg vial (1 ml equals 50 mg). Shake to dissolve; may immerse vial in warm water to dissolve powder. Do not add to IV solutions. (Available as 50 mg/ml solution.)

INCOMPATIBILITIES

Any other drug in syringe or solution; precipitates if pH is altered.

RATE/MODE OF ADMINISTRATION

IV push: 50 mg over 1 min as anticonvulsant; 25 mg over 1 min as antiarrhythmic.

Intermittent: Concentrated preparation/reconstitution over 1 h; dilute solutions 1 g in 1 L over 4–8 h. *Note: Studies have indicated use of 0.9% sodium chloride or lactated Ringer's injection prepared immediately prior to use as an infusion; manufacturer does not recommend.*

Continuous: No.

Filter: Applicable.

NURSING CONSIDERATIONS

Nursing Diagnoses

1. Potential for sensory-perceptual alteration, related to drug side effects.

2. Potential for alteration in skin integrity, related to side effects.
3. Potential for alteration in tissue perfusion, related to drug side effects.
4. Potential for ineffective breathing pattern, related to drug side effects.

Acute Care

Use only a clear solution; discard if hazy or if a precipitate forms. May be light yellow in color. Ensure patency of vein and avoid extravasation. Follow each injection with normal saline flush to reduce local venous irritation and to avoid drug interaction. Capable of many catastrophic drug interactions; monitor patient response carefully.

Precautions

Use caution, lower dosage, and slower rate of administration in the following: the elderly, those with renal/hepatic dysfunction, seriously ill patients. Potentiated by amphetamines, analeptics, anticoagulants, antidepressants, antihistamines, benzodiazepines, chloramphenicol, cimetidine, myocardial depressants, phenothiazines, sulfonamides, valproic acid. Inhibited by alcohol, antineoplastics, antituberculosis drugs, barbiturates, folic acid, theophylline. Potentiates CNS depressants, folic acid antagonists, muscle relaxants. Inhibits corticosteroids, digitalis, diuretics, levodopa. Alters some clinical laboratory test results. Concomitant administration of dopamine and other sympathomimetic antihypertensive drugs causes severe hypotension and bradycardia.

Contraindications

Bradycardia; sinoatrial and second- or third-degree heart block; known sensitivity; Stokes-Adams syndrome.

Side Effects

Neurologic: Ataxia, confusion, dizziness, drowsiness, nervousness, nystagmus, tremors, visual disturbances, tonic seizures.
Cardiovascular: Bradycardia, cardiac arrest, heart block, hypotension, ventricular fibrillation.
Other: Respiratory arrest, skin eruptions, hyperplasia of gums, fever.

Patient/Caregiver Teaching

Instruct patient (1) to report all side effects immediately; (2) to provide accurate medical history and drug profile; and (3) to avoid injury.

Home Care

Not recommended for IV use.

Administration in Other Clinical Settings

Only if closely monitored by physician.

Nursing Interventions

The physician should be notified of all side effects immediately. If they progress, discontinue drug and notify physician. Maintain patent airway; resuscitate as needed. Atropine reverses symptoms of heart block or bradycardia. Hemodialysis may be required.

Physostigmine salicylate

US: Antilirium

Parasympathetic stimulator   pH 3.5–5.0

ACTION

Stimulates parasympathetic nerve stimulation; onset of action is 5 min and lasts 1 h.

INDICATIONS/USES

Used to reverse CNS toxic effects caused by anticholinergic drugs including atropine, antispasmodics, and tricyclic antidepressants.

USUAL DOSE

Adults: 0.5–2.0 mg; repeat with 1–4 mg as needed.
- Postanesthesia: 0.5–1.0 mg; repeat at 10–30-min intervals as needed.

Children (for life-threatening situations only): 0.5 mg; repeat at 5–10-min intervals only if toxic effects exist and patient exhibits no sign of cholinergic effects; maximum total dose is 2 mg.

PREPARATION/RECONSTITUTION

Administer undiluted.

INCOMPATIBILITIES

Unknown. Do not mix with any other drug.

RATE/MODE OF ADMINISTRATION

IV push: 1 mg over 1–3 min.
  • Pediatrics: 0.5 mg over 1 min.
Intermittent: No.
Continuous: No.
Filter: No.

NURSING CONSIDERATIONS

Nursing Diagnoses

1. Potential for alteration in cardiac output, related to effects of drug.
2. Potential for injury, related to disorientation.

Acute Care

Avoid rapid IV administration and subsequent bradycardia, hypersalivation, respiratory distress, and convulsions. Have atropine readily available at all times.

Precautions

Potentiates narcotic analgesics. Antagonizes ganglionic blocking agents and aminoglycoside antibiotics. Potentiated by colistimethate.

Contraindications

Asthma, cardiovascular disease, diabetes, gangrene, vagotonic state, mechanical obstruction of intestinal or urinary tracts.

Side Effects

Cardiovascular: Bradycardia.
Neurologic: Anxiety, coma, delirium, disorientation, hallucinations, hyperactivity, seizures.

Other: Cholinergic crisis, coma, emesis, nausea, salivation, sweating.

Patient/Caregiver Teaching

Instruct patient (1) to report all side effects immediately; (2) to provide accurate medical history and drug profile; and (3) that most side effects are reversible.

Home Care

Not recommended.

Administration in Other Clinical Settings

Not recommended.

Nursing Interventions

The physician must be notified of all side effects immediately. Reduce dose to alleviate sweating or nausea. Discontinue medication for excessive defecation, emesis, salivation, urination. Atropine sulfate, 0.5 mg IV, reverses cholinergic crisis or hypersensitivity reaction. Artificial ventilation, oxygen support, monitoring, and suctioning may be needed.

Phytonadione

US: Aquamephyton, vitamin K1

Vitamin   pH 5-7

ACTION

Fat-soluble vitamin essential for production of prothrombin by the liver. Excreted as metabolized in the urine.

INDICATIONS/USES

Used to treat anticoagulant-induced prothrombin deficiency; hemorrhagic disease of the newborn; hypoprothrombinemia resulting from biliary fistula; sprue; ulcerative colitis; celiac disease; intestinal resection; obstructive jaundice; cystic fibrosis of the pancreas; and regional enteritis.

USUAL DOSE

Adults: 2.5–25.0 mg; up to 50 mg may be given.
Neonates: Not administered IV.

PREPARATION/RECONSTITUTION

Dilute with normal saline for injection or 5% dextrose in saline; add 10 ml of diluent.

INCOMPATIBILITIES

Acid pH barbiturates, ascorbic acid, cyanocobalamin, dextran, pentobarbital, phenobarbital, phenytoin, vancomycin.

RATE/MODE OF ADMINISTRATION

IV push: 1 mg over 1 min or longer.
Intermittent: No.
Continuous: No.
Filter: No.

NURSING CONSIDERATIONS

Nursing Diagnoses

1. Potential for ineffective breathing pattern, related to dyspnea.
2. Potential for sensory perceptual alteration: tactile, related to drug side effects.

Acute Care

Dosage and effect are determined by prothrombin levels; keep physician informed. Discontinue other drugs adversely affecting the clotting cascade. Photosensitive; protect from light in all dilutions. IV route is not preferred. Pain and swelling at injection site are possible.

Precautions

Supplement with whole blood transfusion as required. Use smallest dose possible to achieve desired results. Anticoagulation will require larger doses of same or use of heparin sodium. Use with caution in neonates and premature infants; excessive doses may cause hyperbilirubinemia.

Contraindications

Liver disease if response to initial dose is unsatisfactory; hypersensitivity.

Side Effects

Respiratory: Cyanosis, diaphoresis, dyspnea.
Cardiovascular: Hypotension, tachycardia, anaphylaxis, shock, death.
Neurologic: Peculiar taste sensations.

Patient/Caregiver Teaching

Instruct patient (1) to report all side effects immediately; (2) to provide accurate medical history and drug profile; and (3) to avoid injury.

Home Care

Not recommended.

Administration in Other Clinical Settings

Not recommended.

Nursing Interventions

The physician should be notified of all side effects and the drug should be discontinued. Treat allergic reactions as needed.

Piperacillin sodium

US: Pipracil
CAN: Pipracil (Lederle)

Antibiotic   pH 5.5–7.5

ACTION

Extended spectrum penicillin bactericidal against a variety of gram-positive and gram-negative bacteria including aerobic and anaerobic strains. Excreted in bile and urine. Crosses the placental barrier and is secreted in breast milk.

INDICATIONS/USES

Used in treatment of serious lower respiratory tract infections; infections of intraabdominal, urinary tract, gynecologic, skin and skin structure, bone and joint, gonococcal infections, septicemia. Also used to provide perioperative prophylaxis.

USUAL DOSE

3–4 g in equally divided doses every 4, 6, 8, or 24 h; not to exceed 24 g/24 h.

Perioperative prophylaxis: 2–4 g 30–60 min prior to surgery; repeat every 4–6 h for up to 24 h as needed.

PREPARATION/RECONSTITUTION

Reconstitute each gram of medication with 5 ml sterile water or 0.9% sodium chloride for injection. May further dilute as needed in 50–100 ml 5% dextrose in water, 0.9% sodium chloride solution, or other compatible infusate.

INCOMPATIBILITIES

Aminoglycosides, amphotericin B, chloramphenicol, lincomycin, oxytetracycline, polymyxin B, promethazine, tetracycline, vitamin B with C.

RATE/MODE OF ADMINISTRATION

IV push: Applicable over 3–5 min.
Intermittent: Applicable over 30 min; may temporarily discontinue other fluids at same site.
Continuous: No.
Filter: Applicable.

NURSING CONSIDERATIONS

Nursing Diagnoses

1. Potential for injury, related to side effects.
2. Potential for alteration in nutrition: decreased, related to side effects.

Acute Care

Drug is stable at room temperature for 24 h. Used concurrently with aminoglycosides, but must be administered as separate infusions. Sensitivity studies should be performed to determine susceptibility of the causative organisms. Monitor patient for early signs of allergic reaction. Ensure patency of vein and avoid extravasation or intraarterial injection. Slow infusion rate for pain at the venipuncture site.

Precautions

Avoid prolonged use of drug and subsequent superinfection caused by overgrowth. Evaluate renal, hepatic, and hematopoietic systems and serum potassium in prolonged treatment. Drug has a high sodium content; electrolyte imbalance and cardiac irregularities are possible. Usual duration of treatment is 7–10 days; continue for minimum of 2 days following signs of infection. Risk of bleeding with anticoagulants is increased. Inactivated by chloramphenicol, erythromycin, tetracyclines. Concomitant administration of β-adrenergic blockers may increase risk of anaphylaxis.

Contraindications

Known sensitivity to penicillin or cephalosporins.

Side Effects

Neurologic: Convulsions, dizziness, fatigue, muscle relaxation.
Gastrointestinal: Nausea, diarrhea, vomiting.
Hematologic: Neutropenia, thrombocytopenia, thrombophlebitis, leukopenia.
Other: Increased BUN or creatinine, anaphylaxis, pruritus.

Patient/Caregiver Teaching

Instruct patient (1) to report all side effects immediately; (2) to provide accurate medical history and drug profile; and (3) to learn principles of home self-administration.

Home Care

Appropriate.

Administration in Other Clinical Settings

Appropriate.

Nursing Interventions

The physician should be notified of all side effects immediately. In severe cases, discontinue the drug and treat allergic reactions with antihistamines, epinephrine, and corticosteroids as appropriate. Overdose may be reversed with hemodialysis or peritoneal dialysis.

Plasma protein fraction

US: Plasmanate, Plasmatein, Protenate

Volume expander   pH 6.7–7.3

ACTION

Natural plasma protein containing 88% albumin, 7% alpha globulin, and 5% beta globulin. Contains 130–160 mEq sodium/L. Plasma volume expander.

INDICATIONS/USES

Used in emergency treatment of shock caused by burns, surgery, trauma, infection. Used for temporary treatment of hemorrhage when whole blood is unavailable. Used to treat hypoproteinemia until the cause has been determined and corrective action taken.

USUAL DOSE

Adults: Varies according to intended use, clinical condition of patient, and response to treatment. Range is from 250–1500 ml/24 h.
- Shock: 250–1000 ml.
- Burns: 500–1000 ml.
- Hypoproteinemia: 1000–1500 ml/24 h.

Children: 20–30 ml/kg body wt to treat acute shock.

PREPARATION/RECONSTITUTION

Available as a 5% buffered solution in 250- and 500-ml bottles; Plasmanate is also available in 50-ml bottle; no preparation/reconstitution required.

INCOMPATIBILITIES
Alcohol, norepinephrine.

RATE/MODE OF ADMINISTRATION
IV push: No.
Intermittent: No.
Continuous
- With normal blood volume: Infuse at 1 ml/min.
- Treatment of shock and burns in adult patients: 5–8 ml/min.
- Treatment of shock in infants and children: 5–10 ml/min (do not exceed 10 ml/min.
- Treatment of hypoproteinemia: Single 500-ml dose for 1 h.

Filter: Applicable.

NURSING CONSIDERATIONS
Nursing Diagnoses
1. Potential for alteration in nutrition, related to slight occurrence of nausea.
2. Potential for posttrauma response, related to drug action.

Acute Care
Use immediately after opening and discard any unused portion; contains no preservatives. Do not use solution that is turbid or that has a visible sediment. Administer without regard for blood group or typing. Adjust rate to maintain optimum clinical response. Monitor vital signs, urinary output, and central venous pressure every 5–15 min for 1 h and hourly thereafter. Observe patient for evidence of bleeding.

Precautions
Whole blood may be indicated for large RBC loss or anemia caused by large amounts of plasma protein. Dehydrated patients require additional fluids. Monitor hemoglobin, hematocrit, electrolyte, and serum protein before, during, and after therapy. Alkaline phosphatase level may increase as a result of treatment. Use with caution in renal or hepatic dysfunction.

Contraindications
Cardiopulmonary bypass, cardiac failure, normal or increased intravascular volume, severe anemia, history of allergic reactions.

Side Effects

Gastrointestinal: Slight nausea.
Other: Allergic or pyrogenic reactions; hypotension following rapid
administration.

Patient/Caregiver Teaching

Instruct patient (1) to report bleeding episodes and any side effects
immediately; (2) to provide accurate medical history and drug
profile; and (3) to avoid injury.

Home Care

Not generally recommended.

Administration in Other Clinical Settings

Appropriate if monitoring is available.

Nursing Interventions

The physician should be notified of all side effects immediately.
Discontinue infusion for sudden hypotension. Resuscitate as
needed.

Plicamycin

US: Mithracin, mithramycin

Antineoplastic antibiotic   pH 7

ACTION

An antibiotic antineoplastic drug; cytotoxic to HeLa cell tissue
culture and some animal tumors. Produces hypocalcemia in patients with cancer.

INDICATIONS/USES

Used in treatment of testicular tumors unresponsive to surgery or
radiation and hypercalcemia and hypercalciuria associated with
advanced neoplastic disease.

USUAL DOSE

Testicular tumors: 25–30 μg/kg body wt/24 h; repeat daily for 8–10 days if no toxicity; repeat at monthly intervals.

Hypercalcemia and hypercalciuria: 25 μg/kg/24 h for 3–4 days; repeat weekly as needed to maintain normal calcium levels.

PREPARATION/RECONSTITUTION

Follow manufacturer's guidelines for handling cytotoxic agents; refer to Appendix 14 for handling and precautions. Reconstitute each 2.5-mg vial with 4.9 ml sterile water for injection for a concentration of 0.5 mg/min. Dilute single dose in 1000 ml of 5% dextrose in water for infusion.

INCOMPATIBILITIES

Unavailable. Do not mix with any other drug in syringe or solution.

RATE/MODE OF ADMINISTRATION

IV push: No.

Intermittent: No.

Continuous: Single dose over 4–6 h.

Filter: 5 μ required; smaller pore size causes loss of potency.

NURSING CONSIDERATIONS

Nursing Diagnoses

1. Potential for alteration in nutrition, related to drug side effects.

2. Potential for injury, related to immunosuppression.

Acute Care

Refer to Appendix 14 for guidelines on handling biohazardous waste materials. Ensure patency of vein and avoid extravasation and resultant cellulitis and tissue necrosis. Treat extravasated areas with warm moist heat. Store drug in refrigerator prior to use; reconstitute fresh solution daily and discard any unused portion of drug. Dosage is based on average weight in presence of edema or ascites. Maintain hydration and monitor intake and output. Monitor electrolyte balance and bleeding parameters. Observe patient closely for evidence of infection.

Precautions

Use with caution in renal and hepatic dysfunction. Observe patient closely for possible drug interactions. Prophylactic administration of antiemetics will reduce nausea and vomiting associated with this drug.

Contraindications

Thrombocytopenia, thrombocytopathy, impairment of bone marrow function, lack of appropriate laboratory and inpatient facility, coagulation disorders.

Side Effects

Gastrointestinal: Anorexia, diarrhea, nausea, vomiting, stomatitis.
Dermatologic: Skin rash, flushing.
Hematologic: Elevated bleeding/clotting times, hemoglobin depression, leukopenia, decreased platelet count or PT.
Other: Hematemesis; epistaxis; depression of serum calcium, phosphorus, and potassium.

Patient/Caregiver Teaching

Instruct patient (1) to report all side effects including bleeding episodes immediately; (2) to avoid injury; and (3) to avoid use of straight razor.

Home Care

Appropriate only in well-monitored situation by skilled IV nurse.

Administration in Other Clinical Settings

Appropriate only in well-monitored situation by skilled IV nurse.

Nursing Interventions

The physician should be notified of all side effects immediately. Minor side effects are treated symptomatically. Major side effects require discontinuation of drug and notification of physician. Bleeding episodes can be fatal. LA dexamethasone injected into indurated area with a fine hypodermic needle may help extravasation; apply warm heat.

Polymyxin B sulfate

US: Aerosporin

Antibiotic   pH 5.0–7.5

ACTION

Polypeptide antibiotic bactericidal against many gram-negative organisms. Does not pass the blood–brain barrier. Excreted in the urine.

INDICATIONS/USES

Used in treatment of acute infections caused by susceptible gram-negative organisms, including *Pseudomonas aeruginosa*.

USUAL DOSE

Adults: 15,000–25,000 U/kg body wt/24 h; half of total dose every 12 h (normal renal function required); otherwise, decrease dose from 15,000 U/kg/24 h downward.
Infants: With normal renal function, up to 40,000 U/kg/24 h.

PREPARATION/RECONSTITUTION

Dilute each 500,000 U powder with 5 ml sterile water or normal saline for injection. Each single dose should then be diluted in 300–500 ml of 5% dextrose in water.

INCOMPATIBILITIES

Strong acids and alkalies, amphotericin B, ampicillin, cefazolin, cephalothin, chloramphenicol, chlorothiazide, heparin sodium, magnesium sulfate, prednisolone, tetracycline, ions of cobalt, ferrous, magnesium, manganese.

RATE/MODE OF ADMINISTRATION

IV push: No.
Intermittent: Single dose over 60–90 min.
Continuous: No.
Filter: Applicable.

NURSING CONSIDERATIONS
Nursing Diagnoses
1. Potential for ineffective breathing pattern, related to side effects.
2. Potential for alteration in comfort, related to drug action.

Acute Care
Sensitivity studies should be performed prior to use to determine susceptibility of causative organisms. Refrigerate unused medication after initial dilution; discard after 72 h. Monitor urinary output (decreased); drug may need to be discontinued. Obtain baseline serum levels of BUN, creatinine, and creatinine clearance and evaluate throughout therapy. Maintain good hydration. Avoid superinfection caused by overgrowth.

Precautions
Potentiated by anesthetics, other neuromuscular-blocking antibiotics, antineoplastics, barbiturates, muscle relaxants, phenothiazines, promethazine, procainamide, sodium citrate (apnea may occur).

Contraindications
Known sensitivity; pregnancy.

Side Effects
Neurologic: Ataxia, dizziness, flushing, peripheral paresthesias.
Urinary: Oliguria; increased BUN, nonprotein nitrogen, or creatinine; cylindruria; albuminuria; azotemia.
Other: Apnea, thrombophlebitis.

Patient/Caregiver Teaching
Instruct patient (1) to report all side effects immediately; (2) maintain good hydration; and (3) to learn principles of home self-administration.

Home Care
Appropriate following course of treatment as inpatient; must be given under the direction of a highly qualified IV nurse.

Administration in Other Clinical Settings
Appropriate following course of treatment as inpatient; must be given under the direction of a highly qualified IV nurse.

Nursing Interventions
The physician should be notified of all side effects. Dosage may be reduced or an alternative drug administered. Nephrotoxicity is reversible. Maintain airway and ventilatory response.

Potassium chloride and potassium acetate
US: Potassium acetate injection, Potassium chloride injection

Electrolyte   pH 4–8

ACTION
Maintains osmotic pressure and ion balance. Potassium in the cell increases membrane resting potential and decreases membrane permeability.

INDICATIONS/USES
Used in prophylaxis or treatment of potassium deficiency.

USUAL DOSE
20–50 mEq/24 h; up to 400 mEq/24 h may be given with caution. *Note: Maximum concentration in peripheral infusion is 80 mEq/L; in central infusion, it is 240 mEq/250 ml.*

PREPARATION/RECONSTITUTION
Dilute each dose in 500–1000 ml compatible IV solution.

INCOMPATIBILITIES

Amikacin, amphotericin B, dobutamine, IV fat emulsion 10%, mannitol, penicillin G potassium.

RATE/MODE OF ADMINISTRATION

IV push: No.

Intermittent: No.

Continuous: Applicable; maximum of 10 mEq every hour; with serious depletion, 40 mEq/h may be given to the monitored patient.

Filter: Applicable.

NURSING CONSIDERATIONS

Nursing Diagnoses

1. Potential for alteration in cardiac output, related to drug action.
2. Potential for alteration in nutrition: decreased, related to drug side effects.
3. Potential for ineffective breathing pattern, related to side effects.

Acute Care

Use only clear solution. Do not add potassium to a hanging IV container. Remove container from hook and add potassium by sideport; rotate container to thoroughly mix solution and to avoid bolus of potassium being given. Ensure patency of vein and avoid extravasation and resultant necrosis. Ensure adequate kidney function and urinary output. Continuous cardiac monitoring is required for those receiving more than 10 mEq potassium hourly.

Precautions

Potentiated by spironolactone. Digitalis intoxication may occur with hypokalemia; use caution with patients receiving digitalis preparations. Potassium phosphate is preferred for specific intracellular deficiency not caused by alkalosis. Potassium acetate is preferred for patients with renal tubular acidosis.

Contraindications

Hyperkalemia, adrenal cortex insufficiency, impaired renal function, postoperative oliguria, shock with hemolytic reactions or dehydration, patients on digitalis.

Side Effects

Cardiovascular: Bradycardia, cardiac arrest, ECG changes, ventricular fibrillation, death.
Respiratory: Respiratory distress.
Neurologic: Voluntary muscle paralysis.
Other: Dysphagia, weakness.

Patient/Caregiver Teaching

Instruct patient (1) to report all side effects immediately and (2) to provide accurate medical history and drug profile.

Home Care

Only 20–40 mEq/L for hydration purposes.

Administration in Other Clinical Settings

Only 20–40 mEq/L for hydration purposes.

Nursing Interventions

The physician should be notified of all side effects immediately and drug discontinued. Reverse severe hyperkalemia with IV dextrose, 10% to 20%, with 10 U regular insulin for each 50 g dextrose or 150 ml of ⅙ molar sodium lactate solution. Acidosis may be corrected with administration of sodium bicarbonate. Avoid potassium-containing foods and medications. Monitor ECG constantly. Sodium polystyrene sulfonate (Kayexalate) enemas may be needed to remove potassium from the body. Avoid digitalis toxicity by not removing potassium from the cells of digitalized patients too rapidly; use caution. Resuscitate as needed. Treat extravasation with 1% procaine and hyaluronidase using a 27- or 25-gauge needle; apply warm moist compresses.

Prednisolone sodium phosphate

US: Hydeltrasol, Prednisolone Phosphate

Steroid   pH 7–8

ACTION

Adrenocortical steroid with potent antiinflammatory action. Crosses the placental barrier and is secreted in breast milk.

INDICATIONS/USES

Used as supplementary treatment for severe allergic reactions, adrenocortical insufficiency, shock unresponsive to conventional treatment, acute exacerbations of disease for patients receiving steroids, acute life-threatening infections, to induce remission of some malignancies, thyroid crisis, viral hepatitis.

USUAL DOSE

Adults: 4–60 mg/24 h; 10–20 mg every 3–4 h is sometimes given. Total daily dose should not exceed 400 mg/24 h.
Children: Lesser dose required; 40–250 µg/kg body wt once or twice daily.

PREPARATION/RECONSTITUTION

Administer undiluted. Use a separate syringe.

INCOMPATIBILITIES

Calcium gluceptate and gluconate, dimenhydrinate, metaraminol, methotrexate, polymyxin B, prochlorperazine, promazine, promethazine.

RATE/MODE OF ADMINISTRATION

IV push: 10 mg over 1 min.
Intermittent: Applicable in 0.9% sodium chloride solution or 5% dextrose in water; use within 24 h.

Continuous: No.
Filter: Applicable.

NURSING CONSIDERATIONS
Nursing Diagnoses
1. Potential for alteration in tissue perfusion, related to drug action.
2. Potential for alteration in comfort, related to drug side effects.

Acute Care
Administer single daily dose early in morning (9 am) to reduce suppression of patient's own adrenocortical activity. Drug is sensitive to heat. Hypertension and salt and water retention may occur; monitor patient's salt intake carefully. May mask signs of infection. Abrupt withdrawal may lead to fever; wean patient from drug following long-term use. Patient should be observed, especially under stress, for up to 2 yr. Maintain ulcer regime.

Precautions
May increase insulin needs in diabetics. Use with caution when patient is receiving cyclophosphamide; dosage adjustment may be needed. Inhibits anticoagulants and salicylates. Inhibited by some antihistamines, barbiturates, hydantoins. Potentiates theophyllines and cyclosporine. Monitor serum potassium levels to avoid hypokalemia with digitalis products, amphotericin B, or potassium-depleting diuretics.

Contraindications
Absolute: Hypersensitivity to any product containing sulfites; systemic fungal infections.
Relative: Active or latent peptic ulcer, acute psychoses, chickenpox, diabetes, diverticulitis, fresh intestinal anastomoses, hypertension, ocular herpes simplex, osteoporosis, pregnancy, renal insufficiency, thromboembolic disease, vaccinia, myasthenia gravis, active or healed tuberculosis.

Side Effects
Symptoms of Cushing's syndrome, decrease in spermatozoa, euphoria, fat emboli, fluid and electrolyte imbalances, edema, increased intracranial pressure, menstrual irregularities, protein cata-

bolism with negative nitrogen balance, spontaneous fractures, growth suppression.

Patient/Caregiver Teaching

Instruct patient (1) to report all side effects most of which are reversible immediately; (2) to provide accurate medical history and drug profile; and (3) to limit salt intake.

Home Care

Appropriate.

Administration in Other Clinical Settings

Appropriate.

Nursing Interventions

The physician should be notified of all side effects. Treat symptomatically. Resuscitate as needed. Epinephrine should be available.

Procainamide hydrochloride

US: Pronestyl

Antiarrhythmic   pH 4–6

ACTION

Antiarrhythmic action on the heart with onset of action in 2–3 min. Crosses the placental barrier.

INDICATIONS/USES

Used to treat ventricular and supraventricular dysrhythmias such as extrasystoles and tachycardia; atrial fibrillation; paroxysmal atrial tachycardia.

USUAL DOSE

0.2–1 g; 100 mg every 5 min as an infusion until optimal results are obtained. Initial loading dose of 12 mg/kg body wt may also be given. Follow either regimen with infusion of 6 mg/kg every 3 h.

PREPARATION/RECONSTITUTION

Dilute each 100 mg with 10 ml 5% dextrose in water or sterile water for injection for direct injection. For infusion, add 1 g to 250–500 ml of 5% dextrose in water.

INCOMPATIBILITIES

Phenytoin. Physically compatible with many drugs; do not mix, however, because pronestyl dose requires titration to patient's individual needs.

RATE/MODE OF ADMINISTRATION

IV push: 20 mg over 1 min; administer up to 50 mg over 1 min with great caution.
Intermittent: No.
Continuous: Applicable by electronic infusion device at 2–6 mg/min.
Filter: Applicable.

NURSING CONSIDERATIONS

Nursing Diagnoses

1. Potential for alteration in cardiac output, related to drug action.
2. Potential for alteration in comfort, related to drug side effects.

Acute Care

Protect drug from light to avoid photosensitivity reaction. Solution should be clear; may be light yellow. Discard other discolored solutions. Monitor patient's ECG and blood pressure constantly. Maintain patient in supine position. IV route is for emergency use only.

Precautions

Discontinue IV use when cardiac dysrhythmia is interrupted or when ventricular rate slows. Use with extreme caution in first- and second-degree blocks, ventricular tachycardia following a myocardial infarction, digitalis intoxication, renal/hepatic dysfunction. Potentiates or is potentiated by neuromuscular-blocking antibiotics, anticholinergics, antihypertensive agents, muscle relaxants, cimetidine. Use with care when patient is concomitantly taking digitalis, lidocaine, quinidine; dosage may require adjustment. May increase SGOT levels.

Contraindications

Second- and third-degree AV block unless electrical pacemaker is in place, known sensitivity, myasthenia gravis, systemic lupus erythematosus, complete AV heart block.

Side Effects

Gastrointestinal: Anorexia, nausea, vomiting.
Cardiovascular: Chills, fever, flushing, hypotension, prolonged PR interval, QT interval, and widened QRS complex, ventricular asystole, ventricular tachycardia, ventricular fibrillation.
Other: Agranulocytosis, hallucinations, mental confusion, weakness.

Patient/Caregiver Teaching

Instruct patient (1) to report all side effects immediately and (2) to provide accurate medical history and drug profile.

Home Care

Not recommended.

Administration in Other Clinical Settings

Not recommended in IV form.

Nursing Interventions

The physician should be notified of all side effects immediately. For progression of minor symptoms, discontinue drug and notify physician. Dopamine or phenylephrine corrects hypotension. Treatment is symptomatic. Cardiotoxic effects may be relieved by administration of $1/6$ molar sodium lactate injection. Hemodialysis may be needed to increase renal clearance. Resuscitate as needed; equipment should be readily available.

Prochlorperazine edisylate

US: Compazine
CAN: Stemetil (May & Baker)

Antiemetic   pH 4.2–6.2

ACTION

A potent antiemetic with prompt onset of action. Excreted through the kidneys

INDICATIONS/USES

Used to control nausea, vomiting, and hyperexcitability before, during, and after surgery; treatment of withdrawal symptoms from alcohol, narcotics, barbiturates.

USUAL DOSE

5–10 mg; may repeat in 1–2 h as needed.

PREPARATION/RECONSTITUTION

Dilute 5 mg with 9 ml of normal saline for injection; add 10–20 mg to 1 L of isotonic IV solution.

INCOMPATIBILITIES

Aminophylline, amobarbital, amphotericin B, ampicillin, calcium glucentate and gluconate, chloramphenicol, cephalothin, dexamethasone, dimenhydrinate, epinephrine, erythromycin, heparin sodium, hydrocortisone sodium succinate, hydromorphone, kanamycin, methicillin, oxytetracycline, oxytocin, paraldehyde, penicillin G potassium and sodium, pentobarbital, phenobarbital, phenytoin, prednisolone, secobarbital, tetracycline, thiopental, vancomycin. *Note: Do not mix with any other drug in syringe or solution.*

RATE/MODE OF ADMINISTRATION

IV push: 5 mg over 1 min.
Intermittent: No.
Continuous: Applicable, as ordered, by electronic infusion device.
Filter: Applicable.

NURSING CONSIDERATIONS

Nursing Diagnoses

1. Potential for alteration in nutrition, related to drug side effects.
2. Potential for injury, related to side effects.
3. Potential for sensory-perception alteration: visual, related to side effects.

Acute Care

Administer IV only when necessary. Sensitive to light; slight yellow color does not affect potency of medication. Handle with care to avoid contact dermatitis. Keep patient in supine position; monitor blood pressure and vital signs carefully. May discolor urine pink to reddish brown.

Precautions

May mask diagnosis of brain tumor, drug intoxication, intestinal obstruction. Use with caution in severe hyper- or hypotension, epilepsy, coronary disease. Potentiates CNS depressant effects of narcotics and barbiturates. Contraindicated with epinephrine, thiazide diuretics, quinidine.

Contraindications

Bone marrow depression, children under age 2, hypersensitivity, lactation, pregnancy (except labor and delivery), pediatric surgery, comatose states.

Side Effects

Neurologic: Blurring of vision, dizziness, extrapyramidal symptoms, tightness of throat.
Gastrointestinal: Dysphagia.
Circulatory: Tachycardia, hypotension.
Other: Anaphylaxis, convulsions, tongue discoloration and protrusion.

Patient/Caregiver Teaching
Instruct patient (1) to report all side effects immediately, even though most are transient and (2) to provide accurate medical history and drug profile.

Home Care
Not generally given IV in the home.

Administration in Other Clinical Settings
Appropriate.

Nursing Interventions
Discontinue the drug and notify physician of any side effects. Hypotension may be treated with dopamine and IV fluids. Do not use epinephrine; to do so causes additional hypotension. Convulsions or hyperactivity are relieved by diazepam or phenobarbital. Ventricular dysrhythmias should be treated with phenytoin. Avoid analeptics; resuscitate as needed.

Promazine hydrochloride
US: Norazine, Sparine

Antianxiety agent   pH 4.0–5.5

ACTION
A potent antiemetic and antianxiety drug. Excreted slowly through the kidneys.

INDICATIONS/USES
Used to control nausea, vomiting, and hyperexcitability before, during, and after surgery.

USUAL DOSE
25–50 mg; may repeat as needed after 1 h.

PREPARATION/RECONSTITUTION

Administer undiluted in concentration not to exceed 25 mg/ml. May further dilute 25–50 mg with 9 ml normal saline for injection.

INCOMPATIBILITIES

Aminophylline, amobarbital, ampicillin, atropine, chloramphenicol, dimenhydrinate, epinephrine, heparin sodium, hydrocortisone phosphate, hydrocortisone sodium succinate, methicillin, nafcillin, penicillin G potassium and sodium, phenytoin, prednisolone, sodium bicarbonate, thiopental.

RATE/MODE OF ADMINISTRATION

IV push: 25 mg over 1 min.
Intermittent: No.
Continuous: No.
Filter: No.

NURSING CONSIDERATIONS

Nursing Diagnoses

1. Potential for sensory-perceptual alteration: visual, related to drug side effects.
2. Potential for alteration in nutrition, related to side effects.
3. Potential for injury, related to neurologic side effects.

Acute Care

Administer IV only when essential to do so. Ensure patency of vein and avoid extravasation and intraarterial injection. Handle with care to avoid contact dermatitis. Monitor blood pressure and vital signs frequently. Keep patient in supine position. May discolor urine pink to reddish brown.

Precautions

May mask brain tumor, drug intoxication, intestinal obstruction. Use with caution in cerebral arteriosclerosis, coronary heart disease, hyper- or hypotension. Potentiates CNS depressant effects of narcotics, alcohol, barbiturates. Contraindicated with quinidine, epinephrine, thiazide diuretics. Hypotensive effects are prominent.

Contraindications

Bone marrow depression, children under age 12, pregnancy (except labor and delivery), hypersensitivity to pheonothiazines, comatose patients.

Side Effects

Neurologic: Blurring vision, convulsions, dizziness, extrapyramidal symptoms, excitement, slurred speech.
Other: Tachycardia, anaphylaxis, dysphagia, tightness of throat.

Patient/Caregiver Teaching

Instruct patient (1) to report all side effects immediately, even though many are transient and (2) to provide accurate medical history and drug profile.

Home Care

Generally not given in IV form.

Administration in Other Clinical Settings

Appropriate with supervision.

Nursing Interventions

The physician should be notified of all side effects immediately. Treat symptomatically. Dopamine and IV fluids reverse hypotension. Epincphrine is contraindicated. Phenytoin may reverse ventricular dysrhythmias. Resuscitate as needed.

Promethazine hydrochloride

US: Phenergan, Prometh-25, Prothazine, V-Gan25

Antiemetic   pH 4.0–5.5

ACTION

Potent antihistamine, antiemetic, and amnesic. Readily absorbed and excreted in the urine.

INDICATIONS/USES

Used as prophylaxis for minor transfusion reactions, treatment of hypersensitivity reactions, acute nausea, vomiting, motion sickness, surgical and obstetric sedation.

USUAL DOSE

Adults: 12.5–25 mg; repeat in 4–5 h as needed.
Children: 1 mg/kg body wt every 4–6 h; IV rarely used.

PREPARATION/RECONSTITUTION

Do not exceed concentration of 25 mg/ml; dilute each 25–50 mg with 9 ml normal saline for injection.

INCOMPATIBILITIES

Aminophylline, calcium gluconate, carbenicillin, chloramphenicol, chlordiazepoxide, codeine, dextran, dimenhydrinate, heparin sodium, hydrocortisone sodium succinate, methicillin, methylprednisolone, morphine, penicillin G potassium and sodium, pentobarbital, phenobarbital, phenytoin, secobarbital, thiopental.

RATE/MODE OF ADMINISTRATION

IV push: 25 mg over 2 min.
Intermittent: No.
Continuous: No.
Filter: No.

NURSING CONSIDERATIONS

Nursing Diagnoses

1. Potential for sensory-perceptual alteration: visual, related to drug side effects.
2. Potential for injury, related to side effects.

Acute Care

Refrigerate multidose vials or diluted solutions. Sensitive to light; slight yellow color does not alter potency. Handle with care to avoid contact dermatitis. Ensure patency of vein and avoid extravasation and intraarterial injection. Keep patient in supine position. Monitor blood pressure and vital signs frequently.

Precautions

Potentiates CNS depressant effects of narcotics, barbiturates, alcohol, anesthetics. May produce apnea with neuromuscular-blocking antibiotics. Contraindicated with thiazide diuretics, epinephrine, quinidine. Use with caution in the elderly and in children.

Contraindications

Comatose or depressed states, bone marrow suppression, hypersensitivity, lactation, pregnancy.

Side Effects

Neurologic: Blurring of vision, dizziness, hyperexcitability, spastic movement of upper extremities, coma, convulsions.
Cardiovascular: Cardiac arrest, anaphylaxis, hyper- or hypotension.
Other: Respiratory depression, deep sedation.

Patient/Caregiver Teaching

Instruct patient (1) to report all side effects immediately and (2) to provide accurate medical history and drug profile.

Home Care

Not generally used.

Administration in Other Clinical Settings

Appropriate.

Nursing Interventions

The physician should be notified of all side effects. Discontinue the drug and treat symptomatically. Dopamine and IV fluids reverse hypotension. Epinephrine is contraindicated. Treat convulsions or hyperactivity with diazepam or phenobarbital. Avoid analeptics. Resuscitate as needed.

Propranolol hydrochloride

US: Inderal

β-Adrenergic blocker   pH 2.8–3.5

ACTION

A β-adrenergic blocker with antiarrhythmic effects. Onset of action occurs within 1–2 min and lasts 4 h. Metabolized in the liver; some is excreted in the urine.

INDICATIONS/USES

Used in management of life-threatening cardiac dysrhythmias such as paroxysmal atrial tachycardia, sinus tachycardia, atrial or ventricular extrasystoles, atrial flutter and fibrillation, tachyarrhythmias caused by digitalis intoxication, thyrotoxicosis. Used to reduce blood pressure in systolic hypertension caused by hyperdynamic β-adrenergic circulatory state.

USUAL DOSE

0.5–3.0 mg given 1 mg at a time; if no change, repeat cycle. Wait 4 h before further treatment with propranolol if no effect.

PREPARATION/RECONSTITUTION

Dilute each 1 mg in 10 ml 5% dextrose in water for injection; may further dilute in 50 ml 0.9% sodium chloride solution.

INCOMPATIBILITIES
Any other drug in syringe or solution.

RATE/MODE OF ADMINISTRATION
IV push: 1 mg over 1 min.
Intermittent: No.
Continuous: 1 mg over 10–15 min; allow adequate time for circulation; use electronic flow control device to monitor flow.
Filter: Applicable.

NURSING CONSIDERATIONS
Nursing Diagnoses
1. Potential for alteration in cardiac output, related to drug side effects.
2. Potential for sensory-perceptual defect, related to effects of drug.

Acute Care
Patient requires continuous ECG and pulmonary wedge pressure monitoring. Discontinue drug when rhythm change is noted. Use only when clearly indicated. Monitor vital signs constantly.

Precautions
Potentiated by general anesthetics, cimetidine, furosemide, phenothiazines, promethazine, phenytoin, urethane; may result in death. Antagonizes antihistamines, antiinflammatory agents, isoproterenol, ritodrine. Potentiates antidiabetics, barbiturates. Use with caution in diabetics, asthmatics, those with history of hypoglycemia. Concurrent use of epinephrine is contraindicated. Do not use with verapamil; may potentiate both drugs and lead to depression of myocardium. Discontinue drug 48 h prior to surgery.

Contraindications
Bronchial asthma, allergic rhinitis, bronchospasm, cardiogenic shock, complete heart block, congestive heart failure, COPD, hypersensitivity, right ventricular failure, second-degree heart block, sinus bradycardia, and with all hypertensive drugs including diuretics.

Side Effects

Cardiovascular: Bradycardia, cardiac failure, cardiac standstill, hypotension.

Neurologic: Vertigo, visual disturbances, hallucinations, paresthesias of hands, syncope.

Respiratory: Respiratory distress, laryngospasm.

Patient/Caregiver Teaching

Instruct patient (1) to report all side effects immediately and (2) to provide accurate medical history and drug profile.

Home Care

Not recommended.

Administration in Other Clinical Settings

Not recommended.

Nursing Interventions

The physician should be notified of all side effects immediately. Discontinue drug and treat as needed. Atropine reverses bradycardia; digitalis and diuretics reverse cardiac failure. Treat hypotension with epinephrine; treat bronchospasm with aminophylline and isoproterenol. Resuscitate as needed.

Protamine sulfate

Anticoagulant/heparin antagonist   pH 3

ACTION

An anticoagulant if used alone. In presence of heparin, this drug neutralizes the anticoagulant effect of both drugs.

INDICATIONS/USES

Used to neutralize the anticoagulant effect of heparin in overdosage.

USUAL DOSE

1 mg for every 100 USP U of heparin given; may repeat in 10–15 min. Do not exceed 50 mg in any 10-min period.

PREPARATION/RECONSTITUTION

Reconstitute 50 mg of powder with 5 ml sterile bacteriostatic water for injection; shake vigorously. May further dilute with equal volume of 0.9% sodium chloride or 5% dextrose in water.

INCOMPATIBILITIES

Cephalosporins, penicillins. Do not mix with any other drug in syringe or solution.

RATE/MODE OF ADMINISTRATION

IV push: 20 mg at a concentration of 10 mg/ml over 1–3 min.
Intermittent: No.
Continuous: Applicable over 2–3 h by electronic infusion device.
Filter: Applicable.

NURSING CONSIDERATIONS

Nursing Diagnoses

1. Potential for altered cardiac output, related to side effects.
2. Potential for alteration of thermoregulation, related to side effects.

Acute Care

Refrigerate before dilution; use immediately after reconstitution of drug. Discard remaining medication. Administer promptly to minimize dosage requirements.

Precautions

Dosage is adjusted consistent with coagulation profile. Emergency resuscitative equipment should be readily available, including ability to treat shock. Heparin in rebound may occur following cardiac surgery. Potential for hypersensitivity exists in patients with allergies to fish.

Contraindications

None when used as directed.

Side Effects
Respiratory: Dyspnea.
Cardiovascular: Bradycardia, anaphylaxis.
Other: Hyper- or hypotension, feeling of warmth, flushing.

Patient/Caregiver Teaching
Instruct patient (1) to report all side effects immediately and (2) to provide accurate medical history and drug profile.

Home Care
Not recommended.

Administration in Other Clinical Settings
Not recommended.

Nursing Interventions
The physician should be notified of all side effects. Discontinue drug and resuscitate as needed. Vasopressors reverse hypotension; atropine counteracts bradycardia. Administer oxygen and respiratory support.

Quinidine gluconate injection

Antiarrhythmic   pH 5.5–7.0

ACTION
Antiarrhythmic with a vasodilating effect. Onset of action within 15–30 min and lasts 4–6 h. Mostly excreted in the urine.

INDICATIONS/USES
Used in treatment of cardiac dysrhythmias.

USUAL DOSE
200 mg; repeat as indicated; 330 mg or less is effective in most patients.

PREPARATION/RECONSTITUTION

800 mg in at least 40 ml of 5% dextrose for injection; 1 ml equals 16 mg medication.

INCOMPATIBILITIES

All drugs in syringe or solution. Compatible with bretylium, cimetidine, and verapamil through injection port.

RATE/MODE OF ADMINISTRATION

IV push: No.
Intermittent: No.
Continuous: 1 ml/min by electronic infusion device.
Filter: Appropriate.

NURSING CONSIDERATIONS

Nursing Diagnoses

1. Potential for alteration in cardiac output, related to drug action.
2. Potential for alteration in skin integrity, related to side effects.
3. Potential for alteration in nutrition, related to side effects.
4. Potential for alteration in sensory perception, related to drug side effects.

Acute Care

Requires constant monitoring of blood pressure and ECG. Rapid administration may cause significant drop in arterial pressure. Keep patient in supine position. IV route is not preferred.

Precautions

Use with caution in second- and third-degree blocks, extensive myocardial infarction, liver or hepatic dysfunction, digitalis intoxication. Use with caution in atrial flutter or fibrillation. Test dose of 200 mg IM for idiosyncrasy desired if time permits. Potentiates or is potentiated by neuromuscular-blocking antibiotics, anticholinergics, thiazide diuretics, cimetidine, antihypertensive drugs, muscle relaxants, phenothiazine, anticoagulants, reserpine, urinary alkalizers. Serious cardiac results may occur. May cause increase in urine catecholamines or PT and positive Coombs' test. May cause hypertension (severe) with verapamil in patients with existing hypertrophic cardiomyopathy. Use with caution in the digitalized patient; lower dose of both drugs may be required. Use with caution with procainamide and propranolol; dosage adjustment may be required.

Contraindications

Aberrant impulses and abnormal rhythms due to escape mechanism; known hypersensitivity; lactation; myasthenia gravis; history of thrombocytopenic purpura with quinidine administration; partial AV or complete heart block.

Side Effects

Gastrointestinal: Cramps, nausea, urge to defecate, urge to void, vomiting.
Cardiovascular: Apprehension, AV heart block, cardiac standstill, acute hypotension, prolonged PR or QT intervals, 50% widening of QRS complex, ventricular fibrillation, tachycardia.
Other: Urticaria, diaphoresis, rash, tinnitus, visual disturbances.

Patient/Caregiver Teaching

Instruct patient (1) to report all side effects immediately and (2) to provide accurate medical history and drug profile.

Home Care

Not recommended in IV form.

Administration in Other Clinical Settings

Not recommended in IV form.

Nursing Interventions

The physician should be notified of all side effects immediately. If minor symptoms progress, notify physician and discontinue infusion. Dopamine, metaraminol, or angiotensin corrects hypotension; ¹/₆ molar sodium lactate blocks effects of quinidine on the myocardium. Hemodialysis may be needed. Do not administer any CNS depressants in overdose. Resuscitate as needed; emergency equipment should be readily available.

Ranitidine

US: Zantac

Histamine antagonist   pH 6.7–7.3

ACTION

A histamine hydrogen antagonist that inhibits secretion of gastric acid stimulated by food, histamine, bentazole, and pentagastrin, as well as daytime and nocturnal basal secretion. Excreted in the urine. Crosses the placental barrier and is secreted in breast milk.

INDICATIONS/USES

Used for short-term treatment of intractable duodenal ulcers and pathologic hypersecretory conditions in hospitalized patients.

USUAL DOSE

50 mg every 6–8 h; increase frequency, rather than amount of drug, if needed. Not to exceed 400 mg/day.
- Prevention of pulmonary aspiration during anesthesia. 50 mg 60–90 min prior to induction.

PREPARATION/RECONSTITUTION

Add 50 mg to 20 ml normal saline or other compatible solution for direct injection; for infusion purposes, add 50 mg to 50–100 ml of 5% dextrose in water or other small-volume parenteral.

INCOMPATIBILITIES

Unknown. May be incompatible with aminophylline, amphotericin C, barbiturates, cefamandole, cefazolin, cephalothin.

RATE/MODE OF ADMINISTRATION

IV push: 50 mg over 5 min.
Intermittent: Each 50-mg dose over 15–20 min.
Continuous: No.
Filter: Applicable.

NURSING CONSIDERATIONS

Nursing Diagnoses

1. Potential for alteration in comfort, related to side effects of drug.
2. Potential for alteration in nutrition: decreased, related to side effects.

Acute Care

Rapid administration may precipitate bradycardia, tachycardia, PVCs. Administer as ordered. Inspect solution for color and clarity; slight darkening does not affect potency. Stable at room temperature for 48 h after dilution. May be added to nutritional support formulas; consult with pharmacist regarding compatibility.

Precautions

Concomitant use of antacids will relieve pain. May potentiate warfarin-type anticoagulants; monitor bleeding parameters carefully. In renal impairment, increase intervals between injections to achieve pain relief with less frequent dosage. Use with caution in those with hepatic dysfunction. Potentiates effects of procainamide, sulfonylureas. May inhibit theophyllines. Monitor SGPT if therapy exceeds 400 mg for over 5 days.

Contraindications

Known hypersensitivity.

Side Effects

Gastrointestinal: Abdominal discomfort, constipation, diarrhea, nausea, vomiting.
Neurologic: Headache, agitation, arthralgias, confusion, depression, dizziness, hallucinations, insomnia, somnolence, vertigo.
Cardiovascular: Tachycardia, PVCs, bradycardia.
Other: Bronchospasm, fever, rash, eosinophilia, malaise, hepatitis (reversible).

Patient/Caregiver Teaching

Instruct patient (1) to report all side effects immediately; (2) to avoid injury; and (3) to provide accurate medical history and drug profile.

Home Care
Appropriate.

Administration in Other Clinical Settings
Appropriate.

Nursing Interventions
The physician should be notified of all side effects immediately. Treat symptomatically; hemodialysis or peritoneal dialysis may be indicated in overdose.

Ritodrine hydrochloride
US: Yutopar

β-Adrenergic stimulator   pH 4.8–5.5

ACTION
Inhibits contractility of uterine smooth muscle. Onset prompt, lasting for 2 h. Crosses the placental barrier and is excreted in the urine.

INDICATIONS/USES
Used to arrest preterm labor; temporarily prevents labor during preparation for operative delivery.

USUAL DOSE
0.1 mg/min initially; increase by 0.05 mg/min every 10 min until effect obtained. Continue for 12 h following cessation of contractions; then begin oral medication. Administer first dose of oral medication 30 min before discontinuing the IV.

PREPARATION/RECONSTITUTION
Dilute 150 mg with 500 ml 5% dextrose in water; may use alternative solutions such as 0.9% sodium chloride, Ringer's, or Hartmann's only when dextrose is contraindicated.

INCOMPATIBILITIES
Consider incompatible with any other drug in syringe or solution.

RATE/MODE OF ADMINISTRATION
IV push: No.
Intermittent: No.
Continuous: Applicable by electronic infusion device.
Filter: Applicable.

NURSING CONSIDERATIONS
Nursing Diagnoses
1. Potential for altered cardiac output, related to side effects.
2. Potential for alteration in comfort, related to side effects.

Acute Care
Do not use solution if discolored or contains particulate matter or precipitate; discard solution after 48 h. Obtain maternal baseline ECG to rule out heart disease; monitor uterine contractions, maternal pulse rate, fetal heart rate, blood pressure. Maintain adequate hydration, but avoid fluid overload. Maintain patient in left lateral position during infusion to avoid hypotension.

Precautions
Use with caution if indicated in maternal mild to moderate pre-eclampsia, hypertension, diabetes. Evaluate fetal maturity with ultrasound. Monitor maternal hyperglycemia and treat as needed; may precipitate hypoglycemia in the fetus. Monitor insulin, glucose, and electrolyte levels in patients receiving long-term treatment. Concomitant administration of corticosteroids will precipitate pulmonary edema. Inhibited by β-adrenergic blockers. Potentiated by sympathomimetic amines; do not administer concurrently. Cardiovascular effects are potentiated by concomitant administration of diazoxide, magnesium sulfate, meperidine, general anesthetics. Atropine administered concomitantly may lead to increased hypertension. Allergic reactions intensified with administration of sulfites.

Contraindications
Prior to 20th week of pregnancy, antepartum hemorrhage, cardiac disease, chorioamnionitis, uncontrolled diabetes mellitus, hyper-

thyroidism, hypersensitivity, eclampsia, pulmonary hypertension, hypovolemia, pheochromocytoma, intrauterine fetal death.

Side Effects

Cardiovascular: Chest pain, dysrhythmias, decreased diastolic pressure, elevated systolic pressure, hyperventilation, palpitations, pulmonary edema, widened pulse pressure, tachycardia, tightness of chest.

Neurologic: Anxiety, headache, jitteriness, nervousness, restlessness, tremor.

Other: Vomiting, ileus, glycosuria, erythema, anaphylaxis, constipation, epigastric distress.

Patient/Caregiver Teaching

Instruct patient (1) to report all side effects immediately; (2) to provide accurate medical history and drug profile; and (3) to monitor intake.

Home Care

Not recommended.

Administration in Other Clinical Settings

Not recommended.

Nursing Interventions

The physician should be notified of all side effects immediately. Most may be treated symptomatically. Discontinue drug for marked hypotension, tachycardia, cardiac dysrhythmias, other signs of β-adrenergic stimulation. At first signs of fluid overload and impending pulmonary edema, notify physician and treat as ordered.

Sodium acid carbonate

See Sodium bicarbonate.

Sodium bicarbonate

Alkalizing agent   pH 7–8

ACTION

Alkalizing agent and sodium salt used to maintain osmotic pressure and ion balance; 1% excreted in the urine.

INDICATIONS/USES

Used to correct metabolic acidosis with blood pH below 7.25 caused by circulatory insufficiency (from shock or dehydration), severe renal disease, cardiac arrest, salicylate intoxication, and uncontrolled diabetes with ketoacidosis. Used to treat hyperkalemia and hyponatremia and to relieve bronchospasm in status asthmaticus.

USUAL DOSE

Adjusted according to pH, $PaCO_2$, calculated base deficit, clinical response, fluid limitations. Correction to carbon dioxide level of 20 mEq/L within 24 h usually results in normal pH if cause of acidosis is under control and if kidney function is normal.

PREPARATION/RECONSTITUTION

May be given in prepared solution forms: 4.2% sodium bicarbonate solution (5 mEq/10 ml); 5% solution (297.5 mEq/500 ml); 7.5% solution (44.5 mEq/50 ml); 8.4% solution (50 mEq/50 ml); neut (4% sodium bicarbonate solution with 2.4 mEq/5 ml). The 7.5% and 8.4% solutions should be diluted with equal amounts of water for injection or compatible IV solution; 4.2% solution is preferred for infants and small children.

INCOMPATIBILITIES

5% alcohol with 5% dextrose, amino acids, atropine, calcium chloride and gluconate, carmustine, cefotaxime, chlorpromazine, cisplatin, codeine, corticotropin, dextrose solutions, dobutamine, dopamine, epinephrine, hydromorphone, insulin, ionosol solutions, isoproterenol, lactated Ringer's solution, levarterenol, levophanol, lincomycin, magnesium sulfate, meperidine, methadone, methicillin, metoclopramide, morphine, oxytetracycline, tetracycline, penicillin G potassium, pentobarbital, phenobarbital, procaine, promazine, Ringer's injection, secobarbital, sodium lactate injection, streptomycin, succinylcholine, thiopental, tubocurarine, vancomycin.

RATE/MODE OF ADMINISTRATION

IV push: Up to 1 mEq/kg body wt over 1–3 min in cardiac arrest; repeat half dose in 10 min if indicated by $PaCO_2$ and blood pH.

Intermittent: No.

Continuous: 2–5 mEq/kg over 4–8 h; not to exceed 50 mEq/h. Decreased rate for children and neonates.

Filter: Applicable.

NURSING CONSIDERATIONS

Nursing Diagnoses

1. Potential for impaired gas exchange, related to action of drug.
2. Potential for alteration in comfort, related to drug side effects.

Acute Care

Confirm patency of vein and avoid extravasation resulting in chemical cellulitis, necrosis, sloughing. Flush IV line before and after administration to avoid incompatibilities. Use clear solutions only. Obtain blood pH, PaO_2, $PaCO_2$, PO_2, PCO_2, and electrolyte levels before treatment and several times daily during treatment. Notify physician of all results. Rapid doses or rate in excess of 8 mEq/kg/24 h may cause intracranial hemorrhage. Use only 50-ml ampules in cardiac arrest; smaller doses of 0.5 mEq/kg may be appropriate to arrest and prevent secondary alkalosis.

Precautions

Potentiates amphetamines, ephedrine, quinidine. Inhibits tetracyclines. Rapid or excessive administration may result in alkalosis, hypokalemia, hypocalcemia; cardiac dysrhythmias may result from intracellular shift of potassium. Monitor patient's response to treatment carefully.

Contraindications

Hypertension, hypocalcemia, hypochloremia, impaired renal function, edema, metabolic alkalosis, respiratory alkalosis, respiratory acidosis.

Side Effects

Neurologic: Hyperexcitability, tetany, headache.
Cardiovascular: Congestive heart failure.
Gastrointestinal: Distention, flatulence, nausea, vomiting, cramps.
Metabolic: Alkalosis, hypokalemia.
Respiratory: Respiratory depression.

Patient/Caregiver Teaching

Instruct patient (1) to report all side effects immediately; (2) to provide accurate medical history and drug profile; and (3) not to take over-the-counter drugs unless physician prescribed.

Home Care

Not recommended.

Administration in Other Clinical Settings

Not usually administered.

Nursing Interventions

The physician should be notified of all side effects. Discontinue the medication; sodium and potassium chloride must be supplemented. Administer balanced hypotonic electrolyte solution with sodium and potassium chloride to help excrete bicarbonate ion in the urine. Ammonium chloride may be administered. Treat extravasation of IV site with injection of lidocaine hydrochloride or hyaluronidase using 27- or 25-gauge needle. Raise extremity and apply warm moist compress. Resuscitate as needed; equipment should be readily available.

Sodium nitroprusside
US: Nipride

Antihypertensive   pH 3.5–6.0

ACTION
A rapid-acting antihypertensive agent; effectiveness ends when infusion is stopped. Blood pressure returns to pretreatment levels within 1–10 min. Converted to thiocyanate and excreted in the urine.

INDICATIONS/USES
Used as drug of choice for hypertensive emergency, cardiogenic shock, controlled hypotension during anesthesia.

USUAL DOSE
Adults: 3 μg/kg body wt/min; reduce to 0.5 μg/kg/min in those receiving other antihypertensive medications. Do not exceed 10 μg/kg/min. If desired effect is not obtained with 10 μg/kg/min dosage, discontinue and use alternative agent.
Children: 1.4 μg/kg/min, adjusted to individual response.

PREPARATION/RECONSTITUTION
Dilute 50 mg with 2–3 ml of 5% dextrose in water; further dilute in minimum of 250 ml of 5% dextrose in water.

RATE/MODE OF ADMINISTRATION
IV push: No.
Intermittent: No.
Continuous: Applicable by electronic infusion device; use only 5% dextrose in water as diluent.
Filter: Applicable.

NURSING CONSIDERATIONS
Nursing Diagnoses
1. Potential for alteration in comfort, related to drug side effects.

2. Potential for alteration in cardiac tissue perfusion, related to effects of drug.

Acute Care

Immediately after mixing, wrap infusion bottle in aluminum foil to protect from light. Use only freshly prepared solutions and follow manufacturer's recommendations for maximum hang time of solution (between 4–24 h). Solution should be slightly brown; discard if colored blue, green, or dark red. Avoid extravasation. Monitor IV site carefully.

Precautions

Check blood pressure every minute until desired level is obtained and every 5–15 min thereafter; continuous monitoring is ideal. Do not allow systolic blood pressure to fall below 60 mmHg. Patient with myocardial infarction or congestive heart failure should have pulmonary wedge pressure monitored. Use with caution in hypothyroidism, hepatic or renal dysfunction, the elderly. For long-term use, monitor blood thiocyanate levels daily (not to exceed 10 mg/100 ml). Potentiated by ganglionic blocking agents, liquid anesthesia, circulatory depressants.

Contraindications

Known inadequate cerebral circulation; emergency surgery on moribund patients; compensatory hypertension.

Side Effects

Gastrointestinal: Abdominal pain, nausea.
Respiratory: Dyspnea, diaphoresis.
Cardiovascular: Palpitations, profound hypotension, restlessness, retrosternal discomfort.
Other: Headache, coma, muscle twitching.

Patient/Caregiver Teaching

Instruct patient (1) to report all side effects immediately; (2) to provide accurate medical history and drug profile; and (3) to be aware that most side effects are reversible.

Home Care

Not recommended.

Administration in Other Clinical Settings
Not recommended.

Nursing Interventions
Decrease rate of administration at first sign of side effects. Notify the physician if patient's blood pressure begins to rise or if side effects continue. Thiocyanate levels over 10 mg/100 ml may be reversed with hemodialysis or peritoneal dialysis. If dose must be discontinued, administer amyl nitrite inhalations for 15–30 sec each minute until 3% sodium nitrite solution can be given by IV drip. Administer 2.5–5.0 ml/min of 3% sodium nitrite solution to a total dose of 10–15 ml. Monitor blood pressure and inject 12.5 g sodium thiosulfate in 50 ml of 5% dextrose in water IV over 10 min.

Streptokinase
US: Kabikinase, Streptase

Fibrinolytic agent   pH 6.8

ACTION
Combines with plasminogen and converts it to plasmin, which degrades fibrin clots, fibrinogen, and other plasma proteins. Onset of action prompt, lasting 12–24 h.

INDICATIONS/USES
Used to lyse coronary artery thrombi, acute massive pulmonary emboli involving one or more lobes and unstable hemodynamics, equivalent amount of thrombi in other deep veins, acute arterial thrombi and arterial emboli. Used to clear occluded catheters.

USUAL DOSE
Deep vein thrombosis, pulmonary or arterial embolism, arterial thrombosis
- Loading dose: 250,000 IU.
- Maintenance dose: 100,000 IU/h for 24–72 h.

Arteriovenous cannula occlusion: 250,000 IU into each occluded limb of cannula.

Coronary artery thrombi: 1,500,000 IU direct IV within 6 h of onset of symptoms; or 750,000 direct IV within 3 h of onset of symptoms, followed with 250,000 IU in 30–60 min; or 20,000 IU directly into the coronary artery within 6 h of onset of symptoms, followed with 2,000 IU/min for 60 min.

PREPARATION/RECONSTITUTION

Prepare as follows except for cannula occlusion and direct IV. Reconstitute each vial with 5 ml normal saline for injection or 5% dextrose for injection; add diluent slowly, directing it toward sides of vial; roll and tilt gently to reconstitute. Avoid shaking which may cause foaming. Further slowly dilute each vial to total volume of 45 ml; may be diluted to maximum of 500 ml in 45-ml increments. Discard solution with large amounts of flocculation or solution remaining after 24 h.

Direct IV: Dilute with 5 ml normal saline; further dilute 750,000-IU dose in 50 ml normal saline or 5% dextrose in water. Further dilute 1,500,000-IU dose in 100 ml or more of normal saline or 5% dextrose in water.

Arteriovenous cannula occlusion: Dilute each vial of 250,000 IU with 2 ml sodium chloride for injection. Clamp off limb for 2 h; after treatment, aspirate contents of infused cannula limb, flush saline, and reconnect cannula.

INCOMPATIBILITIES

Consider incompatible with all drugs in syringe or solution.

RATE/MODE OF ADMINISTRATION

IV push

- Coronary artery thrombi: 750,000 IU over 5–10 min; 1,500,000 IU over 60 min.
- Deep vein thrombosis, pulmonary arterial embolism, arterial thrombi: Single dose over 25–30 min.

Intermittent: For clearance of occluded cannula.
Continuous: Applicable by electronic infusion device.
Filter: Use 0.8-μ range.

NURSING CONSIDERATIONS

Nursing Diagnoses

1. Potential for alteration in fluid volume, related to bleeding.
2. Potential for hyperthermia, related to side effects.
3. Potential for injury, related to hypotension.

Acute Care

Refrigerate after initial dilution. Administered only in inpatient environment under direction of a highly qualified physician. Observe patient constantly. Monitor baseline bleeding parameters, vital signs, hemodynamic status. Monitor thrombin time or PT changes in 4 h to determine effectiveness of treatment. Obtain baseline CPK prior to direct IV use. Administer diphenhydramine, 50 mg IV prophylactically as needed. Monitor ECG every 15 min for 4 h. Avoid arterial punctures, venipunctures, and IM injections in this patient. Apply pressure when discontinuing arterial or intravenous infusions.

Precautions

Diagnosis of acute myocardial infarction must be confirmed and site of coronary thrombosis confirmed with selective angiography prior to use of coronary catheter procedure. Concurrent heparin therapy may be needed. Best results are obtained if started within 7 days of onset of emboli. Discontinue drug if PT or other parameters are not above 1.5 times control in 4 h. Do not abruptly reduce or stop treatment. Use with caution in atrial fibrillation; monitor for dysrhythmias during therapy. Avoid use of drugs that may alter platelet function. Avoid blood pressures in lower extremities. Attempt to clear occluded catheters with syringe technique and saline before using this drug. Use caution in the following procedures/conditions: surgical, biopsy, lumbar puncture, thoracentesis, paracentesis, multiple cutdowns, ulcerative wounds, recent trauma, pregnancy, first 10 days postpartum, GI or GU lesion, severe hypertension, hepatic or renal dysfunction, chronic lung disease, hypocoagulable state, subacute bacterial endocarditis, rheumatic valvular disease, obstetric delivery, previous puncture of noncompressible vessels, cerebrovascular disease, diabetic hemorrhagic retinopathy, septic thrombophlebitis.

Contraindications

Active internal bleeding, cerebrovascular accident within past 2 mo, intracranial or intraspinal surgery, hypersensitivity, intracranial neoplasm.

Side Effects

General: Hypersensitivity, anaphylaxis, fever, bleeding.

Patient/Caregiver Teaching

Instruct patient (1) to report all side effects immediately; (2) to avoid use of straight razor; (3) to provide accurate medical history and drug profile; and (4) to avoid injury.

Home Care

Not recommended.

Administration in Other Clinical Settings

Not recommended.

Nursing Interventions

The physician should be notified of all side effects immediately. Treatment may have to be discontinued at sign of bleeding not controlled by local pressure. Whole blood, packed RBC, cryoprecipitate, fresh frozen plasma, and aminocaproic acid may be required. Do not use dextran. Resuscitate as needed. Treat minor allergic reactions symptomatically.

Streptozocin

US: Zanosar

Antineoplastic   pH 3.5–4.5

ACTION

Alkylating agent related to nitrogen mustard with antitumor activity, cell-cycle-phase nonspecific; 20% excreted in the urine.

INDICATIONS/USES

Used to suppress or retard neoplastic growth of metastatic pancreatic islet cell carcinomas. Renal toxicity is dose limiting.

USUAL DOSE

500 mg/m^2 for 5 consecutive days; repeat every 5 wk until maximum benefit or limiting toxicity is observed. Alternatively give 1000 mg/m^2/wk for 2 doses; increase to 1500 mg/m^2 to achieve therapeutic response in absence of toxicities. Overall cumulative dose to onset of response is 2000 mg/m^2; usually maximum response is achieved with 4000 mg/m^2 cumulative dose.

PREPARATION/RECONSTITUTION

Refer to Appendix 14; specific precautions needed to avoid contamination with biohazardous waste materials; use caution in handling this drug or related materials. Reconstitute each gram with 9.5 ml 0.9% sodium chloride or dextrose for injection. May further dilute in 50–250 ml solution if desired.

INCOMPATIBILITIES

Do not mix with any other drug in syringe or solution.

RATE/MODE OF ADMINISTRATION

IV push: Single dose over 5–15 min.
Intermittent: No.
Continuous: Applicable by electronic infusion device.
Filter: Applicable.

NURSING CONSIDERATIONS

Nursing Diagnoses

1. Potential for fluid volume deficit, related to drug side effects.
2. Potential for injury, related to immunosuppression.

Acute Care

Follow guidelines for handling of cytotoxic agents and avoid exposure to skin. Renal toxicity is dose related and can prove to be fatal. Monitor renal function before, weekly during, and for 4 wk after each course of treatment. Store in refrigerator before and after reconstitution; discard within 12 h of dilution (contains no preservatives). Protect from light. Maintain hydration; nausea and vomiting are severe. Observe patient for signs of infection.

Precautions

Monitor CBC and liver function tests weekly. This drug may be administered with other antineoplastic agents in reduced doses to achieve remission. Produces teratogenic effects on fetus; has mutagenic potential. Discontinue breast-feeding.

Contraindications

Hypersensitivity, impaired liver or renal function.

Side Effects

Hematologic: Anemia, thrombocytopenia, leukopenia, decreased platelet count.

Gastrointestinal: Diarrhea, nausea, severe vomiting.

Other: Elevated SGOT and LDH, hepatic toxicity, hypoalbuminemia, hypoglycemia, insulin shock, proteinuria.

Patient/Caregiver Teaching

Instruct patient (1) to report all side effects immediately; (2) to provide accurate medical history and drug profile; and (3) to maintain hydration.

Home Care

May be administered by a highly qualified IV nurse in the home setting under the direction of a physician specialist.

Administration in Other Clinical Settings

May be administered by a highly qualified IV nurse under the direction of a physician specialist.

Nursing Interventions

The physician should be notified of all side effects immediately. May need to reduce dose or discontinue drug for renal toxicity, hematologic changes, nausea, and vomiting.

Succinylcholine chloride

US: Anectine, Quelicin, Sucostrin

Skeletal muscle relaxant   pH 3.0–4.5

ACTION

Skeletal muscle relaxant with onset of action within 1–2 min and lasting 5 min. Complete recovery in about 10 min. Crosses placental barrier.

INDICATIONS/USES

Used to provide skeletal muscle relaxation during operative and manipulative procedures; facilitates management of those undergoing mechanical ventilation.

USUAL DOSE

Adults: 0.3–1.1 mg/kg body wt as initial dose; maintain with 0.04–0.07 mg/kg at appropriate intervals. Use caution: 1 mg/kg is sufficient to cause respiratory paralysis; never exceed 150 mg total dose. Test dose of 0.1 mg may be used.

Children: 2 mg/kg for infants and small children; 1 mg/kg for older children and adolescents.

PREPARATION/RECONSTITUTION

Administer undiluted for short-term muscle relaxation. For infusion, add 1 g to 1 L 5% dextrose in water or isotonic saline.

INCOMPATIBILITIES

Alkaline solutions, barbiturates, amobarbital, pentobarbital, phenobarbital, secobarbital, thiopental, chlorpromazine, nafcillin.

RATE/MODE OF ADMINISTRATION

IV push: Single dose over 30 sec.

Intermittent: Applicable; not to exceed 10 mg/min.

Continuous: Applicable; not to exceed 10 mg/min; use electronic infusion device.

Filter: Not applicable.

NURSING CONSIDERATIONS
Nursing Diagnoses
1. Potential for irregular breathing pattern, related to drug action.
2. Potential for altered cardiac output, related to side effects.

Acute Care
Used under the direction of an anesthesiologist. Produces apnea; artificial respiratory support must be readily available. Use freshly prepared solutions; store in refrigerator. Multidose vial is stable at room temperature for 14 days only. Powder may be stored at room temperature prior to reconstitution. Administer after patient is unconscious to reduce patient discomfort.

Precautions
Use with caution in tissue trauma, fractures, burns, nerve damage, paralysis; hyperkalemia may cause cardiac dysrhythmias. Use with caution in anemia; cardiovascular, hepatic, pulmonary, metabolic, and renal disorders; malnutrition; pregnancy. Observe for early signs of malignant hyperthermic crisis (lack of laryngeal relaxation, rigidity). Potentiated by neuromuscular-blocking antibiotics, β-adrenergic blocking agents, organic phosphate compounds, cimetidine, cyclophosphamide, lidocaine, quinidine, magnesium salts. Inhibited by prior administration of diazepam.

Contraindications
Hypersensitivity, family history of malignant hyperthermia, myopathies associated with elevated CPK values, penetrating eye injuries, acute narrow-angle glaucoma, genetic disorders.

Side Effects
Cardiovascular: Bradycardia, cardiac dysrhythmias.
Neurologic: Muscular twitching.
Other: Prolonged apnea with phase II block, respiratory depression, malignant hyperthermic crisis, prolonged apnea.

Patient/Caregiver Teaching
Instruct patient (1) to report all side effects immediately and (2) to provide accurate family and medical histories and drug profile.

Home Care
Not recommended.

Administration in Other Clinical Settings
Outpatient surgery only.

Nursing Interventions
The physician should be notified of all side effects. Discontinue drug; anesthesiologist should be present. Maintain controlled artificial ventilation and endotracheal intubation or tracheostomy if needed. Confirm diagnosis of phase II block by using peripheral nerve stimulator; presence of muscle twitch must have returned for 20 min. Essential to perform test prior to reversal with anticholinesterase drugs. Bradycardia may be controlled with atropine. Administer IV fluids, restore electrolyte balance, maintain urinary output, and administer sodium bicarbonate as needed. Resuscitate as needed.

Terbutaline sulfate

US: Brethine, Bricanyl
CAN: Bricanyl (Astra)

Sympathomimetic, tocolytic
(uterine relaxant)   pH 3–5

ACTION
Causes bronchodilation and relaxation of pregnant uterus at low dose; at high dose, causes typical sympathomimetic cardiac effects.

INDICATIONS/USES
Used as prophylaxis and treatment of bronchial asthma and reversible bronchospasm that may occur with bronchitis and emphysema; used to inhibit premature labor.

USUAL DOSE

To delay premature labor, 10 μg/min; titrate upward to maximum of 80 μg/min. Maintain at minimum effective dosage for 4 h.

PREPARATION/RECONSTITUTION

Consult product literature.

INCOMPATIBILITIES

Unknown.

RATE/MODE OF ADMINISTRATION

IV push: No.
Intermittent: Applicable by electronic infusion device; see dosing information.
Continuous: No.
Filter: No.

NURSING CONSIDERATIONS

Nursing Diagnoses

1. Potential for injury, related to neurologic side effects.
2. Potential for alteration in tissue perfusion, related to side effects.
3. Potential for alteration in comfort, related to GI side effects.
4. Ineffective airway clearance, related to respiratory effects.

Acute Care

Use only if potential benefit justifies potential risk to fetus. May inhibit labor and can accelerate fetal heartbeat; may cause hypoglycemia, hypokalemia, and pulmonary edema in the mother and hypoglycemia in the neonate. Increased likelihood of cardiac dysrhythmias when given with halothane anesthetic agents.

Precautions

Do not exceed recommended dosage; use minimal doses for minimal periods of time to prevent drug tolerance. Safety for use in lactating mothers not established.

Contraindications

Hypersensitivity to terbutaline; tachycardia caused by digitalis intoxication; unstable vasomotor system disorders; hypertension; history of stroke.

Side Effects

Neurologic: Restlessness, apprehension, anxiety, CNS stimulation, tremors, drowsiness, vertigo.
Cardiovascular: Tachycardia, dysrhythmias, palpitations, PVCs, anginal pain.
Respiratory: Pulmonary edema, coughing, bronchospasm.
Gastrointestinal: Vomiting, heartburn, unusual or bad taste in mouth.

Patient/Caregiver Teaching

Instruct patient (1) to report all side effects immediately; (2) to provide accurate medical history and drug profile; and (3) to avoid use of over-the-counter medications.

Home Care

Not recommended.

Administration in Other Clinical Settings

Not recommended.

Nursing Interventions

Maintain a β-adrenergic blocker on standby in case cardiac dysrhythmias occur. Establish safety precautions if CNS symptoms occur. Reassure patients with acute respiratory distress and provide appropriate therapy for pulmonary toilet.

Tetracycline hydrochloride

US: Achromycin IV
CAN: Acromycin (Lederle)

Antibiotic   pH 2–3

ACTION

Broad-spectrum antibiotic bacteriostatic against many gram-negative and gram-positive organisms. Crosses the placental barrier and is secreted in breast milk.

INDICATIONS/USES

Used in treatment of infections caused by susceptible strains or organisms such as spirochetal agents, viruses, many gram-negative and gram-positive bacteria, rickettsiae.

USUAL DOSE

Adults: 250–500 mg every 24 h; maximum 24-h dose is 500 mg every 6 h. Requires normal renal function.
Children: 12 mg/kg body wt/24 h in 2 divided doses; varies from 10–20 mg/kg/24 h.

PREPARATION/RECONSTITUTION

Reconstitute 250 mg with 5 ml sterile water for injection for a concentration of 50 mg/ml; further dilute with minimum 100 ml 5% dextrose in water or isotonic saline for injection for addition to large-volume parenteral solution.

INCOMPATIBILITIES

Amikacin, aminophylline, amobarbital, amphotericin B, calcium salts and solutions, carbenicillin, cefazolin, cephalothin, cephapirin, chloramphenicol, dimenhydrinate, erythromycin, 10% IV fat emulsion, heparin sodium, hydrocortisone sodium succinate, methicillin, methylprednisolone, methyldopa, metoclopramide, oxacillin, penicillins, pentobarbital, phenobarbital, phenytoin, polymyxin B, prochlorperazine, secobarbital, sodium bicarbonate, thiopental, warfarin.

RATE/MODE OF ADMINISTRATION

IV push: No.

Intermittent: 100 mg over 5 min; must be infused within 12 h of dilution.

Continuous: Applicable; do not hang longer than 12 h.

Filter: Applicable.

NURSING CONSIDERATIONS

Nursing Diagnoses

1. Potential for alteration in skin integrity, related to drug side effects.
2. Potential for alteration in nutrition: decreased, related to side effects.

Acute Care

Store away from heat and light. Check expiration date; outdated medication may cause nephrotoxicity. Sensitivity studies should be done to determine susceptibility of causative organisms. Avoid prolonged use of drug and subsequent superinfection caused by overgrowth. Ensure patency of vein and avoid extravasation and potential thrombophlebitis. Monitor IV site carefully.

Precautions

Use with caution in liver/renal dysfunction, pregnancy, postpartum, lactation. May cause skeletal retardation in fetus and infants and permanent tooth discoloration in patients under age 8. May potentiate digoxin and anticoagulants. May be toxic with sulfonamides. Inhibits bactericidal action of penicillins. Potentiated by alcohol, barbiturates, cimetidine, phenytoin. Inhibited by alkalizing agents.

Contraindications

Known hypersensitivity.

Side Effects

Gastrointestinal: Anorexia, diarrhea, dysphagia, enterocolitis, nausea, vomiting.

Other: Blood dyscrasias, anogenital lesions, skin rash, hypersensitivity, anaphylaxis, photosensitivity, systemic moniliasis, thrombophlebitis.

Patient/Caregiver Teaching

Instruct patient (1) to report all side effects immediately; (2) to realize that photosensitivity reaction may occur; (3) to learn principles of home self-administration; and (4) to report accurate medical history and drug profile.

Home Care

Appropriate.

Administration in Other Clinical Settings

Appropriate.

Nursing Interventions

The physician should be notified of all side effects. Treat symptomatically. Resuscitate as needed.

Theophylline ethylenediamine

US: Aminophylline (79% theophylline)
CAN: Elixophyllin (Bertex Canada)

Muscle relaxant   pH 8.6–9.0

ACTION

Relaxes smooth muscle and bronchial tubes, increasing cardiac output, urinary output, and sodium excretion. Peripheral vasodilator. Crosses the placental barrier and is secreted in breast milk.

INDICATIONS/USES

Used in treatment of bronchial asthma, reversible bronchospasm of chronic bronchitis or emphysema.

USUAL DOSE

Adults: Loading dose (based on lean body weight): 6 mg/kg body wt; follow with infusion of 0.5–0.7 mg/kg/h for first 12 h and 0.1–0.5 mg/kg/h thereafter.

Children: Loading dose: 6 mg/kg; follow with infusion of 1.0–1.2 mg/kg/h for first 12 h and 0.9–1.0 mg/kg/h thereafter.

Neonates

- Apnea and bradycardia in prematurity: 1 mg/kg for each 2 μg/ml serum theophylline concentration desired.

PREPARATION/RECONSTITUTION

Use only 25 mg/ml solution for direct IV use at a rate not exceeding 25 mg/min; further dilute with 100–200 ml compatible diluent (5% dextrose in water) and infuse.

INCOMPATIBILITIES

Acid solutions, amikacin, bleomycin, cephalothin, cephapirin, chloramphenicol, chlorpromazine, cimetidine, clindamycin, codeine, dimenhydrinate, dobutamine, doxapram, doxorubicin, doxycycline, epinephrine, erythromycin, fructose, hydralazine, insulin, invert sugar solutions, isoproterenol, levarterenol, levorphanol, meperidine, methadone, methicillin, methylprednisolone, morphine, nafcillin, oxytetracycline, papaverine, penicillin G sodium and potassium, pentazocine, phenobarbital, phenytoin, prochlorperazine, promazine, promethazine, succinylcholine, sulfisoxazole, tetracycline, vancomycin.

NURSING CONSIDERATIONS

Nursing Diagnoses

1. Potential for injury, related to delirium.
2. Potential for alteration in nutrition: decreased, related to drug side effects.

Acute Care

Use medication designated for IV use only. Minimum dilution is 25 mg/ml; warm to room temperature before using. Avoid rapid administration; will cause ventricular fibrillation or cardiac arrest. Monitor serum levels carefully. Peak serum is measured 15–20 min after initial loading dose. Wait 4–5 h after last IV dose to measure serum levels. Crystals will form if solution pH falls below 8.

Precautions

Use with caution in cardiac disease, congestive heart failure, coronary occlusion, cor pulmonale, renal/hepatic dysfunction, peptic ulcer disease, severe hypertension, hypoxemia, myocardial damage, hyperthyroidism, glaucoma, elderly patients. Use with caution in children; elimination of drug is prolonged in infants, neonates, and children less than 1 yr. Inhibited by β-adrenergic blockers. Potentiated by alcohol, cimetidine, clindamycin, halothane, or ketamine anesthetics. Potentiates erythromycin. Monitor drug profile carefully to avoid drug interactions.

Contraindications

Known hypersensitivity; infants under 6 mo old unless apneic.

Side Effects

Gastrointestinal: Nausea, vomiting.
Neurologic: Convulsions, delirium, dizziness, anxiety.
Other: Ventricular fibrillation, peripheral vascular collapse, cardiac arrest, hyperpyrexia.

Patient/Caregiver Teaching

Instruct patient (1) to report all side effects immediately; (2) to provide accurate medical history and drug profile; and (3) to realize that periodic drug monitoring will be necessary.

Home Care

Not recommended.

Administration in Other Clinical Settings

Only with physician support.

Nursing Interventions

The physician should be notified of all side effects; discontinue drug and treat symptomatically. Maintain adequate ventilation and hydration. Anticonvulsants may reverse grand mal seizure activity. Atrial dysrhythmias may be treated with verapamil; ventricular dysrhythmias may be treated with lidocaine or procainamide. Dopamine reverses hypotension. Resuscitate as needed.

Thiopental sodium

US: Pentothal Sodium

CNS depressant   pH 10−11

ACTION

Short-acting barbiturate and CNS depressant and potent anticonvulsant. Onset of action prompt, lasting 15−30 min. Crosses the placental barrier and is secreted in breast milk.

INDICATIONS/USES

Used to control convulsive states.

USUAL DOSE

75−125 mg for convulsions; may require maximum of 250 mg.

PREPARATION/RECONSTITUTION

Reconstitute each 500 mg ampule of powder with 20 ml sterile water for injection (supplied), or use manufacturer's prepared solution. Soluble only in isotonic saline or 5% dextrose in water for infusion.

INCOMPATIBILITIES

Acid solutions, amikacin, aminophylline, arginine, benzquinamide, calcium salts, cephalothin, cephapirin, cimetidine, clindamycin, chlorpromazine, codeine, dimenhydrinate, diphenydramine, ephedrine, hydromorphone, insulin, lavarterenol, levorphanol, magnesium sulfate, meperidine, metaraminol, methadone, methylprednisolone, morphine, penicillins, prochlorperazine, promazine, promethazine, Ringer's solutions, solutions with greater than 5% dextrose, tetracycline, tubocurarine, sodium bicarbonate.

RATE/MODE OF ADMINISTRATION

IV push: No.
Intermittent: Applicable in a 2.5%−5.0% solution.
Continuous: Applicable in a 0.2% or 0.4% concentration.
Filter: Applicable consistent with institutional policy.

NURSING CONSIDERATIONS

Nursing Diagnoses

1. Potential for ineffective breathing pattern, related to side effects.
2. Potential for altered cardiac output, related to side effects.

Acute Care

Administer under the direction of a physician. Use only freshly prepared solutions that are clear. Ensure patency of vein to avoid extravasation and intraarterial injection. Avoid rapid injection and subsequent overdose. Monitor vital signs every 3–5 min. Have resuscitative equipment readily available.

Precautions

Use with caution in cardiovascular disease, hypotension, shock, impaired hepatic/renal function, Addison's disease, increased intracranial pressure, asthma, myasthenia gravis; reduction in dosage is indicated. Use with caution if other CNS depressants have been administered. Inhibits effectiveness of propranolol, corticosteroids, doxycycline, quinidine, theophylline, oral anticoagulants, oral contraceptives. Monitor phenytoin and barbiturate levels when given concurrently. Furosemide may increase orthostatic hypotension. Children and elderly patients may develop paradoxical excitement.

Contraindications

Known hypersensitivity, porphyria, status asthmaticus.

Side Effects

Respiratory: Asthma, bronchospasm, neonatal apnea, respiratory depression, cough reflex depression, laryngospasm.
Neurologic: Coma, flat EEG, sluggish or absent reflexes.
Cardiovascular: Facial edema, fever, hypotension, dysrhythmias, hypothermia, pulmonary edema.
Other: Renal shutdown, thrombocytopenic purpura.

Patient/Caregiver Teaching

Instruct patient (1) to report all side effects immediately and (2) to provide accurate medical history and drug profile.

Home Care
Not recommended.

Administration in Other Clinical Settings
Not recommended.

Nursing Interventions
The physician should be notified of all side effects immediately. Keep patient dry and warm. Administer IV fluids and volume expanders to maintain circulatory status. Promote elimination of drug with diuretics or hemodialysis. Maintain blood pressure with vasopressors. Treat extravasation with local injection of 1% procaine and apply local heat.

Ticarcillin disodium/ clavanate potassium
US: Ticar
CAN: Ticar (Beecham)

Penicillin antibiotic   pH 6–8

ACTION
Extended spectrum penicillin bactericidal against many gram-positive, gram-negative, and anaerobic organisms. Crosses the placental barrier and is secreted in breast milk.

INDICATIONS/USES
Used in treatment of bacterial septicemia, acute and chronic infections of respiratory tract, skin and soft tissue, female pelvis, genital tract, urinary tract, intraabdominal area.

USUAL DOSE
Adults: 150–300 mg/kg body wt/24 h every 3, 4, 6 h in divided doses; maximum dose is 24 g/24 h.

Children under 40 kg: 50–300 mg/kg/24 h in divided doses every 4, 6, 8 h.

Neonates

- Under 2 kg and up to 7 days: 75 mg/kg/every 12 h.
- Under 2 kg and over 7 days: 75 mg/kg every 8 h.
- Over 2 kg and up to 7 days: 75 mg/kg/every 8 h.
- Over 2 kg and over 7 days: 100 mg/kg every 8 h.

PREPARATION/RECONSTITUTION

Reconstitute each gram with 4 ml sterile water for injection for a concentration of 200 mg/ml. Further dilute with 10–20 ml additional sterile water for injection, 5% dextrose in water, or 0.9% sodium chloride solution for direct or intermittent infusion. May use 5% dextrose in 0.2% sodium chloride, 5% dextrose in 0.45% sodium chloride, or lactated Ringer's solution.

INCOMPATIBILITIES

Amikacin, gentamicin, kanamycin, netilmicin, tobramycin.

RATE/MODE OF ADMINISTRATION

IV push: Applicable slowly and at concentration of 50 mg/ml or less.
Intermittent: Applicable in appropriate small volume parenteral over 30–120 min.
Continuous: Applicable.
Filter: Applicable.

NURSING CONSIDERATIONS

Nursing Diagnoses

1. Potential for injury, related to bleeding.
2. Potential for alteration in skin integrity, related to drug side effects.

Acute Care

Stable at room temperature for 48 h. Sensitivity studies should be done to determine susceptibility of causative organisms. Avoid superinfection caused by overgrowth. Administer slowly to avoid pain along venous wall.

Precautions

Reduce daily dose consistent with degree of renal impairment. Evaluate renal, hepatic, and hematopoietic systems regularly. Electrolyte imbalance and cardiac irregularities are possible due to high sodium content. Inactivates aminoglycosides; may administer gentamicin and tobramycin concurrently, but in separate infusions. Inactivated by chloramphenicol, erythromycin, tetracyclines. Risk of bleeding increased with anticoagulants.

Contraindications

Known penicillin or cephalosporin sensitivity.

Side Effects

Hematologic: Abnormal clotting time and PT, anemia, eosinophilia, leukopenia, neutropenia, thrombocytopenia.
Gastrointestinal: Nausea, vomiting.
Neurologic: Convulsions.
Other: Anaphylaxis, elevated SGOT and SGPT, fever, pruritus, skin rash, urticaria.

Patient/Caregiver Teaching

Instruct patient (1) to report all side effects immediately; (2) to provide accurate medical history and drug profile; (3) to avoid injury; and (4) to learn principles of home self-administration.

Home Care

Appropriate.

Administration in Other Clinical Settings

Appropriate.

Nursing Interventions

The physician should be notified of all side effects immediately. Treat symptomatically. For severe symptoms, discontinue the drug and treat allergic reactions. Resuscitate as needed.

Tobramycin sulfate

US: Nebcin

Aminoglycoside antibiotic   pH 6–8

ACTION

Aminoglycoside antibiotic bactericidal against specific gram-positive and gram-negative bacilli, including *Escherichia coli*, *Klebsiella*, *Proteus*, *Pseudomonas*. Crosses the placental barrier and is excreted by the kidneys.

INDICATIONS/USES

Used in short-term treatment of serious infections such as meningitis, peritonitis, septicemia; used when penicillin and other drugs are ineffective or contraindicated.

USUAL DOSE

Adults: 3 mg/kg body wt/24 h in 3 or 4 equally divided doses; normal renal function required. Dosage based on lean body weight plus 40% for obese patient.

Children: 6.0–7.5 mg/kg/24 h in 3 or 4 equally divided doses every 6 or 8 h.

Neonates of 1 wk or less: 4 mg/kg/24 h in 2 equal doses every 12 h; refer to manufacturer's product literature for additional information on administration to those with immature kidney function.

PREPARATION/RECONSTITUTION

Prepared solution contains 10 or 40 mg/ml; further dilute each dose in 50–100 ml 5% dextrose in water or 0.9% sodium chloride solution; use less volume for children.

INCOMPATIBILITIES

All other drugs in syringe or solution; cefamandole; heparin.

RATE/MODE OF ADMINISTRATION

IV push: No.
Intermittent: Applicable over 20–60 min.

Continuous: Applicable over 2 h.
Filter: Applicable.

NURSING CONSIDERATIONS

Nursing Diagnoses

1. Potential for injury, related to side effects.
2. Potential for reduced urinary elimination, related to side effects.
3. Potential for sensory-perceptual alteration, related to toxicity.

Acute Care

Sensitivity studies should be performed to determine susceptibility of causative organisms. Use with caution if treatment is to extend beyond 7–10 days. Use with caution in existing renal impairment; adjust dose accordingly. Monitor urine output, rising BUN and serum creatinine levels and declining creatinine clearance level. Evaluate hearing routinely. Monitor peak and trough concentrations to avoid peak serum concentrations above 12 μg/ml and trough concentrations above 2 μg/ml; therapeutic ranges are peak, 4 μg/ml, and trough, 8 μg/ml.

Precautions

Potentiated by anesthetics, antineoplastics, other neuromuscular-blocking antibiotics, cephalosporins, muscle relaxants, phenothiazines, sodium citrate; apnea can occur. Avoid superinfection caused by overgrowth of susceptible organisms. Ototoxicity may be increased by administration of loop diuretics. Synergistic in combination with penicillins and cephalosporins; adjust dosing accordingly. Maintain adequate hydration.

Contraindications

Known tobramycin and aminoglycoside sensitivities.

Side Effects

Neurologic: Dizziness, lethargy, roaring in the ears, vertigo, neuromuscular blockage, hearing loss, tinnitus.
Gastrointestinal: Vomiting.
Other: Urticaria, itching, rash, fever, headache, apnea, blood dyscrasias, elevated BUN and nonprotein nitrogen, increased creatinine, oliguria.

Patient/Caregiver Teaching

Instruct patient (1) to report all side effects immediately; (2) to maintain adequate hydration; (3) to learn principles of home self-administration; and (4) to provide accurate medical history and drug profile.

Home Care

Appropriate.

Administration in Other Clinical Settings

Appropriate.

Nursing Interventions

The physician should be notified of all side effects immediately. Treat symptomatically. Discontinue drug for major side effects, including ototoxicity and nephrotoxicity. Hemodialysis may be needed. Exchange transfusion in the newborn may be required. Reverse neuromuscular blockade with calcium salts or neostigmine. Resuscitate as needed.

Triethylene thiophosphoramide

US: Tespa, Thiotepa, TSPA

Antineoplastic agent   pH 7.6

ACTION

Alkylating agent related to nitrogen mustard with antitumor potential. Cell-cycle-phase nonspecific. Excreted unchanged in the urine.

INDICATIONS/USES

Used to suppress or retard neoplastic growth in Hodgkin's disease, non-Hodgkin's lymphoma, retinoblastoma, adrenocarcinoma of breast and ovaries.

USUAL DOSE

0.3–0.4 mg/kg body wt; maintenance adjusted according to blood levels and administered at 1- to 4-wk intervals.

PREPARATION/RECONSTITUTION

Use precautions as provided in Appendix 14. Avoid exposure to biohazardous waste materials; handle and dispose of safely. Reconstitute each 15 mg of drug with 1.5 ml sterile water for injection for a final concentration of 5 mg/0.5 ml. Shake gently and allow to stand until clear. May add to IV solutions.

INCOMPATIBILITIES

Do not mix with other medications in syringe or solution.

RATE/MODE OF ADMINISTRATION

IV push: Applicable over 1 min.
Intermittent: Applicable.
Continuous: Applicable.
Filter: Applicable.

NURSING CONSIDERATIONS

Nursing Diagnoses

1. Potential for injury, related to dizziness.
2. Potential for alteration in comfort, related to side effects.
3. Potential for alteration in nutrition, related to side effects.

Acute Care

Refer to Appendix 14 for guidelines for handling biohazardous waste associated with cytotoxic agents. Refrigerate before and after reconstitution of drug; potent for 5 days after dilution. Do not use solution if precipitate is evident. Monitor blood cell parameters daily during treatment and weekly thereafter until 3 wk following completion of treatment cycle. Dosage is based on average weight in presence of edema/ascites. Prophylactic administration of antiemetics may ease discomfort.

Precautions

Use with caution in leukopenia, thrombocytopenia, infection, recent radiation therapy. Allow complete recovery of cells before using a second antineoplastic agent. Monitor patient for signs/

symptoms of infection. Produces mutagenic effects on fetus; has mutagenic potential and should be used with caution in those of childbearing age. Combined with urokinase to treat bladder carcinoma. May be administered into tumor mass if indicated; dosing is site specific.

Contraindications

Known hypersensitivity; hepatic or renal dysfunction; bone marrow depression.

Side Effects

Gastrointestinal: Anorexia, nausea, vomiting.

Hematologic: Bone marrow depression, hemorrhage, leukopenia, thrombocytopenia.

Other: Amenorrhea, fever, headache, hives, hyperuricemia, pain at injection site, throat tightness, anaphylaxis, septicemia.

Patient/Caregiver Teaching

Instruct patient (1) to report all side effects immediately; (2) to avoid injury; (3) to provide accurate medical history and drug profile.

Home Care

Appropriate.

Administration in Other Clinical Settings

Appropriate.

Nursing Interventions

The physician should be notified of all side effects immediately. Treatment is symptomatic. Discontinue drug if platelet count is below 150,000/mm^3 or WBC is below 3000/mm^3. May require administration of whole blood, platelets, leukocytes.

Trifluopromazine hydrochloride

US: Vesprin

Antianxiety agent   pH 4.5—5.2

ACTION

An antianxiety agent affecting the central, autonomic, and peripheral nervous systems. A potent antiemetic. Slow excretion through the kidneys.

INDICATIONS/USES

Used as a pre- and postoperative tranquilizer; used to relieve nausea and vomiting after ventriculograms, encephalograms, and administration of antineoplastic agents.

USUAL DOSE

1 mg; may repeat in 4 h; not to exceed 3 mg/24 h.

PREPARATION/RECONSTITUTION

Dilute each 10 mg of drug with 9 ml normal saline for injection.

INCOMPATIBILITIES

Ethacrynic acid, pentobarbital, posterior pituitary extract; many others are possible.

RATE/MODE OF ADMINISTRATION

IV push: 1 mg over 2 min.
Intermittent: No.
Continuous: No.
Filter: No.

NURSING CONSIDERATIONS

Nursing Diagnoses

1. Potential for bleeding, related to side effects.
2. Potential for alteration in comfort, related to side effects.

Acute Care

Handle drug carefully; may cause contact dermatitis. Monitor patient's blood pressure and pulse before, during, and between doses. Keep patient in supine position. Slight yellow color to drug does not affect potency. May discolor urine pink to reddish brown. Possibility of photosensitivity reaction.

Precautions

May mask diagnosis of brain tumor, drug intoxication, intestinal obstruction. Use with caution in those with hypertension, coronary disease, epilepsy. Potentiates narcotics; reduce narcotic dosage by half. Also potentiates other CNS depressants, insulin, anticholinergics, antihypertensives, hypnotics, muscle relaxants. Capable of a number of drug interactions.

Contraindications

Known hypersensitivity; blood dyscrasias, cerebral arteriosclerosis, circulatory collapse, coronary disease, hypo- or hypertension, Parkinson's disease, subcortical brain damage.

Side Effects

Hematologic: Agranulocytosis, leukopenia.
Cardiovascular: Hypotension.
Other: Extrapyramidal symptoms; overdose may result in hallucinations, convulsions, death.

Patient/Caregiver Teaching

Instruct patient (1) to report all side effects immediately and (2) to provide accurate medical history and drug profile.

Home Care

Not recommended.

Administration in Other Clinical Settings

Not recommended unless for outpatient surgery with physician in attendance.

Nursing Interventions

The physician should be notified of all side effects and the drug should be discontinued. Dopamine and IV fluids reverse hypotension; treat allergic reactions with antihistamines. Do not administer epinephrine; further hypotension will result. Diazepam relieves convulsions. Resuscitate as needed.

Trimethoprim sulfamethoxazole

US: Bactrim, Co-Trimoxazole, Septra

Antibacterial   pH 10

ACTION

Broad-spectrum antibacterial and antiprotozoal agent with action against gram-negative and gram-positive organisms. Prompt onset of action with serum levels maintained up to 10 h. Metabolized in the liver; up to 60% is excreted in the urine in 24 h. Crosses placental barrier and is secreted in breast milk.

INDICATIONS/USES

Used in treatment of severe urinary tract infections, *Pneumocystis carinii* pneumonitis, shigellosis, prophylaxis in neutropenic patients.

USUAL DOSE

Severe urinary tract infection (UTI)/shigellosis: 8–10 mg/kg body wt every 6, 8, 12 h for 14 days (UTI); or 5 days (shigellosis); use equally divided doses.

P. carinii *pneumonitis:* 15–20 mg/kg every 5 or 8 h in equally divided doses for 14 days.

Prophylaxis in neutropenic patients: 800 mg sulfamethoxazole and 160 mg trimethoprim every 12 h.

PREPARATION/RECONSTITUTION

Dilute each 5-ml (80 mg of drug) ampule with 125 ml 5% dextrose in water for infusion; may use 75 ml of diluent if fluid restriction required. Use within 5 h; or use less concentrated solution within 2 h of reconstitution. Discard if crystals are present or solution is cloudy. Individual doses are 80–160 mg/250 ml.

INCOMPATIBILITIES

Do not mix in syringe or solution with any other drug.

RATE/MODE OF ADMINISTRATION

IV push: No.
Intermittent: Applicable over 60–90 min; flush all lines after infusion.
Continuous: No.
Filter: Yes.

NURSING CONSIDERATIONS

Nursing Diagnoses

1. Potential for injury, related to neurologic side effects.
2. Potential for alteration in nutrition: decreased, related to GI side effects.

Acute Care

Avoid extravasation and intraarterial puncture; may cause phlebitis. Stable at room temperature; do not refrigerate. Maintain adequate hydration. Sensitivity studies should be obtained to determine susceptibility of organisms. Obtain baseline CBC before treatment and repeat during therapy. Obtain urinalysis and renal function tests; reduce dosage for creatinine clearance between 15–30 ml/min to half usual dose. Observe patient for sensitivity reactions.

Precautions

Use with caution in those with renal/hepatic dysfunction. Use with caution in those hypersensitive to furosemide, thiazide diuretics, sulfonylureas, carbonic anhydrase inhibitors. Inhibits bactericidal action of penicillins and renal excretion of methotrexate. Inhibits cyclosporine and increases nephrotoxicity. May potentiate warfarin, phenytoin. Inhibited by alkalizing agents and thiopental. Increase in side effects in patients with HIV infection; may not respond to this medication.

Contraindications

Known hypersensitivity; megaloblastic anemia from folate deficiency, pregnancy, lactation, streptococcal pharyngitis, creatinine clearance below 15 ml/min; infants less than 2 mo old.

Side Effects

Gastrointestinal: Nausea, vomiting.
Neurologic: Tremors, convulsions, ataxia.
Respiratory: Respiratory depression.
Hematologic: Megaloblastic anemia, thrombocytopenia, leukopenia.

Patient/Caregiver Teaching

Instruct patient (1) to report all side effects immediately; (2) to provide accurate medical history and drug profile; and (3) to learn principles of home self-administration.

Home Care

Appropriate.

Administration in Other Clinical Settings

Appropriate.

Nursing Interventions

The physician should be notified of all side effects. Discontinue treatment for major side effects or bone marrow depression. Leucovorin 3–5 mg IM daily for 3 days activates normal hematopoiesis. Treat anaphylaxis with epinephrine, corticosteroids, antihistamines, vasopressors as needed.

Tubocurarine chloride

US: Curare

Skeletal muscle relaxant   pH 2.5–5.0

ACTION
Skeletal muscle relaxant with onset of action within 2–3 min, lasting up to 60 min. Crosses the placental barrier.

INDICATIONS/USES
Used to provide muscle relaxation in severe muscle contraction or convulsion; to diagnose myasthenia gravis; to facilitate management of those undergoing mechanical ventilation; and as an adjunct to a general anesthetic.

USUAL DOSE
To control respirations: 16.5 μg/kg body wt; adjust as needed.
Muscle contraction/convulsions: 0.15 mg/kg minus 3 mg; repeat as needed.
Diagnosis of myasthenia gravis: 4–33 μg/kg.

PREPARATION/RECONSTITUTION
Administer undiluted in 3 mg/ml concentration. For myasthenia gravis testing, dilute single dose to 4 ml with normal saline for injection, or 100 mg/100 ml with maximum concentration of 200 mg/100 ml.

INCOMPATIBILITIES
Barbiturates; do not mix with any other drug in syringe or solution.

RATE/MODE OF ADMINISTRATION
IV push: Applicable over 60–90 sec; avoid too rapid injection and resultant histamine release and bronchospasms/hypotension.
  • For myasthenia testing: 0.5 mg diluted drug over 2 min.
Intermittent: No.
Continuous: No.
Filter: No.

NURSING CONSIDERATIONS
Nursing Diagnoses
1. Potential for ineffective breathing pattern, related to drug side effects.
2. Potential for injury, related to side effects.
3. Potential for decreased tissue perfusion, related to cardiovascular side effects.

Acute Care
Administered by or under direction of anesthesiologist; controlled artificial ventilation and oxygen must be continuous and patient must be observed constantly. Maintain patent airway. Confirm potassium level prior to use; may need to withhold diuretics for 4 days before elective surgery. Use peripheral nerve stimulator to monitor effectiveness of treatment. Use only clear solutions; faint discoloration does not alter potency.

Precautions
Use with caution in impaired renal/hepatic function. Use caution in pregnancy, lactation. Potentiated by inhalant anesthetics, neuro-muscular-blocking antibiotics, digitalis, diuretics, diazepam, other muscle relaxants, MAO inhibitors, propranolol, lidocaine, quinidine, tetracyclines, succinylcholine. Antagonized by acetylcholines, anticholinesterases, potassium; hyperkalemia may cause cardiac dysrhythmias and increase paralysis.

Contraindications
Known sensitivity.

Side Effects
Respiratory: Airway closure following relaxation of epiglottis, pharynx, and tongue muscles; respiratory depression; severe bronchospasm.
Circulatory: Shock, profound hypotension, anaphylaxis.
Other: Histamine release.

Patient/Caregiver Teaching
Instruct patient (1) to expect that he may be conscious and unable to communicate and (2) to provide accurate medical history and drug profile.

Home Care
Not recommended.

Administration in Other Clinical Settings
Only with anesthesiologist present.

Nursing Interventions
The physician should be notified of all side effects which are considered medical emergencies. Treat symptomatically providing controlled artificial respiration at all times. Reverse muscle relaxation by administration of edrophonium or neostigmine methylsulfate. Resuscitate as needed.

Urokinase

US: Abbokinase, Abbokinase Open-Cath

Fibrinolytic agent   pH 6.0–7.5

ACTION
Converts plasminogen to plasmin, degrading fibrin clots, fibrinogen, and other plasma proteins. Onset of action prompt; lasts up to 12–24 h.

INDICATIONS/USES
Used to lyse acute massive pulmonary emboli involving one or more lobes and if hemodynamic status is unstable; used to lyse coronary artery thrombi and to restore patency of IV catheters.

USUAL DOSE
Pulmonary embolism: 4400 IU/kg body wt as priming dose over 10 min; follow with infusion of 4400 IU/kg/h for 12 h (do not exceed total volume of 200 ml); then flush with normal saline or 5% dextrose in water using volume equal to the volume of the

catheter (refer to manufacturer's recommendations). Maintain patency of line by keeping it open with the flush solution at 15 ml/h.

Coronary artery thrombi: Bolus of heparin 2500–10,000 IU into coronary artery. (Heparin administered within previous 4–5 h should be considered in calculating total dose). Infuse drug directly into coronary artery at 4 ml/min (6000 IU/min) for 2 h. Continue for 15–30 min following initial breakthrough. Obtain coagulation profile and reinitiate heparin sodium therapy.

IV catheter clearance: 5000 IU (prepackaged diluted solution) equal to the volume capacity of the catheter in place.

PREPARATION/RECONSTITUTION

Dilute each 250,000-IU vial with 5.2 ml of sterile water for injection without preservatives. Add diluent slowly, reaching sides of the vial; roll and tilt gently without shaking. Filter before administration.

Pulmonary embolism: Further dilute each dose with sufficient 0.9% sodium chloride solution to administer a total infusion of 195 ml.

Lysis of coronary artery thrombi: Dilute 3 vials as described and add contents of all three to 500 ml of 5% dextrose in water.

Catheter clearance: Add 1 ml of reconstituted drug to 9 ml sterile water for injection without preservatives. Prepare immediately prior to use and discard unused solution in vial.

INCOMPATIBILITIES

Do not mix with any other drug in syringe or solution.

RATE/MODE OF ADMINISTRATION

IV push: No.
Intermittent: No.
Continuous

- Pulmonary embolism: Initial dose over 10 min; follow with infusion of calculated total dose over 12 h by electronic infusion device.
- Lysis of coronary artery thrombi: 4 ml/min.
- IV catheter clearance: Confirm occlusion by attempting to aspirate. Inject premeasured amount of urokinase into cathe-

ter by tuberculin syringe. Connect a 5-ml syringe to hub and wait 5 min; gently aspirate to remove clot. Repeat aspiration every 5 min until clot clears or 30 min have passed. If unsuccessful, recap catheter and wait for 30–60 min. Attempt to aspirate again; a second dose of urokinase may be administered and procedure repeated. If successful, irrigate catheter with 10 ml normal saline solution and reconnect to IV infusion.

Filter: Applicable for initial reconstitution and infusion purposes.

NURSING CONSIDERATIONS

Nursing Diagnoses
1. Potential for injury, related to bleeding disorders.
2. Potential for alteration in skin integrity, related to side effects.

Acute Care
All applications other than catheter clearance should be performed in inpatient environment only with physician and laboratory support readily available. Observe patient continuously. Monitor bleeding parameters before treatment. Thrombin time and activated PTT should be less than twice normal control value before treatment. Monitor every 4 h and during therapy. Keep physician informed of parameters. Confirm diagnosis prior to use. Use care in handling patient to avoid injury, avoid arterial punctures, venipuncture, IM injection. Perform Valsalva maneuver during tubing change. Drug contains no preservatives; reconstitute immediately prior to use to produce a clear, colorless solution. Discard unused portions. Unit dose form available for catheter clearance.

Precautions
Avoid force when attempting to clear catheters. Do not take blood pressure in lower extremities; thrombi may dislodge. Use with caution in the following: surgical procedures, biopsy, lumbar puncture, thoracentesis, paracentesis, intraarterial diagnostic procedures within 10 days, ulcerative wounds, multiple cutdowns, visceral malignancy, pregnancy, first 10 days postpartum, intracranial malignancy, lesion of GI or GU tract with potential for bleeding, renal insufficiency, uncontrolled hypocoagulable state,

subacute bacterial endocarditis, recent cerebral embolism, chronic lung disease with cavitation, rheumatic valvular heart disease.

Contraindications

Cerebral vascular accident within past 2 mo, active internal bleeding, intracranial or intraspinal surgery, intracranial neoplasm, hypersensitivity, liver failure, subacute bacterial endocarditis, visceral malignancy.

Side Effects

Hematologic: Bleeding.
Respiratory: Bronchospasm.
Cardiovascular: Reperfusion, atrial and ventricular dysrhythmias.
Other: Skin rash.

Patient/Caregiver Teaching

Instruct patient (1) to report all side effects immediately; (2) to provide accurate medical history and drug profile; (3) to call home care nurse for emergency situations; and (4) to recognize catheter occlusion in the home.

Home Care

Appropriate for use by a qualified IV nurse for IV catheter clearance only.

Administration in Other Clinical Settings

Appropriate for use by a qualified IV nurse for IV catheter clearance only.

Nursing Interventions

The physician should be notified of all side effects immediately. Note any bleeding tendency; treatment may need to be discontinued. Whole blood, packed RBC, cryoprecipitate, fresh frozen plasma, and aminocaproic acid may relieve serious bleeding and subsequent blood loss. Treat minor symptoms symptomatically. Resuscitate as needed.

Vancomycin hydrochloride

US: Vancocin, Vancoled

Bactericidal antibiotic   pH 2.4–4.5

ACTION

Bactericidal against gram-positive cocci. Limited use due to oto-toxic and nephrotoxic tendency. Excreted in the urine.

INDICATIONS/USES

Used for treatment of life-threatening gram-positive infections un-responsive to penicillins or cephalosporins. Used to treat endocar-ditis caused by *Streptococcus viridans* or *S. bovis* concurrently with an aminoglycoside antibiotic. Used as prophylaxis against endocar-ditis in dental, upper respiratory, GI, and GU procedures.

USUAL DOSE

Adults: 500 mg every 6 h or 1 g/12 h; maximum dose of 3–4 g/24 h used only in very severe infections. Patient should have normal renal function.

- Prevention of subacute bacterial endocarditis in penicillin-allergic patients undergoing dental procedures, upper respi-ratory tract surgery, instrumentation: Over 27 kg, 1 g IV 1 h before procedure; under 27 kg, 20 mg/kg 1 h before pro-cedure. May repeat in 8–12 h.

- Prevention of subacute bacterial endocarditis in penicillin-allergic patients having GU or GI surgery or instrumentation: Over 27 kg, 1 g IV 1 h before procedure; under 27 kg, 20 mg/kg 1 h before procedure. May repeat in 8–12 h.

Note: Concomitant administration of gentamicin in prescribed dose is indicated for the above.

Children: 40 mg/kg/24 h in 4 equal doses; not to exceed 2 g in 24 h.

Infants: 15 mg/kg as initial dose; follow with 10 mg/kg every 12 h for those up to 1 mo old and at 8-h intervals for those over 1 mo old.

Premature and full-term neonates: Use with caution due to incompletely developed renal function. Initial dose of 15 mg/kg followed by 10 mg/kg every 12 h in first week of life.

PREPARATION/RECONSTITUTION

Reconstitute each 500 mg of powder preparation in 10 ml sterile water for injection for a concentration of 50 mg/ml. Further dilute by adding to 100 ml 0.9% sodium chloride solution or 5% dextrose in water. Minimum dilution is 12.5–5.0 mg per ml of infusate.

INCOMPATIBILITIES

Aminophylline, amobarbital, chloramphenicol, dexamethasone, heparin sodium, hydrocortisone sodium succinate, methicillin, penicillins, pentobarbital, phenobarbital, phenytoin, prochlorperazine, secobarbital, sodium bicarbonate.

RATE/MODE OF ADMINISTRATION

IV push: No.
Intermittent: Applicable over 60 min minimum to avoid red man syndrome (see Precautions).
Continuous: Applicable following initial dose; subsequent doses given over 12 h.
Filter: Yes.

NURSING CONSIDERATIONS

Nursing Diagnoses

1. Potential for sensory-perceptual defect, related to drug side effects.
2. Potential for injury, related to side effects.

Acute Care

Store diluted preparation in refrigerator; potency maintained for 2 wk. Sensitivity studies should be performed to determine susceptibility of organisms to vancomycin. Avoid superinfection and subsequent overgrowth. Monitor IV sites and rotate carefully to avoid phlebitis. Ensure patency of vein and avoid extravasation; necrosis and sloughing will result.

Precautions

Ototoxic and nephrotoxic; use with caution. Reduce total daily dose if renal function is impaired. Monitor blood levels, auditory testing, renal function during use. Use with caution with dimenhydrinate; may mask ototoxicity. Potentiated by neuromuscular-blocking antibiotics, other nephrotoxic or ototoxic drugs, cisplatin, ethacrynic acid. Rapid injection causes histamine release with transient blotching (red man syndrome) of face, neck, chest, and extremities, as well as hypotension and cardiac arrest; avoid rapid injection. Observe for furry tongue, diarrhea, foul-smelling stools. Monitor blood pressure during infusion.

Contraindications

Known hypersensitivity.

Side Effects

Cardiovascular: Chills, fever, anaphylaxis, cardiac arrest, hypotension, thrombophlebitis.
Neurologic: Tinnitus.
Other: Eosinophilia, hearing loss, macular rashes, pain at injection site, urticaria.

Patient/Caregiver Teaching

Instruct patient (1) to report all side effects immediately; (2) to provide accurate medical history and drug profile; and (3) to learn principles of home self-administration.

Home Care

Appropriate; monitor first several infusions closely.

Administration in Other Clinical Settings

Appropriate; monitor first several infusions closely.

Nursing Interventions

The physician should be notified of all side effects. Treat symptomatically. Hearing loss may progress when drug is discontinued. Fluids, antihistamines, corticosteroids, and vasopressors may be needed for severe reactions. Resuscitate as needed.

Verapamil hydrochloride
US: Calan, Isoptin
CAN: Isoptin Parenteral (Knoll)

Calcium channel blocker   pH 4.1–6.0

ACTION
A calcium channel blocker that reduces myocardial contractility, afterload, arterial pressure, vascular tone, and oxygen demand within 1–5 min. Hemodynamic effects last 20 min; antiarrhythmic effects last 6 h. Crosses the placental barrier and is secreted in breast milk.

INDICATIONS/USES
Used in treatment of supraventricular tachyarrhythmias and temporary control of rapid ventricular rate in atrial flutter and fibrillation.

USUAL DOSE
Adults: 5–10 mg; may repeat in 30 min if needed.
Children
- Up to 1 yr: 0.1–0.2 mg/kg body wt; repeat in 30 min if needed.
- One to 15 yr: 0.1–0.3 mg/kg; repeat in 30 min if needed. Do not exceed 5 mg.

PREPARATION/RECONSTITUTION
Administer undiluted through Y-site of ongoing infusion of compatible infusate.

INCOMPATIBILITIES
Albumin, amphotericin B, dobutamine, hydralazine, nafcillin, sodium bicarbonate, trimethoprim sulfamethoxazole.

RATE/MODE OF ADMINISTRATION
IV push: Applicable as single dose over 2 min; extend to 3 min in elderly patients.

Intermittent: No.
Continuous: No.
Filter: Not applicable in less than 1-ml dose.

NURSING CONSIDERATIONS

Nursing Diagnoses

1. Potential for alteration in comfort, related to side effects.
2. Potential for alteration in cardiac output, related to drug action.

Acute Care

Monitor ECG during administration. Monitor blood pressure carefully. Protect vials from light; do not use if solution is discolored. Maintain emergency resuscitative drugs and equipment at bedside. Monitor side effects when used concurrently with digitalis. Abrupt withdrawal may precipitate rebound angina; wean patient from drug.

Precautions

Before using this drug, treat heart failure with digitalis and diuretics. Monitor for side effects. Do not administer disopyramide within 48 h before or 24 h after use of this drug. Potentiates cyclosporine, carbamazepine, nondepolarizing muscle relaxants. Use with caution in renal/hepatic dysfunction. Discontinue breast-feeding. May cause excessive hypotension when used concurrently with other antihypertensive drugs.

Contraindications

Congestive heart failure, cardiogenic shock, second- or third-degree AV block, severe hypotension, patients receiving IV β-adrenergic blocking drugs within 2–4 h, ventricular tachycardia.

Side Effects

Gastrointestinal: Abdominal discomfort, nausea.
Cardiovascular: Anaphylaxis, asystole, bradycardia, heart failure, hypotension, premature ventricular contractions, tachycardia.
Neurologic: Dizziness, headache.

Patient/Caregiver Teaching

Instruct patient (1) to report all side effects immediately and (2) to provide accurate medical history and drug profile.

Home Care
Not recommended.

Administration in Other Clinical Settings
Only with full medical support.

Nursing Interventions
The physician should be notified of all side effects. Calcium chloride may be used in toxicity. Cardioversion, procainamide, and lidocaine should reverse rapid ventricular response in atrial flutter and fibrillation. Atropine, isoproterenol, and pacing should be used to treat bradycardia. Resuscitate as needed.

Vidarabine
US: Vira-A
CAN: Vira-A (P.D.)

Antiviral agent   pH 5.0–6.2

ACTION
An antiviral drug that changes quickly to Ara-Hx, a metabolite that is distributed in the tissues. Plasma and tissue levels maintained by slow IV infusion; excreted in the urine.

INDICATIONS/USES
Used in the treatment of herpes simplex virus encephalitis; investigationally used to reduce complications associated with herpes zoster in immunocompromised patients.

USUAL DOSE
15 mg/kg body wt for 10 days.

PREPARATION/RECONSTITUTION
Add 2.22 ml of compatible infusate to each 1 mg of drug; may be diluted with most IV solutions except biologic and colloidal fluids.

Shake drug well prior to measuring dose. Warm diluent to 35–40°C to facilitate reconstitution. Administer a clear solution.

INCOMPATIBILITIES
Blood and blood products, protein solutions.

RATE/MODE OF ADMINISTRATION
IV push: No.
Intermittent: No.
Continuous: Applicable; follow preparation requirements.
Filter: Applicable.

NURSING CONSIDERATIONS
Nursing Diagnoses
1. Potential sensory-perceptual alteration, related to neurologic effects.
2. Potential fluid volume excess, related to large volume of drug infusate.

Acute Care
Administer by slow infusion only; avoid bolus or rapid injection. More than 1 L of solution may be required to dissolve each dose of medication. Carefully monitor IV site and avoid extravasation of infusate. Monitor for signs of fluid overload (increased central venous pressure, edema).

Precautions
Confirm diagnosis by cell culture from brain biopsy. For IV infusion only. Reduce dose if renal function is impaired. Use with caution in cerebral edema or fluid overload. Must be initiated within 72 h of onset of herpes zoster. Use only freshly prepared solution; stable at room temperature for 48 h.

Contraindications
Known allergy to vidarabine; hepatic dysfunction; congestive heart failure; pregnancy and lactation.

Side Effects
Neurologic: Tremors, psychoses, malaise, dizziness, confusion, irritability.

Dermatologic: Rash, pruritus, pain at injection site.
Gastrointestinal: Nausea, vomiting, anorexia, diarrhea.

Patient/Caregiver Teaching

Instruct patient (1) to report all side effects immediately and (2) to provide accurate medical history and drug profile.

Home Care

Appropriate in well-monitored setting.

Administration in Other Clinical Settings

Appropriate in well-monitored setting.

Nursing Interventions

The physician should be notified of all side effects immediately. Monitor hematologic, renal, and hepatic functions. Treat allergic reactions as indicated; resuscitate as needed.

Vinblastine sulfate

US: Velban, VLB
CAN: Velbe (Lilly)

Antineoplastic agent   pH 3.5–5.0

ACTION

Cell cycle specific for M phase; alkaloid with antitumor activity. Some excretion through bile and urine.

INDICATIONS/USES

Used to suppress or retard neoplastic growth in Hodgkin's disease, non-Hodgkin's lymphomas, renal cell and breast malignancies.

USUAL DOSE

Adults: 3.7 mg/m^2 once every 7 days, increasing dose to specific amounts (5.5, 7.4, 9.25 mg/m^2) until WBC is decreased to 3000 cells/ml, remission is obtained, or maximum dose of 18.5 mg/m^2 is attained.

- Maintenance: one step lower than any dose causing leuko-penia (usually 5.5–7.4 mg/m^2) once every 7–14 days.

Children: 2.5 mg/m^2 initially. Same procedure as adult dosing using 3.75, 5.0, 6.25, 7.5 mg/m^2.

PREPARATION/RECONSTITUTION

Use precautions for handling biohazardous waste; see Appendix 14. Reconstitute each 10 mg with 10 ml sodium chloride for injection for a concentration of 1 mg/ml. Do not add to IV solutions.

INCOMPATIBILITIES

Do not mix with any other drug in syringe or solution.

RATE/MODE OF ADMINISTRATION

IV push: Applicable by sideport of freely flowing infusion.
Intermittent: No.
Continuous: No.
Filter: No.

NURSING CONSIDERATIONS

Nursing Diagnoses

1. Potential for alteration in self-concept, related to alopecia.
2. Potential for injury, related to myelosuppression.
3. Potential alteration in nutrition, related to GI side effects.

Acute Care

Refer to Appendix 14 for guidelines on handling antineoplastics and their disposal. Usually administered under direction of a highly qualified physician specialist. Refrigerate before and following preparation/reconstitution; potent for 30 days following reconstitution. Ensure patency of vein and avoid extravasation; cellulitis may result. Rinse syringe and needle with venous blood before withdrawing from vein. Avoid contact with eyes; corneal ulceration may occur. Monitor WBC prior to each dose to ensure level greater than 4000 cells/ml. Dosage based on average weight in presence of ascites or edema. Maintain hydration. Provide prophylactic anti-emetics to increase comfort level.

Precautions

May produce teratogenic effects on fetus; is mutagenic and should be given with caution to those of childbearing age. Potentiated by other antineoplastics. Potentiates anticoagulants. Inhibited by some amino acids. Use with caution if patient has ulcerated skin areas; use with caution in hepatic dysfunction.

Contraindications

Leukopenia below 3000 cells/ml; bacterial infection.

Side Effects

(Usually dose-related)

Hematologic: Hemorrhage, myelosuppression, leukopenia.
Neurologic: Peripheral neuritis, reflex depression, convulsions, dizziness, malaise, mental depression, numbness, paresthesias.
Gastrointestinal: Nausea, vomiting, weakness, oral lesions, diarrhea.
Other: Gonadal suppression, ileus, skin lesions, thrombophlebitis, tumor site pain.

Patient/Caregiver Teaching

Instruct patient (1) to report all side effects immediately; (2) to be aware that side effects are dose related and not always reversible; and (3) to avoid injury due to potential for bleeding.

Home Care

Appropriate for use by highly qualified IV nurse.

Administration in Other Clinical Settings

Appropriate for use by highly qualified IV nurse.

Nursing Interventions

The physician should be notified of all side effects. Treat extravasation with hyaluronidase injected locally into area using fine hypodermic needle; apply moist heat. Treat side effects symptomatically.

Vincristine sulfate

US: LCR, Oncovin, VCR
CAN: Oncovin (Lilly)

Antineoplastic alkaloid   pH 3.5–4.5

ACTION
Alkaloid with antitumor activity; cell cycle specific for M phase.

INDICATIONS/USES
Used to suppress or retard neoplastic growth in Hodgkin's disease, oat cell, lymphosarcoma, leukemia.

USUAL DOSE
Adults: 1.4 mg/m^2 every 7 days; 0.05 to 1.0 mg/m^2 in hepatic dysfunction.
Children: 2 mg/m^2. If child weighs less than 10 kg or has body surface area less than 1 m^2, administer 0.05 mg/kg once a week.

PREPARATION/RECONSTITUTION
See Appendix 14 for guidelines on handling biohazardous waste materials. Diluent is provided by manufacturer; or dilute 1 mg with 10 ml sterile water or normal saline for injection. Do not add to IV solutions.

INCOMPATIBILITIES
Do not mix with any other drug in syringe or solution. Incompatible with all solutions except 0.9% sodium chloride solution and 5% dextrose in water.

RATE/MODE OF ADMINISTRATION
IV push: Applicable by sideport of freely flowing IV.
Intermittent: No.
Continuous: No.
Filter: No.

NURSING CONSIDERATIONS
Nursing Diagnoses
1. Potential for alteration in comfort, related to side effects.
2. Potential for injury, related to immunosuppression.
3. Potential for alteration in nutrition, related to GI side effects.

Acute Care
Avoid contact; follow guidelines for handling biohazardous waste. Usually administered under direction of a highly qualified physician specialist. Refrigerate before and after preparation/reconstitution; label vial with milligram to milliliter conversion. Ensure patency of vein and avoid extravasation; cellulitis may result. Dosage is based on average weight in presence of ascites or edema. Avoid contact with eye; flush with water immediately. Maintain adequate hydration. Prophylactic administration of antiemetics may increase patient comfort level.

Precautions
Use with caution in bone marrow suppression. Acute pulmonary reactions may occur with mitomycin-C. Use with caution when patient is receiving radiation therapy. Mutagenic potential; give with caution to those of childbearing age. Discontinue breast-feeding. Potentiates anticoagulants. Potentiated by calcium channel blockers. Inhibits digoxin. Stool softener may be required to prevent impactions.

Contraindications
None absolute.

Side Effects
Gastrointestinal: Constipation, abdominal pain, diarrhea, nausea, vomiting, weight loss, upper colon impaction, paralytic ileus.
Neurologic: Ataxia, convulsions, footdrop, headache, tingling and numbness of extremities, paresthesias, sensory impairment, neuritic pain, cranial nerve damage.
Respiratory: Bronchospasm.
Cardiovascular: Thrombophlebitis, hyper- or hypotension.
Other: Alopecia, cellulitis, dysuria, gonadal suppression, leukopenia, muscle wasting.

Patient/Caregiver Teaching

Instruct patient (1) to report all side effects immediately and (2) to provide accurate medical history and drug profile.

Home Care

Appropriate for administration by a highly qualified IV nurse.

Administration in Other Clinical Settings

Appropriate for administration by a highly qualified IV nurse.

Nursing Interventions

The physician should be notified of all side effects. Treat symptomatically. Discontinue drug for inappropriate ADH secretion or hyponatremia. Overdose may be reversed by administration of folinic acid: 100 mg every 3 h for 24 h; then every 6 h for 48 h. For extravasation, inject hyaluronidase into extravasated area using fine hypodermic needle and apply moist heat.

Warfarin

US: Coumadin
CAN: Coumadin sodium (DuPont)

Anticoagulant   pH 7.2–8.3

ACTION

Anticoagulant; depresses formation of prothrombin and other factors. Metabolized in the liver and excreted in changed form in the urine. Crosses the placental barrier and is secreted in breast milk.

INDICATIONS/USES

Used in prevention and treatment of thromboses and emboli.

USUAL DOSE

40–50 mg initial dose; maintenance dose is 2–10 mg.

PREPARATION/RECONSTITUTION

Diluent is provided. Reconstitute each 50 mg of powder with 2 ml for a concentration of 25 mg/ml; rotate vial to dissolve completely. Do not mix with infusates.

INCOMPATIBILITIES

Amikacin, ammonium chloride, dextrose, epinephrine, metaraminol, oxytocin, promazine, vancomycin, tetracycline. *Note: Compatible in syringe with heparin; may be given concomitantly.*

RATE/MODE OF ADMINISTRATION

IV push: 25 mg over 1 min.
Intermittent: No.
Continuous: No.
Filter: No.

NURSING CONSIDERATIONS

Nursing Diagnoses

1. Potential for injury, related to bleeding.
2. Potential for alteration of skin integrity, related to drug side effects.

Acute Care

Obtain PT level before initial injection; repeat daily throughout treatment. Draw blood for PT just before concomitant administration of heparin. Dosage is adjusted consistent with prothrombin activity; desired level is 20% of normal (21–35 sec, with a control of 14 sec). Wean patient rather than withdraw medication abruptly. Skin necrosis may occur.

Precautions

Use with caution in the following: hepatic or renal dysfunction, trauma, extensive surgical interventions, hypertension, the elderly, diabetes, history of allergies or sensitivity reactions. Potentiated by acidifying agents, alcohol, analgesics, anesthetics, antibiotics, antineoplastics, salicylates, skeletal muscle relaxants; severe bleeding may result. Inhibited by barbiturates, corticosteroids, digitalis. Potentiates anticonvulsants, insulin. Do not use concurrently with streptokinase or urokinase.

Contraindications

Active bleeding episodes, anesthesia, blood dyscrasias, inadequate laboratory facilities, lactation, pregnancy, recent surgery, extensive trauma, subacute bacterial endocarditis, threatened abortion, continuous GI suctioning.

Side Effects

General: Alopecia, bruising, epistaxis, hematuria, PT lower than 20% activity.

Patient/Caregiver Teaching

Instruct patient (1) to report all side effects immediately; (2) to avoid injury; (3) to avoid over-the-counter medications without physician approval; and (4) to provide accurate medical history and drug profile.

Home Care

Not recommended.

Administration in Other Clinical Settings

Not recommended.

Nursing Interventions

The physician should be notified of all side effects. Phytonadione is a warfarin antagonist and should be used to treat overdose.

BIBLIOGRAPHY

AHFS drug information '89. Bethesda: American Society of Hospital Pharmacy, 1989.

Alfaro R. Application of nursing process: a step-by-step guide. 2nd ed. Philadelphia: JB Lippincott, 1986.

Batastini PH, Davidson JK. Pharmacological calculations for nurses. New York: John Wiley & Sons, 1985.

Caplik JF, Walters JK. Guidelines for the preparation of intravenous admixture solutions. Berkeley: Cutter Medical, 1980.

Dorr RT, Fritz WL. Cancer chemotherapy handbook. New York: Elsevier, 1982.

Fischer DS, Knobf MT. The cancer chemotherapy handbook. 3rd ed. Chicago: Yearbook Medical Publishers, 1989.

Greenblatt DJ, Shader RI. Pharmacokinetics in clinical practice. Philadelphia. WB Saunders, 1985.

Hansten PD. Drug interactions. 3rd ed. Philadelphia: Lea & Febiger, 1976.

Johnson GE. Blue book of pharmacologic therapeutics. Philadephia: WB Saunders, 1985.

Karch AM, Boyd EH. Handbook of drugs and the nursing process. Philadelphia: JB Lippincott, 1989.

Katcher BS, Young LY, Koda-Kimble MA. Applied therapeutics. the clinical use of drugs. New York: Applied Therapeutics, 1984.

Krough CME, ed. Compendium of pharmaceuticals and specialities. 24th ed. Toronto: Southam Murray Publishers, 1989.

Maddox RR, John JF. Effect of inline filtration on post-infusion phlebitis. Clin Pharm 1983;21(1).

Marder VJ, Francis CW. Thrombolytic therapy for acute transmural myocardial infarction: intracoronary versus intravenous. Am J Med 1984;77(5).

Mark LC. The "puff technic" for intravenous diazepam. Anesthesiology 1984;61(5).

Rapp RP, Ermesling DP. Guidelines for the administration of commonly used intravenous drugs. Drug Intell Clin Pharm 1984;18(3).

Sager DP, Bomar SK. Quick reference to intravenous drugs. Philadelphia: JB Lippincott, 1980.

Trissel LA. ASHP handbook on injectable drugs. 4th ed. Bethesda: American Society of Hospital Pharmacy, 1986.

Weil MH. Current understanding of mechanisms and treatment of circulatory shock caused by bacterial infections. Ann Clin Res 1977:9:181.

Weinberger M, et al. Decreased theophylline clearance due to cimetidine. N Engl J Med 1981;304:672.

Weinstein S. Biohazards of antineoplastic agents. Home Healthcare Nurse 1987;5:30.

Weinstein S. Use of investigational drugs. J IV Nurs 1987;1:336.

Weinstein S. Math calculations for IV nurses. J IV Nurs 1990;4.

Weiss HJ. Antiplatelet drugs: a new pharmacologic approach to the prevention of thrombosis. Am Heart J 1976;92:86.

Winter ME. Basic clincial pharmacokinetics. San Francisco: Applied Therapeutics, 1980.

Zimmerman HJ. Hepatotoxicity: adverse effects of drugs and other chemicals on the liver. New York: Appleton-Century-Crofts, 1978.

Appendices

APPENDIX 1. IV Infusion Solutions

The following tables summarize the composition and characteristics of the commercially available intravenous infusion solutions. All of the information presented was provided by the manufacturers of the various products. In some cases, the requested information was not supplied. The tables are as complete as possible using the data that were supplied. Where both glass and plastic containers are indicated for a particular solution, not all sizes are necessarily available in both container types.

Abbott Laboratories has introduced Aminosyn II products as replacements for much of the Aminosyn and Aminosyn (pH 6) product lines. Information on all of these products is included in this table because the transition may take some time to complete entirely.

Amino Acid Injections

LVP NAME	MFR	VOLUME (ml)					APPROX. pH	mOsm/ L
		150	250	500	1000	OTHER		
Aminess 5.2%	KV					400	6.4	416
Aminosyn 3.5%	AB			×			5.3	357
Aminosyn 3.5% M	AB			×			5.3	477
Aminosyn 4.25%	AB				×			
Aminosyn 5%	AB	×	×	×			5.3	500
Aminomysin 7%	AB			×			5.3	700
Aminosyn 7% with electrolytes	AB			×			5.3	1013
Aminosyn 7% (pH 6)	AB			×	×		6.0	711
Aminosyn 8.5%	AB			×	×		5.3	850
Aminosyn 8.5% with electrolytes	AB			×			5.3	1160
Aminosyn 8.5% (pH 6)	AB			×	×		6.0	856
Aminosyn 10%	AB			×	×		5.3	1000
Aminosyn 10% (pH 6)	AB			×	×		6.0	993
Aminosyn II 3.5%	AB				×		5.0–6.5	308
Aminosyn II 3.5% M	AB				×		5.0–6.5	425
Aminosyn II 5%	AB	×	×	×			5.0–6.5	438

CALORIC VALUE/ L	Na	K	Ca	Mg	Cl	Acet	Lact	OTHER	GLASS	PLASTIC
						50			×	
						46		Amino acids 3.5%	×	×
144	47	13		3	40	58		Phosphate 3.5 mM, amino acids 3.5%	×	
								Amino acids 4.2%		×
202		5.4				86		Amino acids 5%	×	
279		5.4				105		Amino acids 7%	×	
	70	66		10	96	124		Phosphate 30 mM, amino acids 7%	×	
		2.7				78		Amino acids 7%	×	
		5.4			35	90		Amino acids 8.5%	×	
	70	66		10	98	142		Phosphate 30 mM, amino acids 8.5%	×	
		2.7			11.7	90		Amino acids 8.5%	×	
394		5.4				148		Amino acids 10%	×	
		2.7				111		Amino acids 10%	×	
	16.3					25.2		Amino acids 3.5%	×	
	36	13		3	37	25		Phosphate 3.5 mM, amino acids 3.5%	×	
	19.3					35.9		Amino acids 5%	×	

(continued)

| | | VOLUME (ml) | | | | | APPROX. | mOsm/ |
LVP NAME	MFR	150	250	500	1000	OTHER	pH	L
Aminosyn II 7%	AB			×	×		5.0–6.5	612
Aminosyn II 7% with electrolytes	AB			×			5.0–6.5	869
Aminosyn II 8.5%	AB			×	×		5.0–6.5	742
Aminosyn II 8.5% with electrolytes	AB			×			5.0–6.5	999
Aminosyn II 10%	AB			×	×		5.0–6.5	873
Aminosyn II 10% with electrolytes	AB				×		5.0–6.5	1130
Aminosyn-HBC 7%	AB			×	×		5.2	665
Aminosyn-PF 7%	AB		×	×			5.4	586
Aminosyn-RF 5.2%	AB					300	5.2	475
BranchAmin 4%	TR			×			6.0	316
FreAmine III 3% with electrolytes	MG				×		6.8	400
FreAmine III 8.5%	MG			×	×		6.5	810
FreAmine III 10%	MG			×	×		6.5	950
FreAmine HBC 6.9%	MG					750	6.5	620
HepatAmine	MG			×			6.5	785
NephrAmine	MG		×				6.5	435
Novamine 11.4%	TR			×	×		5.6	1057
Novamine 15%	TR			×	×		5.2–6.0	1388
ProcalAmine	MG				×		6.8	735
RenAmine	TR		×				6.0	600
Travasol 3.5% with electrolytes	TR			×	×		6.0	450
Travasol 5.5% with electrolytes	TR			×	×	2000	6.0	850
Travasol 5.5% without electrolytes	TR			×	×	2000	6.0	575
Travasol 8.5% with electrolytes	TR			×	×	2000	6.0	1160
Travasol 8.5% without electrolytes	TR			×	×	2000	6.0	890

* *Nonprotein calories.*

CALORIC VALUE/L	mEq/L							OTHER	GLASS	PLASTIC
	Na	K	Ca	Mg	Cl	Acet	Lact			
	31.3					50.3		Amino acids 7%	×	
	76	66		10	86	50		Phosphate 30 mM, amino acids 7%	×	×
	33.3					61.1		Amino acids 8.5%	×	×
	80	66		10	86	61		Phosphate 30 mM, amino acids 8.5%	×	×
	45.3					71.8		Amino acids 10%	×	×
	87	66		10	86	72		Phosphate 30 mM, amino acids 10%	×	
	7				40	72		Amino acids 7%	×	
	3.4					32.5		Amino acids 7%	×	
		5.4				105		Amino acids 5.2%	×	
								Amino acids 4%		×
	35	24.5		5	40	44		Phosphate 3.5 mM, amino acids 3%	×	
	10				<3	72		Phosphate 10 mM, amino acids 8.5%	×	
	10				<3	89		Phosphate 10 mM, amino acids 10%	×	
	10				<3	57		Amino acids 6.9%	×	
	10				<3	62		Phosphate 10 mM, amino acids 8%	×	
	5				<3	44		Essential amino acids 5.4%	×	
						114		Amino acids 11.4%	×	
						151		Amino acids 15%	×	
130*	35	24	3	5	41	47		Phosphate 3.5 mM, amino acids 3%, glycerin 3%	×	
					31	60		Amino acids 6.5%	×	
	25	15		5	25	54		Phosphate 7.5 mM, amino acids 3.5%	×	
	70	60		10	70	100		Phosphate 30 mM, amino acids 5.5%	×	×
					22	48		Amino acids 5.5%	×	×
	70	60		10	70	141		Phosphate 30 mM, amino acids 8.5%	×	×
					34	73		Amino acids 8.5%	×	×

(continued)

LVP NAME	MFR	VOLUME (ml)					APPROX. pH	mOsm/L
		150	250	500	1000	OTHER		
Travasol 10% without electrolytes	TR		×	×	×	2000	6.0	1000
TrophAmine	MG			×			5.5	525

Dextran Injections

LVP NAME	MFR	VOLUME (ml)					APPROX. pH	mOsm/L
		150	250	500	1000	OTHER		
Dextran 75 6% in dextrose 5%	AB			×			4.0	253
Dextran 75 6% in sodium chloride 0.9%	AB			×			4.5	309
Dextran 70 6% in dextrose 5%	PH*			×			3.5–7.0	287
Dextran 70 6% in sodium chloride 0.9%	MG			×			5.7	310
	PH*			×			4.7–7.0	300
	TR†			×			5.0	308
Dextran 40 10% in dextrose 5%	AB‡			×			3.0–7.0	255
	MG			×			4.6	250
	PH§			×			3.7	309
	TR†			×			4.5	252
Dextran 40 10% in sodium chloride 0.9%	AB‡			×			4.5	310
	MG			×			5.5	310
	PH§			×			3.5–7.0	317
	TR†			×			5.0	308

* Macrodex injections.
† Gentran injections.
‡ LMD injections.
§ Rheomacrodex injections.

Dextrose-Saline Injections

LVP NAME	MFR	VOLUME (ml)					APPROX. pH	mOsm/L
		150	250	500	1000	OTHER		
Dextrose 2½% in water	AB				×		5.1	126
	TR				×		4.0	126
Dextrose 2½% in sodium chloride 0.45%	AB		×	×	×		4.5	280
	MG		×	×	×		4.6	280
	TR			×	×		4.0	280

CALORIC VALUE/ L	Na	K	Ca	Mg	Cl	Acet	Lact	OTHER	GLASS	PLASTIC
				40	87			Amino acids 10%	×	
	5				<3	56		Amino acids 6%	×	

CALORIC VALUE/ L	Na	K	Ca	Mg	Cl	Acet	Lact	OTHER	GLASS	PLASTIC
170									×	
	154				154				×	
200									×	×
	154				154				×	
	154				154				×	×
	154				154					×
170									×	
									×	
200									×	×
170										×
	154				154				×	
	154				154				ʍ	
	154				154				×	
	154				154				×	×
										×

CALORIC VALUE/ L	Na	K	Ca	Mg	Cl	Acet	Lact	OTHER	GLASS	PLASTIC
85									×	
85									×	
85	77				77				×	×
85	77				77				×	×
85	77				77					×

(continued)

LVP NAME	MFR	VOLUME (ml)					APPROX. pH	mOsm/ L
		150	250	500	1000	OTHER		
Dextrose 5% in water	AB	×	×	×	×	50,100,400	5.0	253
	MG	×	×	×	×	25,50,100,200		
	TR	×	×	×	×	25,50,100	4.0	252
Dextrose 5% in sodium chloride 0.11%	MG			×	×		4.3	290
Dextrose 5% in sodium chloride 0.2%	AB		×	×	×		4.4	330
	MG		×	×	×	25	4.3	320
	TR		×	×	×		4.0	321
Dextrose 5% in sodium chloride 0.3%	AB		×	×	×		4.4	355
	MG		×	×	×		4.3	365
	TR		×	×	×		4.0	365
Dextrose 5% in sodium chloride 0.45%	AB		×	×	×		4.2	407
	AB		×	×	×		4.4	407
	MG		×	×	×		4.3	405
	TR		×	×	×		4.0	406
Dextrose 5% in sodium chloride 0.9%	AB		×	×	×		4.2	561
	AB		×	×	×		4.4	561
	MG		×	×	×		4.3	560
	TR		×	×	×		4.0	560
Dextrose 7.7% in water	MG					650	4.7	390
Dextrose 10% in water	AB		×	×	×		4.6	505
	MG		×	×	×	50,750	4.6	505
	TR		×	×	×		4.0	505
Dextrose 10% in sodium chloride 0.2%	MG		×	×			4.4	575
Dextrose 10% in sodium chloride 0.45%	MG			×			4.4	660
Dextrose 10% in sodium chloride 0.9%	AB			×	×		4.4	813
	MG				×		4.4	815
	TR			×	×		4.0	813
Dextrose 11.5% in water	MG					650		
Dextrose 20% in water	AB			×			4.4	1010
	MG			×			4.6	1010
	TR			×	×		4.0	1010
Dextrose 30% in water	AB			×				
	MG			×			4.7	1515
	TR			×	×		4.0	1510
Dextrose 38% in water	MG					650	4.7	1920

CALORIC VALUE/L	Na	K	Ca	Mg	Cl	Acet	Lact	OTHER	GLASS	PLASTIC
170									×	×
									×	×
170									×	×
170	19				19				×	×
170	38.5				38.5				×	×
170	34				34				×	×
170	34				34					×
170	51				51				×	×
170	56				56				×	×
170	56				56					×
170	77				77				×	
170	77				77					×
170	77				77				×	×
170	77				77					×
170	154				154				×	
170	154				154					×
170	154				154				×	×
170	154				154					×
260									×	
340									×	×
340									×	×
340									×	×
	34				34				×	
340	77				77				×	×
340	154				154				×	
340	154				154				×	×
340	154				154					×
									×	
680									×	×
680									×	
680									×	×
1020									×	×
1020									×	
									×	×
1290									×	

(continued)

LVP NAME	MFR	VOLUME (ml)					APPROX. pH	mOsm/ L
		150	250	500	1000	OTHER		
Dextrose 40% in water	AB			×				
	MG			×			4.7	2020
	TR			×	×		4.0	2020
Dextrose 50% in water	AB			×	×		4.2	2526
	MG			×	×	2000	5.0	2525
	TR			×	×	2000	4.0	2520
Dextrose 60% in water	AB			×				
	MG			×	×		5.0	3030
	TR			×			4.0	3020
Dextrose 70% in water	AB			×	×	70		
	MG		×	×	×		5.0	3530
	TR			×	×	2000	4.0	3530
Sodium chloride 0.45%	AB			×	×		5.3	154
	AB			×	×		4.8	154
	MG			×	×		5.3	155
	MG			×	×		5.0	155
	TR			×	×		5.0	154
Sodium chloride 0.9%	AB	×	×	×	×	50,100	5.7	308
	AB	×	×	×	×	50,100	4.8	308
	MG	×	×	×	×	25,50,100	5.3	310
	MG			×	×	50,100	4.9	310
	TR	×	×	×	×	25,50,100	5.0	308
Sodium chloride 3%	MG			×			5.8	1030
	TR			×			5.0	1026
Sodium chloride 5%	AB			×			5.6	1711
	MG			×			6.0	1710
	TR			×			5.0	1710

Electrolyte Injections

LVP NAME	MFR	VOLUME (ml)					APPROX. pH	mOsm/ L
		150	250	500	1000	OTHER		
Acetated Ringer's	MG				×		6.7	275
Acetated Ringer's with dextrose 5%	MG				×		4.7	540
Dextrose 2½% in half-strength lactated Ringer's	AB				×		5.0	263
	MG		×				5.1	265
	TR			×			5.0	263
Dextrose 4% in modified lactated Ringer's	MG		×				5.0	255
Dextrose 5% in Electrolyte #48	TR		×	×	×		5.0	347

CALORIC VALUE/L	mEq/L								GLASS	PLASTIC
	Na	K	Ca	Mg	Cl	Acet	Lact	OTHER		
									×	×
1360									×	
1360									×	×
1700									×	×
1700									×	
1700									×	×
									×	×
2040									×	
2040									×	
									×	×
2380									×	
2380									×	
	77				77				×	
	77				77					×
	77				77				×	
	77				77					×
	77				77				×	×
	154				154				×	
	154				154					×
	154				154				×	
	154				154					×
	154				154				×	×
	513				513				×	
	513				513					×
	855				855				×	
	855				855				×	
	855				855					×

CALORIC VALUE/L	mEq/L								GLASS	PLASTIC
	Na	K	Ca	Mg	Cl	Acet	Lact	OTHER		
	131	4	3		109	28			×	
170	131	4	3		122	28				×
89	65	2	1.4		54		14		×	
85	65	2	1		55		14		×	
85	65.5	2	1.5		55		14		×	
135	26	<1	<1		22		6		×	
	25	20		3	24		23	Phosphate 3		×

(continued)

| LVP NAME | MFR | VOLUME (ml) | | | | | APPROX. pH | mOsm/ L |
		150	250	500	1000	OTHER		
Dextrose 5% in Electrolyte #75	TR		×	×	×		5.0	402
Dextrose 5% in lactated Ringer's	AB			×	×		5.3	527
	AB			×	×		4.9	525
	MG		×	×	×		4.7	530
	TR			×	×		5.0	525
Dextrose 5% in Ringer's	AB			×	×		4.0	562
	AB			×	×		4.6	562
	MG				×		4.6	560
	MG				×		4.1	560
	TR			×	×		4.5	561
Dextrose 38% with electrolyte pattern T	MG					650	5.0	2125
Dextrose 50% with electrolyte pattern A	MG			×			4.7	2800
Dextrose 50% with electrolyte pattern B, no K+	MG			×			4.7	2615
Dextrose 50% with electrolyte pattern N	MG			×			4.8	2875
Dextrose 50% with electrolytes and acetate 60 mEq/L	MG			×			5.0	2810
Dextrose 50% with electrolytes	AB			×			4.7	2917
Ionosol B in dextrose 5% in water	AB			×	×		5.8	423
	AB			×	×		5.2	427
Ionosol B with invert sugar 10%	AB				×		4.4	719
Ionosol D with invert sugar 10%	AB				×		4.8	804
Ionosol MB in dextrose 5% in water	AB			×	×		4.7	350
	AB		×	×	×		5.0	350
Ionosol T in dextrose 5% in water	AB		×	×	×		4.7	406
	AB		×	×	×		5.0	415
Isolyte E	MG				×		6.0	310
Isolyte E with dextrose 5%	MG				×		5.8	565
Isolyte G with dextrose 5%	MG				×		3.3	555
Isolyte G with dextrose 10%	MG				×		3.5	805

CALORIC VALUE/L	Na	K	Ca	Mg	Cl	Acet	Lact	OTHER	GLASS	PLASTIC
					mEq/L					
170	40	35			48		20	Phosphate 15		×
179	130	4	3		109		28		×	
179	130	4	3		109		28			×
170	130	4	3		112		28		×	×
170	130	4	3		109		28		×	×
170	147.5	4	4.5		156				×	
170	147	4	4		155					×
170	147	4	4		156				×	
170	147	4	4		156					×
170	147.5	4	4.5		156					×
840	49	46		7.7	54	37		Phosphate 35	×	
850	84	40	10	16	115			Gluconate 13, sulfate 16	×	
850	32		9	16	32			Gluconate 4.2, sulfate 16	×	
	90	80		16	150			Phosphate 28, sulfate 16	×	
850	80	40	9.6	16	70	60		Gluconate 9.6, sulfate 16	×	
850	100	80		16	140	36		Phosphate 24	×	
170	57	25		5	49		25	Phosphate 13	×	
170	57	25		5	49		25	Phosphate 7 mM		×
375	54	25		5	49		22	Phosphate 13	×	
375	80	36	5	3	64		60		×	
170	25	20		3	22		23	Phosphate 3	×	
170	25	20		3	22		23	Phosphate 3		×
170	40	35			40		20	Phosphate 15	×	
170	40	35			40		20	Phosphate 15		×
	140	10	5	3	103	49		Citrate 8	×	×
170	141	10	5	3	103	49		Citrate 8	×	×
170	65	17			149			NH_4 70	×	
340	65	17			149			NH_4 70	×	

(continued)

LVP NAME	MFR	VOLUME (ml)					APPROX. pH	mOsm/L
		150	250	500	1000	OTHER		
Isolyte H, 960 cal	MG				×		4.4	1910
Isolyte H with dextrose 5%	MG				×		5.4	370
Isolyte M with dextrose 5%	MG		×	×	×		5.6	400
Isolyte P with dextrose 5%	MG		×	×	×		5.5	350
Isolyte R with dextrose 5%	MG				×		5.6	380
Isolyte S	MG				×		5.8	295
	MG				×		6.8	295
Isoltye S with dextrose 5%	MG				×		5.3	555
Isolyte S, pH 7.4	MG			×	×		7.4	295
Lactated Ringer's	AB		×	×	×		6.7	273
	AB		×	×	×		6.3	273
	MG		×	×	×		6.3	275
	TR		×	×	×		6.5	273
Normosol M in dextrose 5% in water	AB			×	×		5.2	368
Normosol M, 900 cal	AB				×		4.0	1890
Normosol R	AB			×	×		6.4	295
Normosol R, pH 7.4	AB			×	×		7.4	295
Normosol R in dextrose 5% in water	AB			×	×		5.4	552
	AB			×	×		5.2	547
Plasma-Lyte A	TR			×	×		7.4	294
Plasma-Lyte M in dextrose 5%	TR			×	×		5.0	376
Plasma-Lyte R	TR				×		5.5	312
Plasma-Lyte R in dextrose 5%	TR				×		5.0	564
Plasma-Lyte 56 in dextrose 5%	TR			×	×		5.0	362
Plasma-Lyte 56 in water	TR				×		5.5	110
Plasma-Lyte 148 in dextrose 5%	TR			×	×		5.0	547

CALORIC VALUE/ L	mEq/L									
	Na	K	Ca	Mg	Cl	Acet	Lact	OTHER	GLASS	PLASTIC
960	43	13		3	49	16			×	
170	42	13		3	39	17			×	×
170	38	35			44	20		Phosphate 15	×	×
170	25	20		3	23	23		Phosphate 3	×	×
170	41	16	5	3	40	24			×	×
	140	5		3	98	27		Gluconate 23	×	
	140	5		3	98	27		Gluconate 23		×
170	142	5		3	98	30		Gluconate 23	×	×
	141	5		3	98	27		Gluconate 23, phosphate 1		×
9	130	4	3		109		28		×	
9	130	4	3		109		28			×
	130	4	3		110		28		×	×
	130	4	3		109		28		×	×
170	40	13		3	40	16			×	×
957	40	13		3	40	16		Alcohol 40 ml, dextrose 50 g, fructose 150 g	×	
15	140	5		3	98	27		Gluconate 23	×	×
15	140	5		3	98	27		Gluconate 23	×	×
185	140	5		3	98	27		Gluconate 23	×	
185	140	5		3	98	27		Gluconate 23		×
	140	5		3	98	27		Gluconate 23	×	×
170	40	16	5	3	40	12	12			×
	140	10	5	3	103	47	8			×
170	140	10	5	3	103	47	8		×	
170	40	13		3	40	16				×
	40	13		3	40	16				×
170	140	5		3	98	27		Gluconate 23		×

(continued)

LVP NAME	MFR	VOLUME (ml)					APPROX. pH	mOsm/L
		150	250	500	1000	OTHER		
Plasma-Lyte 148 in water	TR			×	×		5.5	294
Ringer's injection	AB			×	×		5.8	309
	AB			×	×		6.0	309
	MG			×	×		6.1	310
	MG			×	×		5.9	310
	TR			×	×		6.0	309

Fat Emulsion, Intravenous

LVP NAME	MFR	VOLUME (ml)					APPROX. pH	mOsm/L
		150	250	500	1000	OTHER		
Intralipid 10%	BA TR		×	×		50,100	8.0	260
Intralipid 20%	BA TR		×	×		50,100	8.0	268
Liposyn II 10%	AB			×		25,50,100,200	8.0	276
Liposyn II 20%	AB			×		25,50,200	8.3	258
NutriLipid 10%	MG		×	×			6.0–7.9	280
NutriLipid 20%	MG		×	×			6.0–7.9	315
Soyacal 10%	AT		×	×			6.0–7.9	280
Soyacal 20%	AT		×	×			6.0–7.9	315
Travamulsion 10%	TR			×			5.5–9.0	270
Travamulsion 20%	TR			×			5.5–9.0	300

Invert Sugar Injections

LVP NAME	MFR	VOLUME (ml)					APPROX. pH	mOsm/L
		150	250	500	1000	OTHER		
Invert sugar 5% and Electrolyte #2	TR*				×		5.0	449
Invert sugar 10% and Electrolyte #2	TR*				×		5.0	725
Invert sugar 10% in water	MG TR*				× ×		4.4 4.0	555 555
Multiple Electrolyte #2 with invert sugar 5%	MG				×		4.6	445

* *Travert products.*

CALORIC VALUE/L	Na	K	Ca	Mg	Cl	Acet	Lact	OTHER	GLASS	PLASTIC
	140	5		3	98	27		Gluconate 23		×
	147.5	4	4.5		156				×	
	147	4	4		155					×
	147	4	4.5		156				×	
	147	4	4.5		156					×
	147.5	4	4.5		156					×

CALORIC VALUE/L	Na	K	Ca	Mg	Cl	Acet	Lact	OTHER	GLASS	PLASTIC
1.1									×	
2.0									×	
1.1									×	
2.0									×	
1.1									×	
2.0									×	
1.1									×	
2.0									×	
1.1									×	
2.0									×	

CALORIC VALUE/L	Na	K	Ca	Mg	Cl	Acet	Lact	OTHER	GLASS	PLASTIC
187.5	56	25		6	56		25	Phosphate 12.5	×	
375	56	25		6	56		25	Phosphate 12.5	×	
340									×	
375										)(
200	57	25		6	46		25	Phosphate 13	×	

(continued)

LVP NAME	MFR	VOLUME (ml)					APPROX. pH	mOsm/ L
		150	250	500	1000	OTHER		
Multiple Electrolyte #1 with invert sugar 10%	MG				×		4.8	800
Multiple Electrolyte #2 with invert sugar 10%	MG				×		4.7	720

Mannitol Injections

LVP NAME	MFR	VOLUME (ml)					APPROX. pH	mOsm/ L
		150	250	500	1000	OTHER		
Mannitol 5% in water	AB				×		5.6	274
	MG				×		6.0	275
	TR*				×		6.0	274
Mannitol 10% in water	AB				×		5.6	549
	MG				×		6.0	550
	TR*			×	×		6.0	549
Mannitol 15% in water	AB			×			5.7	823
	MG	×					6.0	825
	TR*			×			6.0	823
Mannitol 20% in water	AB			×			5.7	1098
	MG		×	×			6.0	1100
	TR*		×	×			6.0	1098

* *Osmitrol products.*

Premixed Potassium Chloride Injections

LVP NAME	MFR	VOLUME (ml)					APPROX. pH	mOsm/ L
		150	250	500	1000	OTHER		
Dextrose 5% in Ringer's injection, lactated, with potassium chloride 20 mEq	TR				×		5.0	565
Dextrose 5% in Ringer's injection, lactated, with potassium chloride 40 mEq	TR				×		5.0	605

CALORIC VALUE/L	mEq/L								GLASS	PLASTIC
	Na	K	Ca	Mg	Cl	Acet	Lact	OTHER		
400	80	36	5	3	60		60		×	
400	57	25		6	46		25	Phosphate 13	×	

CALORIC VALUE/L	mEq/L								GLASS	PLASTIC
	Na	K	Ca	Mg	Cl	Acet	Lact	OTHER		
									×	
									×	
										×
									×	
									×	
										×
									×	
									×	
										×
									×	
									×	
										×

CALORIC VALUE/L	mEq/L								GLASS	PLASTIC
	Na	K	Ca	Mg	Cl	Acet	Lact	OTHER		
	130	24	3		129		28			×
	130	44	3		149		28			×

(continued)

LVP NAME	MFR	VOLUME (ml)					APPROX. pH	mOsm/L
		150	250	500	1000	OTHER		
Dextrose 5% in	AB				×		4.5	350
sodium chloride	AB				×		4.8	349
0.2% with	MG				×		4.1	340
potassium chloride	TR				×		4.0	341
10 mEq								
Dextrose 5% in	AB				×		4.5	370
sodium chloride	MG		×	×	×		4.6	360
0.2% with	MG				×		4.2	360
potassium chloride	TR			×	×		4.0	361
20 mEq								
Dextrose 5% in	AB				×		4.5	390
sodium chloride	AB				×		4.8	389
0.2% with	MG				×		4.6	380
potassium chloride	MG				×		4.2	380
30 mEq	TR				×		4.0	381
Dextrose 5% in	AB				×		4.5	410
sodium chloride	AB				×		4.8	409
0.2% with	MG				×		4.6	400
potassium chloride	MG				×		4.2	400
40 mEq	TR				×		4.0	401
Dextrose 5% in	MG				×		4.6	405
sodium chloride	TR			×	×		4.0	405
0.33% with								
potassium chloride								
20 mEq								
Dextrose 5% in	MG				×		4.6	425
sodium chloride	TR				×		4.0	425
0.33% with								
potassium chloride								
30 mEq								
Dextrose 5% in	MG				×		4.6	445
sodium chloride	TR				×		4.0	445
0.33% with								
potassium chloride								
40 mEq								
Dextrose 5% in	AB				×		4.5	427
sodium chloride	AB				×		4.8	426
0.45% with	MG				×		4.7	425
potassium chloride	MG				×		4.2	425
10 mEq	TR				×		4.0	426
Dextrose 5% in	AB				×		4.5	447
sodium chloride	MG			×	×		4.7	445
0.45% with	MG				×		4.2	445
potassium chloride	TR			×	×		4.0	446
20 mEq								

CALORIC VALUE/L	Na	K	Ca	Mg	Cl	Acet	Lact	OTHER	GLASS	PLASTIC
170	38.5	10			48.5				×	
170	38.5	10			48.5					×
	34	10			44					×
	34	10			44					×
170	38.5	20			58.5				×	×
170	34	20			54				×	
170	34	20			54					×
	34	20			54					×
170	38.5	30			68.5				×	
170	38.5	30			68.5					×
170	34	30			64				×	
170	34	30			64					×
	34	30			64					×
170	38.5	40			78.5				×	
170	38.5	40			78.5					×
170	34	40			74				×	
170	34	40			74					×
	34	40			74					×
	56	20			76				×	×
	56	20			76					×
	56	30			86				×	
	56	30			86					×
	56	40			96				×	
	56	40			96					×
170	77	10			87				×	
170	77	10			87					×
170	77	10			87				×	
170	77	10			87					×
	77	10			87					×
170	77	20			97				×	×
170	77	20			97				×	
170	77	20			97					×
	77	20			97					×

(continued)

LVP NAME	MFR	VOLUME (ml)					APPROX. pH	mOsm/L
		150	250	500	1000	OTHER		
Dextrose 5% in	AB				×		4.5	467
sodium chloride	AB				×		4.8	467
0.45% with	MG				×		4.7	465
potassium chloride	MG				×		4.2	465
30 mEq	TR				×		4.0	466
Dextrose 5% in	AB				×		4.5	487
sodium chloride	MG				×		4.7	485
0.45% with	MG				×		4.2	485
potassium chloride	TR				×		4.0	486
40 mEq								
Dextrose 5% in sodium chloride 0.9% with potassium chloride 20 mEq	TR				×		4.0	601
Dextrose 5% in sodium chloride 0.9% with potassium chloride 40 mEq	TR				×		5.0	641
Dextrose 5% in water with potassium chloride 10 mEq	TR				×		4.0	272
Dextrose 5% in	AB				×		4.5	293
water with	MG				×		4.2	290
potassium chloride	TR				×		4.0	292
20 mEq								
Dextrose 5% in	AB				×		4.5	313
water with	MG				×		4.2	310
potassium chloride	TR				×		4.0	312
30 mEq								
Dextrose 5% in	AB				×		4.5	333
water with	MG				×		4.2	330
potassium chloride	TR				×		4.0	332
40 mEq								
Dextrose 10% in sodium chloride 0.2% with potassium chloride 20 mEq	MG		×				4.6	615
Sodium chloride 0.9% with potassium chloride 20 mEq	TR				×		5.0	348

CALORIC VALUE/L	mEq/L								GLASS	PLASTIC
	Na	K	Ca	Mg	Cl	Acet	Lact	OTHER		
170	77	30			107				×	
170	77	30			107					×
170	77	30			107				×	
170	77	30			107				·	×
	77	30			107					×
170	77	40			117				×	×
170	77	40			117				×	
170	77	40			117					×
	77	40			117					×
	154	20			174					×
	154	40			194					×
		10			10					×
170		20			20				×	
		20			20				×	×
		20			20					×
170		30			30				×	
		30			30				×	×
		30			30					×
170		40			40				×	
		40			40				×	×
		40			40					×
	34	20			54				×	
	154	20			174					×

(continued)

LVP NAME	MFR	VOLUME (ml)					APPROX. pH	mOsm/L
		150	250	500	1000	OTHER		
Sodium chloride 0.9% with potassium chloride 40 mEq	TR			×			5.0	388

Other Injections

LVP NAME	MFR	VOLUME (ml)					APPROX. pH	mOsm/L
		150	250	500	1000	OTHER		
Alcohol 5% in dextrose 5% in water	AB				×		4.4	1114
	MG				×		5.0	1125
	TR				×		4.5	1114
Alcohol 10% in dextrose 5% in water	MG				×			
Fructose 10% in water	AB				×		3.8	555
	MG				×		4.0	555
Hespan 6% hetastarch in sodium chloride 0.9%	ACC		×				5.5	310
Plegisol (buffered)*	AB				×		7.8	280
R-Gene 10	KA VT					300	5.0–6.5	950
Sodium bicarbonate 5%	AB		×				7.8	1203
	MG		×				8.0	1190
	TR		×				8.0	1190
Sodium lactate, 1/6 molar	AB		×	×			6.9	333
	MG		×	×			6.3	335
	TR		×	×			6.5	334
Sterile water for injection	AB	×	×	×			5.7	
	AB		×	×			5.2	
	MG	×	×	×			5.5	
	TR	×	×	×				

AB, Abbott; ACC, American Critical Care; AD, Adria; BA, Baxter; KV, Kabi-Vitrum; MG, Kendall-McGaw; PH, Pharmacia; TR, Travenol.
* *After addition of 10 mEq of sodium bicarbonate.*

CALORIC VALUE/L	mEq/L							OTHER	GLASS	PLASTIC
	Na	K	Ca	Mg	Cl	Acet	Lact			
	154	40			194					×

CALORIC VALUE/L	mEq/L							OTHER	GLASS	PLASTIC
	Na	K	Ca	Mg	Cl	Acet	Lact			
450									×	
450									×	
150									×	
									×	
375									×	
340									×	
	154				154				×	
	120	16	2.4	32	160			HCO₃ 10		×
					475			Arginine HCl 10%	×	
	595							HCO₃ 595	×	
	595							HCO₃ 595	×	
	595							HCO₃ 595	×	
55	167						167		×	×
	167						167		×	×
54	167						167			×
									×	
										×
									×	×
									×	×

APPENDIX 2. Calculation of IV Medications

DRUGS ADMINISTERED IN μg/kg/min

First: *Convert the amount of drug in solution to micrograms:*

$$\text{mg of drug} \times 1000 - \mu g$$

Then: *Determine number of milliliters equal to 1 μg by setting up a proportion, as follows:*

$$\frac{\mu g \text{ of drug in IV}}{ml \text{ of IV}} = \frac{1 \ \mu g}{X \ ml}$$

X ml = ml in IV ÷ μg of drug in solution.

Next: *Calculate the rate (μg/min or ml/h) for 1 μg/kg/min:*

Rate for 1 μg/kg/min = ml in 1 μg × patient weight in kg × 60

Note: Multiply by 60 because, if using an electronic infusion device that delivers ml/h, you need to multiply the milliliters in one μg/kg/min times 60 min; *or,* if using a microdrip set, you must multiply the milliliters in one μg/kg/min times 60 microdrops.

Then: *Determine the IV rate for the prescribed dosage:*
Multiply result times dose ordered, *or*
Determine dose when IV rate is known by dividing current infusion rate by the result obtained in the last step.

Example
A patient is to receive 5 μg/kg/min of dopamine (Intropin) and the patient weighs 80 kg. What is the appropriate rate of flow?

Add 400 mg dopamine to 500 ml of infusate. Convert the amount of drug in solution to micrograms:

$$400 \text{ mg} \times 1000 = 400{,}000 \text{ } \mu g$$

Determine the number of milliliters equal to 1 μg:

$$\frac{400{,}000 \text{ } \mu g}{500 \text{ ml}} = \frac{1 \text{ } \mu g}{X \text{ ml}}$$

$$X = 500 \div 400{,}000$$

$$= 0.00125 \text{ ml}$$

Calculate the rate for 1 μg/kg/min:

$$0.00125 \text{ ml} \times 80 \text{ kg} \times 60$$

Rate − 6 ml/h or 5 microdrops/min

Determine IV rate for prescribed dose for this patient:

$$5 \text{ } \mu g \times 6 = 30$$

Rate = 30 ml/h or 30 μg/min.

QUICK CALCULATION OF DRUGS ORDERED IN μg/min:

Dopamine

400 mg/500 ml	Multiply kg by 0.075
800 mg/500 ml	0.040
1200 mg/500 ml	0.025
1600 mg/500 ml	0.020

Nitroprusside

50 mg/500 ml	Multiply kg by 0.6
50 mg/250 ml	0.3

Dobutamine

250 mg/500 ml	Multiply kg by 0.12
250 mg/250 ml	0.06
500 mg/250 ml	0.03

APPENDIX 3. Calculation of IV Flow Rates

Any of the following formulas may be used to determine the flow rate of an infusion:

$$\frac{\text{drops/ml; of set}}{60^*} \times \text{total hourly volume} = \text{drops/min}$$

$$\frac{\text{ml/h} \times \text{drop factor of set}}{60^*} = \text{drops/min}$$

For pediatric set, drops/min equals ml to be delivered:

$$\frac{\text{ml/h} \times \text{drop factor}}{60^*} = \text{drops/min}$$

Minutes in 1 hour.

APPENDIX 4. IV Dilution and Stability Chart

DRUG	RECOMMENDED DILUENT VOLUME
Ampicillin	Sterile, bacteriostatic water
	125 mg–1.2 ml
	250 mg–1.0 ml
	500 mg–1.8 ml
	5 ml water 125–500 mg
	5 ml water 125–500 mg
	10 ml water 1–2 g
Amikin	In solution, D5/W, D5½, D5¼, NS, LR
Bactrim	In solution
Carbenicillin	2 ml/g sterile water
	7 ml/g sterile water
	10 ml/g

ROUTE	DELIVERY RATE	STABILITY	DILUTION
IM			
IM		1 h	Per table
IM			
IVP	125–500 mg over 3–5 min		
IV	15–30 min	4–8 h	
IV	15–30 min		
IV	30–60 min	24 h	500 mg/100–200 ml
IV	60–90 min	24 h. Do not mix with other drugs.	5 ml/125 ml D5U/W
IM			At least 1 g/20 ml NS,
IVP			D5/W, LR, D5/½, D5/¼
IV	30–60 min	24 h	

(continued)

DRUG	RECOMMENDED DILUENT VOLUME
Cefazolin	10 ml sterile water
Cefizox	Sterile water: 10 ml/g of NS, D5/W, D5/NS, D5/$\frac{1}{4}$, D5/$\frac{1}{2}$
Cefobid	Sterile, bacteriostatic water: 2.2 ml/g 5 ml/g Allow to stand until foam is gone.
Chloromycetin	10 ml sterile water/g
Cleocin	In solution
Erythromycin	10 ml sterile water/500 mg
Gentamicin	In solution
Mandol	10 ml sterile water/g D5/W, NS, D5/NS, D5/$\frac{1}{2}$, D5/$\frac{1}{4}$
Mefoxin	Sterile water, 10 ml/g
Methicillin	IVP: Add 25 ml sterile NaCl to each ml of IV dilution. IV: 1.5 ml/g sterile water
Minocin	5 ml sterile water, D5/W, NS, D5/NS, LR

ROUTE	DELIVERY RATE	STABILITY	DILUTION
IV IVP	20 min/500 mg 3–5 min	24 h	50–100 ml NS, D5/W, D10/W, D5/RL, D5/NS, D5/$^1/_2$, D5/$^1/_4$
IV	IVP over 3–5 min, IV over 30–60 min	8 h	50–100 ml
IM IV	15–30 min	24 h	25–50 ml/g D5/W, D5/RL, D5/NS, D5/$^1/_2$, D10/W
IV	IVP 100 mg/ml over 1 min, IVPB 20 min/g	24 h	50 ml/g
IV	30 mg/min	24 h	300 mg/50 ml D5/W, NS, LR
IV	20–60 min/500 mg	Administer within 8 h of reconstitution.	1–5 mg/ml NS, LR
IV	30–120 min	24 h	50–200 ml NS or D5/W
IVP IV	3–5 min 30–60 min	24 h	100 ml/1–2 g
IVP IV	3–5 min 30–60 min	24 h	50–100 ml of NS, D5/W, D5/NS, LR, D5/$^1/_2$, D5/$^1/_4$
IVP IV	10 ml/min	24 h	Concentration of 10–30 mg/ml of D5/W, NS, D5/NS, LR
IV	Over 2–24 h	24 h	500–1000 ml

(continued)

DRUG	RECOMMENDED DILUENT VOLUME
Nebcin	In solution
Netromycin	In solution, NS, D5/W, D10/W, LR, D5/NS
Oxacillin	10 ml/g NS, D5/W, D5/NS, LR
Penicillin	Sterile water, 1.6 ml/g
Piperacillin	5 ml bacteriostatic water or saline/g
Tetracycline	5 ml sterile water/250 mg NS, D5/W, D5/NS, LR
Ticar	Bacteriostatic NaCl, 2 ml/g 4 ml/g sterile water or bacteriostatic water/saline
Unipen	15–30 ml sterile water D5/W, NS, D5/$\frac{1}{2}$
Vancomycin	500 mg/10 ml sterile water D5/W, NS
Vibramycin	10 ml sterile water/100 mg; D5/W, NS, D5/LR, D5/$\frac{1}{2}$
Zinacef	9 ml sterile water/750 mg (use 8 ml) NS, D5/W, D5/NS, D5/$\frac{1}{2}$
Zovirax	10 ml sterile water 50 mg/ml

ROUTE	DELIVERY RATE	STABILITY	DILUTION
IV	20–60 min	24 h	1 mg/ml of NS, D5/W
IV	15–120 min	72 h	50–200 ml
IVP IV	Over 10 min 30–60 min	24 h	0.5–2.0 mg/ml
IV	20–30 min	24 h	1,000,000 U/50 ml D5/W, NS, D5/NS
IVP IV	3–5 min Over 30 min	24 h	50 ml/g D5/W, NS, D5/NS, LR
IV	1–6 h	12 h	100–1000 ml NS, D5/W, D5/NS, LR
IM IV	Immediately 30–120 min	24 h	1 g/20 ml minimum
IV IVP	30–60 min	24 h at 2–40 mg/ml concentration	To make concentration of 2–40 mg/ml
IV	20–30 min	6 h	100–200 ml of NS, D5/W
IV	1–4 h	12 h	Minimum of 100 ml/100 mg
IV IVP	30–60 min Over 3–5 min	24 h	1–30 mg/ml of NS, D5/W, D5/NS, D5/¹/₂
IV	60 min	12 h	Less than 2 mg/ml

D5¹/₄, 0.2% dextrose in water; D5¹/₂, 5% dextrose in 0.45% sodium chloride; D5/LR, 5% dextrose in lactated Ringer's solution; D5NS, 5% dextrose in 0.9% sodium chloride; D5/W, 5% dextrose in water; D10/W, 10% dextrose in water; LR, lactated Ringer's solution; NaCl, sodium chloride; NS, 0.9% sodium chloride.

(Adapted from St. Mary's Hospital, Richmond, VA, Department of Pharmacy.

APPENDIX 5. Metric and Apothecaries' Systems*

METRIC	APOTHECARIES
Conversion Factors	
1 mg	1/64 gr
64.79 mg	1 gr (65 mg)
1 g	15.43 gr (15 g)
1 ml	16 minims
3.888 ml or g	1 dram (4 ml or g)
31.103 ml or g	1 oz (30 ml or g)
473.167 ml	1 pint (500 ml)

Weights

0.0001 g =	0.1 mg =	1/640 gr (1/600 gr)
0.0002 g =	0.2 mg =	1/320 gr (1/300 gr)
0.0003 g =	0.3 mg =	1/210 gr (1/200 gr)
0.0004 g =	0.4 mg =	1/150 gr
0.0005 g =	0.5 mg =	1/120 gr
0.0006 g =	0.6 mg =	1/100 gr
0.0007 g =	0.7 mg =	1/90 gr
0.0008 g =	0.8 mg =	1/80 gr
0.0009 g =	0.9 mg =	1/75 gr
0.001 g =	1 mg =	1/64 gr (1/60 gr)
0.0011 g =	1.1 mg =	1/60 gr
0.0013 g =	1.3 mg =	1/50 gr (1.2 mg)
0.0014 g =	1.4 mg =	1/48 gr
0.0016 g =	1.6 mg =	1/40 gr (1.5 mg)
0.0018 g =	1.8 mg =	1/36 gr
0.0020 g =	2 mg =	1/32 gr (1/30 gr)
0.0022 g =	2.2 mg =	1/30 gr
0.0026 g =	2.6 mg =	1/25 gr
0.003 g =	3 mg =	1/20 gr
0.004 g =	4 mg =	1/16 gr (1/15 gr)
0.005 g =	5 mg =	1/12 gr
0.006 g =	6 mg =	1/10 gr
0.007 g =	7 mg =	1/9 gr
0.008 g =	8 mg =	1/8 gr
0.009 g =	9 mg =	1/7 gr
0.01 g =	10 mg =	1/6 gr
0.013 g =	13 mg =	1/5 gr (12 mg)
0.016 g =	16 mg =	1/4 gr (15 mg)

METRIC						APOTHECARIES
0.02	g =	20	mg =		$^1/_3$	gr
0.025	g =	25	mg =		$^3/_8$	gr
0.03	g =	30	mg =		$^2/_5$	gr ($^1/_2$ gr)
0.032	g =	32	mg =		$^1/_2$	gr (30 mg)
0.04	g =	40	mg =		$^3/_5$	gr ($^2/_3$ gr)
0.043	g =	43	mg =		$^2/_3$	gr (40 mg)
0.05	g =	50	mg =		$^3/_4$	gr
0.057	g =	57	mg =		$^7/_8$	gr
0.06	g =	60	mg =		$^9/_{10}$	gr (1 gr)
0.065	g =	65	mg =	1		gr (60 mg)
0.07	g =	70	mg =	1	$^1/_{20}$	gr
0.08	g =	80	mg =	1	$^1/_5$	gr
0.09	g =	90	mg =	1	$^1/_3$	gr
0.097	g =	97	mg =	1	$^1/_2$	gr (0.1 g)
0.12	g =	120	mg =	2		gr
0.2	g =	200	mg =	3		gr
0.24	g =	240	mg =	4		gr (0.25 g)
0.3	g =	300	mg =	4	$^1/_2$	gr
0.33	g =	330	mg =	5		gr (0.3 g)
0.4	g =	400	mg =	6		gr
0.45	g =	450	mg =	7		gr
0.5	g =	500	mg =	7	$^1/_2$	gr
0.53	g =	530	mg =	8		gr
0.6	g =	600	mg =	9		gr
0.65	g =	650	mg =	10		gr (0.6 g)
0.73	g =	730	mg =	11		gr
0.80	g =	800	mg =	12		gr (0.75 g)
0.86	g =	860	mg =	13		gr
0.93	g =	930	mg =	14		gr
1.0	g =	1000	mg =	15		gr
1.06	g =	1060	mg =	16		gr
1.13	g =	1130	mg =	17		gr
1.18	g =	1180	mg =	18		gr
1.26	g =	1260	mg =	19		gr
1.30	g =	1300	mg =	20		gr
1.50	g =	1500	mg =	22		gr
2.0	g =	2000	mg =	30		gr ($^1/_2$ dram)
4.0	g		=	1		dram (60 gr)
5.0	g		=	75		gr
8.0	g		=	2		drams (7.5 g)

(continued)

METRIC			APOTHECARIES	
10.0	g	=	2 ¹/₂	drams
15.0	g	=	4	drams
30.0	g	=	1	oz

Liquid Measures

0.03	ml	=		¹/₂ minim
0.05	ml	=		³/₄ minim
0.06	ml	=	1	minim
0.1	ml	=	1 ¹/₂	minims
0.2	ml	=	3	minims
0.25	ml	=	4	minims
0.3	ml	=	5	minims
0.5	ml	=	8	minims
0.6	ml	=	10	minims
0.75	ml	=	12	minims
1.0	ml	=	15	minims
2.0	ml	=	30	minims
3.0	ml	=	45	minims
4.0	ml	=	1	fluid dram
5.0	ml	=	1 ¹/₄	fluid drams
8	ml	=	2	fluid drams
10	ml	=	2 ¹/₂	fluid drams
15	ml	=	4	fluid drams
20	ml	=	5 ¹/₂	fluid drams
25	ml	=		⁵/₆ fluid oz
30	ml	=	1	fluid oz
50	ml	=	1 ³/₄	fluid oz
60	ml	=	2	fluid oz
100	ml	=	3 ¹/₂	fluid oz
120	ml	=	4	fluid oz
200	ml	=	7	fluid oz
250	ml	=	8	fluid oz
360	ml	=	12	fluid oz
500	ml	=	1	pint
1000	ml	=	1	quart

g, grams; gr, grains; mg, milligram; ml, milliliter; oz, ounce.
* *Approved* approximate *dose equivalents are enclosed in parentheses. Use* exact *equivalents in calculations.*
(Adapted from Culver VM. Modern bedside nursing. Philadelphia: WB Saunders, 1969.)

APPENDIX 6. Comparative Scales of Measures, Weights, and Temperatures

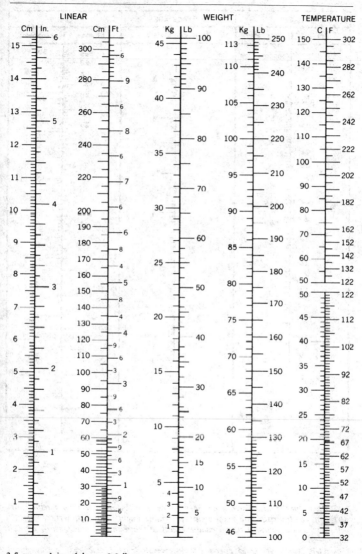

2.5 cm = 1 in.; 1 kg = 2.2 lb.
(Brunner LS, Suddarth DS. Lippincott manual of nursing practice, 4th ed. Philadelphia: JB Lippincott, 1986:1527–1529.)

APPENDIX 7. Nomogram for Estimating Surface Area of Infants and Young Children*

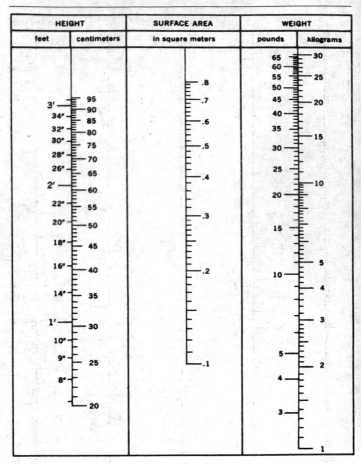

* To determine the surface area of the patient, draw a straight line from the point representing height on the left vertical scale to the point representing weight on the right vertical scale. The point at which this line intersects the middle vertical scale represents the patient's surface area in square meters.

(Sager DP, Bomar SK. Quick reference to intravenous drugs. Philadelphia: JB Lippincott, 1983.)

APPENDIX 8. Nomogram for Estimating Surface Area of Older Children and Adults

HEIGHT		SURFACE AREA	WEIGHT	
feet	centimeters	in square meters	pounds	kilograms

			440	200
			420	190
			400	180
			380	170
			360	160
			340	150
	220	3.00	320	140
7'	215	2.90	300	
10"	210	2.80	290	130
8"	205	2.70	280	
6"	200	2.60	270	120
4"	195	2.50	260	
2"	190	2.40	250	110
6'	185	2.30	240	
10"	180	2.20	230	
	175	2.10	220	100
8"	170	2.00	210	95
6"	165	1.95	200	90
4"	160	1.90	190	85
2"	155	1.85	180	80
5'	150	1.80	170	75
10"	145	1.75	160	
8"	140	1.70	150	70
6"	135	1.65	140	65
4"	130	1.60	130	60
2"	125	1.55	120	55
4'	120	1.50	110	50
10"	115	1.45	100	45
8"	110	1.40	90	40
6"	105	1.35	80	35
4"	100	1.30		
2"	95	1.25	70	30
3'	90	1.20	60	25
10"	85	1.15	50	20
8"	80	1.10		
6"	75	1.05		

(Sager DP, Bomar SK. *Quick reference to intravenous drugs.* Philadelphia: JB Lippincott, 1983.)

Blood, Plasma, or Serum Values

DETERMINATION	REFERENCE RANGE	
	CONVENTIONAL	SI
Acetoacetate plus acetone	Negative	
Aldolase	1.3–8.2 U/L	22–137 nmol · sec^{-1}/L
Ammonia	12–55 μmol/L	12–55 μmol/L
Amylase	4–25 U/ml	4–25 arb. unit
Ascorbic acid	0.4–1.5 mg/100 ml	23–85 μmol/L
Bilirubin	Direct: Up to 0.4 mg/100 ml Total: Up to 1 mg/100 ml	Up to 7 μmol/L Up to 17 μmol/L
Blood volume	8.5%–9.0% kg body wt	80–85 ml/kg
Calcium	8.5–10.5 mg/100 ml (slightly higher in children)	2.1–2.6 mM/L
Carbon dioxide content	24–30 mEq/L	24–30 mM/L
Carbamazepine	4–12 μg/ml	17–51 μmol/L
Carbon monoxide	Less than 5% of total hemoglobin	
Carotenoids	0.8–4.0 μg/ml	1.5–7.4 μmol/L
Ceruloplasmin	27–37 mg/100 ml	1.8–2.5 μmol/L
Chloramphenicol	10–20 μg/ml	31–62 μmol/L

MINIMAL MI REQUIRED	NOTE	METHOD
1-B		Behre. J Lab Clin Med 1928;13:770 (modified).
2-S	Use unhemolyzed serum	Beisenherz et al. Z Naturforsch 1963:86:555.
2-B	Collect in heparinized tube; deliver *immediately* packed in ice	Da Fonseca-Wolheim. J Clin Chem Clin Biochem 1973;11:421.
1-S		Zinterhofer et al. Clin Chim Acta 1973;43:5.
7-B	Collect in heparinized tube before any food is given	Roe, Kuether. J Biol Chem 1943;147:399.
1-S		Gambino. Standard Methods Clin Chem 1965:5:55.
		Isotope dilution technique with I-131 albumin
1-S		Spectrophotometry using cresolphthalein complexone
1-S	Fill tube to top	By CO_2 electrode
		Liquid chromatography
3-B	Fill tube to top	Multi-wave length spectrophotometry
3-S	Vitamin A may be done on same specimen	Natelson. Microtechniques of clinical chemistry, 2nd ed. 1961, p. 454.
2-S		Ravin. J Lab Clin Med. 1961;58:161.
0.2-S		Liquid chromatography

(continued)

DETERMINATION	REFERENCE RANGE	
	CONVENTIONAL	SI
Chloride	100–106 mEq/L	100–106 mM/L
CK isoenzymes	5% MB or less	
Copper	Total: 100–200 μg/100 ml	16–31 μmol/L
Creatine kinase	Female: 10–79 U/L Male: 17–148 U/L	167–1317 nmol • sec⁻¹/L 283–2467 nmol • sec⁻¹/L
Creatinine	0.6–1.5 mg/100 ml	53–133 μmol/L
Ethanol	0 mg/100 ml	0 mM/L
Glucose	Fasting: 70–110 mg/100 ml	3.9–5.6 mM/L
Iron	50–150 μg/100 ml (higher in males)	9.0–26.9 μmol/L
Iron-binding capacity	250–410 μg/100 ml	44.8–73.4 μmol/L
Lactic acid	0.6–1.8 mEq/L	0.6–1.8 mM/L
Lactic dehydrogenase	45–90 U/L	750–1500 nmol • sec⁻¹/L
Lead	50 μg/100 ml or less	Up to 2.4 μmol/liter
Lipase	2 U/ml or less	Up to 2 arb. unit
Lipids Cholesterol	120–220 mg/100 ml	3.10–5.69 mM/L
Triglycerides	40–150 mg/100 ml	0.4–1.5 g/L

MINIMAL MI REQUIRED	NOTE	METHOD
1-S		Cotlove. Standard Methods Clin Chem 1961:3:81.
0.2-S		Electrophoresis
1-S		Atomic-absorption spectrophotometry
1-S		Szasz. Clin Chem 1976:22:650.
1-S		Fabiny, Ertingshausen. Clin Chem 1971:17:696.
2-B	Collect in oxalate and refrigerate	Gas-liquid chromatography
1-P	Collect with oxalate-fluoride mixture	Bergmeyer. Methods of enzymatic analysis. 1965, p. 117.
1-S		Spectrophotometry using Ferrozine
1-S		Spectrophotometry using Ferrozine
2-B	Collect with oxalate-fluoride; deliver immediately packed in ice	Hadjivassiliou, Rieder. Clin Chim Acta 1968:19:357.
1-S	Unsuitable if hemolyzed	Gay, McComb, Bowers. Clin Chem 1968:14:740.
2-B	Collect with oxalate-fluoride mixture	Berman. Atom Absorp Newslett 1964:3:9 (modified).
1-S		Zinterhofer. Clin Chim Acta 1973:44:173.
1-S	Fasting	Siedel. J Clin Chem Clin Biochem 1981:19:838.
1-S	Fasting	Ziegenhorn. Clin Chem 1975:21:1627.

(continued)

	REFERENCE RANGE	
DETERMINATION	CONVENTIONAL	SI
Lipoprotein electrophoresis		
Lithium	0.5–1.5 mEq/L	0.5–1.5 mM/L
Magnesium	1.5–2.0 mEq/L	0.8–1.3 mM/L
5' Nucleotidase	1–11 U/L	17–183 nmol • sec^{-1}/L
Osmolality	280–296 mOsm/kg water	280–296 mM/kg
Oxygen saturation (arterial)	96%–100%	0.96–1.00
PCO_2	35–45 mmHg	4.7–6.0 kPa
pH	7.35–7.45	Same
PO_2	75–100 mmHg (dependent on age) while breathing room air; above 500 mmHg while on 100% O_2	10.0–13.3 kPa
Phenobarbital	15–50 μg/ml	65–215 μmol/L
Phenytoin (Dilantin)	5–20 μg/ml	20–80 μmol/L
Phosphatase (acid)	Male, total: 0.13–0.63 sigma U/ml Female, total: 0.01–0.56 sigma U/ml Prostatic: 0–0.5 Fishman-Lerner U/100 ml	36–175 nmol • sec^{-1}/L 2.8–156 nmol • sec^{-1}/L

MINIMAL MI REQUIRED	NOTE	METHOD
2-S	Fasting, do not freeze serum	Less, Hatch. J Lab Clin Med 1963:61:518.
1-S		Pybus, Bowers. Clin Chem 1970:16:139.
1-S		Willis. Clin Chem 1965:11:251 (modified).
1-S		Arkesteijn. J Clin Chem Clin Biochem 1976:14:155.
1-S		Osmometry using freezing-point depression
3-B	Deliver in sealed heparinized syringe packed in ice	Gordy, Drabkin. J Biol Chem 1957:227:285.
2-B	Collect and deliver in sealed heparinized syringe	By CO_2 electrode
2-B	Collect without stasis in sealed heparinized syringe; deliver packed in ice	Glass electrode
2-B		Oxygen electrode
1-S		Liquid chromatography
1-S		Liquid chromatography
1-S	Must always be drawn just before analysis or stored as frozen serum; avoid hemolysis	Bessey et al. J Biol Chim 1946:164:321. Babson et al. Clin Chim Acta 1966:13:264.

(continued)

	REFERENCE RANGE	
DETERMINATION	CONVENTIONAL	SI
Phosphatase (alkaline)	13–39 U/L; infants and adolescents up to 104 U/L	217–650 nmol • sec^{-1}/L, up to 1.26 mol • sec^{-1}/L
Phosphorus (inorganic)	3.0–4.5 mg/100 ml (infants in first year up to 6.0 mg/100 ml)	1.0–1.5 mM/L
Potassium	3.5–5.0 mEq/L	3.5–5.0 mM/L
Primidone (Mysoline)	4–12 μg/ml	18–55 μmol/L
Procainamide	4–10 μg/ml	17–42 μmol/L
Protein		
Total	6.0–8.4 g/100 ml	60–84 g/L
Albumin	3.5–5.0 g/100 ml	35–50 g/L
Globulin	2.3–3.5 g/100 ml	23–35 g/L
Electrophoresis	(% of total protein)	
Albumin	52–68	
Globulin		
α$_1$	4.2–7.2	
α$_2$	6.8–12.0	
β	9.3–15.0	
γ	13–23	
Pyruvic acid	0–0.11 mEq/L	0–0.11 mM/L
Quinidine	1.2–4.0 μg/ml	3.7–12.3 μmol/L
Salicylate	0	
Therapeutic	20–25 mg/100 ml; 25–30 mg/100 ml to age 10 given 3 h post dose	1.4–1.8 mM/L 1.8–2.2 mM/L
Sodium	135–145 mEq/L	135–145 mM/L

MINIMAL MI REQUIRED	NOTE	METHOD
1-S		Stevens, Thomas. Clin Chim Acta 1972:37:541.
1-S		Daly, Ertingshausen. Clin Chem 1972:18:263.
1-S	Serum must be separated promptly from cells	Ion-selective electrode
1-S		Enzyme immunoassay
1-S		Liquid chromatography
1-S		Weichselbaum. Am J Clin Pathol 1946:16:40.
1-S		Doumas et al. Clin Chim Acta 1971:31:87.
	Globulin equals total protein minus albumin	
1-S	Quantitation by densitometry	Kunkel, Tiselius. J Gen Physiol 1951:35:89. Durrum. J Am Chem Soc 1950:72:2943.
2-B	Collect with oxalate fluoride; deliver immediately packed in ice	Hadjivassiliou, Rieder. Clin Chim Acta 1968:19:357.
1-S		Liquid chromatography
2-P		Keller. Am J Clin Pathol 1947:17:415.
1-S		Ion-selective electrode

(continued)

	REFERENCE RANGE	
DETERMINATION	CONVENTIONAL	SI
Sulfonamide	5–15 mg/100 ml	
Transaminase		
SGOT (aspartate aminotransferase)	7–27 U/L	117–450 nmol • sec^{-1}/L
SGPT (alanine aminotransferase)	1–21 U/L	17–350 nmol • sec^{-1}/L
Urea nitrogen	8–25 mg/100 ml	2.9–8.9 mM/L
Uric acid	3–7 mg/100 ml	0.18–0.42 mM/L
Vitamin A	0.15–0.6 μg/ml	0.5–2.1 μmol/L

Special Endocrine Tests

Steroid Hormones

Aldosterone	Excretion: 5–19 μg/24 h	14–53 nmol/day
	Supine: 48 ± 29 pg/ml	133 ± 80 pmol/L
	Upright (2 h): 65 ± 23 pg/ml	180 ± 64 pmol/L
	Supine: 107 ± 45 pg/ml	279 ± 125 pmol/L
	Upright (2 h): 239 ± 123 pg/ml	663 ± 341 pmol/L
	Supine: 175 ± 75 pg/ml	485 ± 208 pmol/L
	Upright (2 h): 532 ± 228 pg/ml	1476 ± 632 pmol/L

MINIMAL MI REQUIRED	NOTE	METHOD
2-P		Bratton, Marshall. J Biol Chem 1939:128:537.
1-S		Karmen et al. J Clin Invest 1955:34:126.
1-S		Henry et al. Am J Clin Pathol 1960:34:381.
1-S		Paulson et al. Clin Chem 1971:17:644
1-S		Spectrophotometry using uricase
3-S		Natelson. Microtechniques of clinical chemistry, 2nd ed. 1961, p. 451.

5/day	Keep specimen cold	Bayard et al. J Clin Endocrinol Metab 1970:31:507.
3-S, P	Fasting, at rest, 210-mEq sodium diet Upright, 2 h, 210-mEq sodium diet Fasting, at rest, 110-mEq sodium diet Upright, 2 h, 110-mEq sodium diet Fasting, at rest, 10-mEq sodium diet Upright, 2 h, 10-mEq sodium diet	Poulson et al. Clin Immunol Immunopathol 1974:2:373.

(continued)

DETERMINATION	REFERENCE RANGE	
	CONVENTIONAL	SI
Cortisol	8 am: 5–25 μg/100 ml	0.14–0.69 μmol/L
	8 pm: Below 10 μg/100 ml	0–0.28 μmol/L
	4-h ACTH test: 30–45 μg/100 ml	0.83–1.24 μmol/L
	Overnight suppression test: Below 5 μg/100 ml	0.14 nmol/L
	Excretion: 20–70 μg/24 h	55–193 nmol/day
Dehydroepi-androsterone (DHEA)	Male: 0.5–5.5 ng/ml	1.7–19 nmol/L
	Female:	
	1.4–8.0 ng/ml	4.9–28 nmol/L
	0.3–4.5 ng/ml	1.0–15.6 nmol/L
Dehydroepi-androsterone sulfate (DHEA-S)	Male: 151–446 μg/100 ml	3.9–11.4 μmol/L
	Female	2.2–11.1 μmol/L
	84–433 μg/100 ml	0.04–4.5 μmol/L
	1.7–177 μg/100 ml	
11-Deoxycortisol	Responsive: Over 7.5 μg/100 ml	>0.22 μmol/L
Estradiol	Male: <50 pg/ml	<184 pmol/L
	Female	
	23–361 pg/ml	84–1325 pmol/L
	<30 pg/ml	<110 pmol/L
	<20 pg/ml	<73 pmol/L
Progesterone	Male: <1.0 ng/ml	<3.2 nmol/L
	Female	
	0.2–0.6 ng/ml	0.6–1.9 nmol/L
	0.3–3.5 ng/ml	0.95–11 nmol/L
	6.5–32.2 ng/ml	21–102 nmol/L

MINIMAL MI REQUIRED	NOTE	METHOD
1-P	Fasting	Catt, Tregear. Science 1967:158:1670.
1-P	At rest	
1-P	20 U ACTH, IV per 4 h	
1-P	8 AM sample after 0.5 mg dexamethasone by mouth at midnight	
2/day	Keep specimen cold	
2-S, P		Sekihara, Ohsawa. Steroids. 1974:24:317.
	Adult	
	Postmenopausal	
2-S, P		Buster, Abraham. Anal Lett 1972:5:543.
	Adult	
	Postmenopausal	
1-P	8 am sample, preceded by 4.5 g/24 h of metyrapone by mouth or by single dose of 2.5 g by mouth at midnight	Mahajan et al. Steroids 1972:20:609.
5-S, P		Mikhail et al. Steroids 1970:15:333.
	Adult	
	Postmenopausal	
	Prepubertal	
5-S, P		Furuyama, Nugent. Steroids 1971:17:663.
	Follicular phase	
	Midcycle peak	
	Postovulatory	

(continued)

	REFERENCE RANGE	
DETERMINATION	CONVENTIONAL	SI
Testosterone	Adult male: 300–1100 ng/100 ml	10.4–38.1 nmol/L
	Adolescent male: Over 100 ng/100 ml	>3.5 nmol/L
	Female: 25–90 ng/100 ml	0.87–3.12 nmol/L
Unbound testosterone	Adult male: 3.06–24.0 ng/100 ml	106–832 pmol/L
	Adult female: 0.09–1.28 ng/100 ml	3.1–44.4 pmol/L

Polypeptide Hormones

Adrenocortico-tropin (ACTH)	15–70 pg/ml	3.3–15.4 pmol/L
α subunit	<0.5–2.5 mg/ml	<0.4–2.0 nmol/L
	<0.5–5.0 ng/ml	<0.4–4.0 nmol/L
Calcitonin	Male: 0–14 pg/ml	0–4.1 pmol/L
	Female: 0–28 pg/ml	0–8.2 pmol/L
	>100 pg/ml in medullary carcinoma	>29.3 pmol/L
Follicle-stimulating hormone	Male: 3–18 mU/ml	3–18 arb. unit
	Female:	
	4.6–22.4 mU/ml	4.6–22.4 arb. unit
	13–41 mU/ml	13–41 arb. unit
	30–170 mU/ml	30–170 arb. unit
Growth hormone	Below 5 ng/ml	<233 pmol/L
	Children: Over 10 ng/ml	>465 pmol/L
	Female: Up to 30 ng/ml	0–1395 pmol/L
	Below 5 ng/ml	<233 pmol/L
Insulin	6–26 μU/ml	43–187 pmol/L
	Below 20 μU/ml	<144 pmol/L
	Up to 150 μU/ml	0–1078 pmol/L

MINIMAL MI REQUIRED	NOTE	METHOD
1-P	am sample	Catt, Tregear. Science 1967:158:1670.
2-P	am sample	Forest et al. Steroids 1968:12:323
5-P	Place specimen on ice and send promptly to laboratory. Use EDTA tube only	Gonzales. Clin Chem 1980:26:1228.
2-S	Adult male or female Postmenopausal female	Kourides et al. Endocrinology 1974:94:1411.
5-S	Test done only on known or suspected cases of medullary carcinoma of the thyroid	Deftos et al. Metabolism 1971:20:1129. Deftos et al. Metabolism 1971:20:428.
5-S, P	Same sample may be used for LH Pre- or postovulatory Midcycle peak Postmenopausal	Midgley. J Clin Endocrinol Metab 1967:27:295.
1-S	Fasting, at rest After exercise After glucose load	Glick et al. Nature 1963:199:784.
1-S	Fasting During hypoglycemia After glucose load	Morgan, Lazarow. Proc Soc Exp Biol Med 1962:110:29.

(continued)

	REFERENCE RANGE	
DETERMINATION	CONVENTIONAL	SI
Luteinizing hormone	Male: 3–18 mU/ml	3–18 arb. unit
	Female:	
	2.4–34.5 mU/ml	2.4–34.5 arb. unit
	43–187 mU/ml	43–187 arb. unit
	30–150 mU/ml	30–150 arb. unit
Parathyroid hormone	<25 pg/ml	<2.94 pmol/L
Prolactin	2–15 ng/ml	0.08–6.0 nmol/L
Renin activity	Supine: 1.1 ± 0.8 ng/ml/h	0.9 ± 0.6 nmol/L/h
	Upright: 1.9 ± 1.7 ng/ml/h	1.5 ± 1.3 nmol/L/h
	Supine: 2.7 ± 1.8 ng/ml/h	2.1 ± 1.4 nmol/L/h
	Upright: 6.6 ± 2.5 ng/ml/h	5.1 ± 1.9 nmol/L/h
	Diuretics: 10.0 ± 3.7 ng/ml/h	7.7 ± 2.9 nmol/L/h
Somatomedin C (Sm-C, IGF-1)	0.08–2.8 U/ml	0.08–2.8 arb. unit
	0.9–5.9 U/ml	0.9–5.9 arb. unit
	0.34–1.9 U/ml	0.34–1.9 arb. unit
	0.45–2.2 U/ml	0.45–2.2 arb. unit
Thyroid Hormones		
Thyroid-stimulating hormone	0.5–5.0 µU/ml	0.5–5.0 arb. unit
Thyroxine-binding globulin capacity	15–25 µg T_4/100 ml	193–322 nmol/L
Total triiodo-thyronine (T_3)	75–195 ng/100 ml	1.16–3.00 nmol/L

MINIMAL MI REQUIRED	NOTE	METHOD
5-S, P	Same sample may be used for FSH. Pre- or postovulatory Midcycle peak Postmenopausal	Odell et al. J Clin Invest 1967:46:248.
5-P	Keep blood on ice, or plasma must be frozen if it is to be sent any distance; am sample	Stewart et al. N Engl J Med 1982:306:1136.
2-S		Sinha et al. J Clin Endocrinol Metab 1973:36:509.
4-P	EDTA tubes, on ice, normal diet	Haber et al. J Clin Endocrinol Metab
	Low-sodium diet	1969:29:1349.
2-P	EDTA plasma, prepubertal During puberty Adult males Adult females	Furlanetto et al. J Clin Invest 1977:60:648.
2-S		Ridgway et al. J Clin Invest 1973:52:2785.
2-S		Levy et al. J Clin Endocrinol Metab 1971:32:372.
2-S		Larsen et al. J Clin Invest 1972:51:1939.

(continued)

	REFERENCE RANGE	
DETERMINATION	CONVENTIONAL	SI
Reverse triiodo-thyronine (rT3)	13–53 ng/ml	0.2–0.8 nmol/L
Total thyroxine by RIA (T_4)	4–12 μg/100 ml	52–154 nmol/L
T_3 resin uptake	25%–35%	0.25–0.35
Free thyroxine index (FT_4I)	1–4	

Vitamin D Derivatives

1,25-Dihydroxy-vitamin D	26–65 pg/ml	62–155 pmol/L
25-Hydroxy-vitamin D	8–55 ng/ml	19.4–137 nmol/L

Hematologic Values

Coagulation Factors

Factor I (fibrinogen)	0.15–0.35 g/100 ml	4.0–10.0 μmol/L
Factor II (prothrombin)	60%–140%	0.60–1.40
Factor V (accelerator globulin)	60%–140%	0.60–1.40
Factor VII-X (proconvertin-Stuart)	70%–130%	0.70–1.30
Factor X (Stuart factor)	70%–130%	0.70–1.30

MINIMAL MI REQUIRED	NOTE	METHOD
2-S		Cooper et al. J Clin Endocrinol Metab 1982:54:101.
1-S		Chopra. J Clin Endocrinol Metab 1972:34:938.
2-S		Taybearn et al. J Nucl Med 1967:8:739.
2-S		Sarin, Anderson. Arch Intern Med 1970:126:631.
1-S		Reinhardt et al. J Clin Endocrinol Metab 1984:58:91
1-S		Preece et al. Clin Chim Acta 1974:54:235.
4.5-P	Collect in Vacutainer containing sodium citrate	Ratnoff, Menzies. J Lab Clin Med 1951:37:316.
4.5-P	Collect in platic tubes with 3.8% sodium citrate	Owren, Aas. Scand J Clin Lab Invest 1951:3:201.
4.5-P	Collect as in factor II determination	Lewis, Ware. Proc Soc Exp Biol Med 1953:84:640.
4.5-P	Collect as in factor II determination	Same as factor II
4.5-P	Collect as in factor II determination	Bachman et al. Thromb Diath Haemorrh 1958:2:29.

(continued)

	REFERENCE RANGE	
DETERMINATION	CONVENTIONAL	SI
Factor VIII (anti-hemophilic globulin)	50%–200%	0.50–2.0
Factor IX (plasma thromboplastic cofactor)	60%–140%	0.60–1.40
Factor XI (plasma thromboplastic antecedent)	60%–140%	0.60–1.40
Factor XII (Hageman factor)	60%–140%	0.60–1.40

Coagulation Screening Tests

Bleeding time (Simplate)	3.0–9.5 min	180–570 sec
Prothrombin time	Less than 2-sec deviation from control	Less than 2-sec deviation from control
Partial thromboplastin time (activated)	25–38 sec	25–38 sec
Whole-blood clot lysis	No clot lysis in 24 h	0/day

Fibrinolytic Studies

Euglobin lysis	No lysis in 2 h	0/2 h
Fibrinogen split products	Negative reaction at >1:4 dilution	0 (at 1:4 dilution)
Thrombin time	Control ± 5 sec	Control ± 5 sec

MINIMAL MI REQUIRED	NOTE	METHOD
4.5-P	Collect as in factor II determination	Tocantins, Kazal. Blood coagulation, hemorrhage and thrombosis, 2nd ed. 1964.
4.5-P	Collect as in factor II determination	*Ibid*
4.5-P	Collect as in factor II determination	*Ibid*
4.5-P	Collect as in factor II determination	*Ibid*
		Simplate Bleeding Time Device (General Diagnostics)
4.5-P	Collect in Vacutainer containing 3.8% sodium citrate	Colman et al. Am J Clin Pathol 1975:64:108.
4.5-P	Collect in Vacutainer containing 3.8% sodium citrate	Babson, Babson. Am J Clin Pathol 1974:62:856.
2.0-whole blood	Collect in sterile tube and incubate at 37°C	Page, Culver. Syllabus, laboratory examination and clinical diagosis. 1960, p. 207.
4.5-P	Collect as in factor II determination	Sherry et al. J Clin Invest 1959:38:810
4.5-S	Collect in special tube containing thrombin and epsilon aminocaproic acid	Carvalho. Am J Clin Pathol 1974:62:107.
4.5-P	Collect as in factor II determination	Stefanini, Dameshel. Hemorrhagic disorders. 1962, p. 492.

(continued)

	REFERENCE RANGE	
DETERMINATION	CONVENTIONAL	SI

Complete Blood Count

Hematocrit	Male: 45%–52% Female: 37%–48%	Male: 0.45–0.52 Female: 0.37–0.48
Hemoglobin	Male: 13–18 g/100 ml Female: 12–16 g/100 ml	Male: 8.1–11.2 mM/L Female: 7.4–9.9 mM/L
Leukocyte count	4300–10,800/mm^3	4.3–10.8×10^9/L
Erythrocyte count	4.2–5.9 10^6/mm^3	4.2–5.9×10^{12}/L
Mean corpuscular volume (MCV)	86–98 μm^3/cell	86–98 fl
Mean corpuscular hemoglobin (MCH)	27–32 pg/RBC	1.7–2.0 pg/cell
Mean corpuscular hemoglobin concentration (MCHC)	32%–36%	0.32–0.36
Erythrocyte sedimentation rate	Male: 1–13 mm/h Female: 1–20 mm/h	Male: 1–13 mm/h Female: 1–20 mm/h

Erythrocyte Enzymes

Glucose-6-phosphate dehydrogenase	5–15 U/g Hgb	5–15 U/g
Pyruvate kinase	13–17 U/g Hgb	13–17 U/g
Ferritin (serum)		
Iron deficiency	0–12 ng/ml 13–20 borderline	0–4.8 nmol/L 5.2–8 nmol/L borderline
Iron excess	>400 ng/liter	>160 nmol/L

MINIMAL MI REQUIRED	NOTE	METHOD
1-B	Use EDTA as anti-coagulant; the seven listed tests are performed automatically on the Ortho ELT 800, which directly determines cell counts, hemoglobin (as the cyanmethemoglobin derivative), and MCV and computes hematocrit, MCH, and MCHC	
5-B	Use EDTA as anticoagulant	Modified Westergren method. Gambino et al. Am J Clin Pathol 1965;35:173.
9-B	Use special anticoagulant (ACD solution)	Beck. J Biol Chem 1958;232:251.
8-B	Use special anticoagulant (ACD solution)	Beutler. Red cell metabolism, 2nd ed. 1975, p. 60. Addison et al. J Clin Pathol 1972;25:326.

(continued)

	REFERENCE RANGE	
DETERMINATION	CONVENTIONAL	SI
Folic acid		
Normal	>3.3 ng/ml	>7.3 nmol/L
Borderline	2.5–3.2 ng/ml	5.75–7.39 nmol/L
Haptoglobin	40–336 mg/100 ml	0.4–3.36 g/L

Hemoglobin Studies

Electrophoresis for abnormal hemoglobin		
Electrophoresis for A_2 hemoglobin	3%	0.015–0.035
Borderline	0.3–3.5%	0.03–0.035
Hemoglobin F (fetal hemoglobin)	Less than 2%	<0.02
Hemoglobin, met- and sulf-	0	0
Serum hemoglobin	2–3 mg/100 ml	1.2–1.9 μmol/L
Thermolabile hemoglobin	0	0
Lupus anticoagulant	0	0

Leukocyte Alkaline Phosphatase

Qualitative method	Males: 33–188 U	33–188 U
	Female (off contraceptive pill): 30–160 U	30–160 U
Muramidase	Serum, 3–7 μg/ml	3–7 mg/L
	Urine, 0–2 μg/ml	0–2 mg/L

MINIMAL MI REQUIRED	NOTE	METHOD
1-S		Waxman, Schreiber. Blood 1973:42:281.
1-S		
1-S		Behring Diagnostic Reagent Kit
5-B	Collect with anticoagulant	Singer. Am J Med 1955:18.633.
5-B	Use oxalate as anticoagulant	Abraham. Hemoglobin 1976:1:27.
5-B	Collect with anticoagulant	Maile. Laboratory medicine—hematology, 2nd ed. 1962, p. 845.
5-B	Use heparin as anticoagulant	Michel, Harris. J Lab Clin Med 1940:29:445.
2-S		Hunter et al. Am J Clin Pathol 1950:20:429.
1-B	Any anticoagulant	Dacie et al. Br J Haematol 1964:10:388.
4.5-P	Collect as in factor II determination	Boxer et al. Arthritis Rheum 1976:19:1244.
20-Isolated blood leukocytes	Special handling of blood necessary	Valentine, Beck. J Lab Clin Med 1951:38:39.
Smear-B		Kaplow. Am J Clin Pathol 1963:39:439.
1-S 1-U		Osserman, Lawlor. J Exp Med 1966:124:921.

(continued)

	REFERENCE RANGE	
DETERMINATION	CONVENTIONAL	SI
Osmotic fragility of erythrocytes	Increased if hemolysis occurs in over 0.5% NaCl; decreased if hemolysis is incomplete in 0.3% NaCl	
Peroxide hemolyis	Less than 10%	0.10
Platelet count	150,000–350,000/mm³	150–350 × 10⁹/L

Lupus Erythematosus Preparation

Method I	0	0
Method II	0	0

Platelet Function Tests

Clot retraction	50%–100%/2 h	0.50–1.00/2 h
Platelet aggregation	Full response to ADP, epinephrine, and collagen	1
Platelet factor 3	33–57 sec	33–57 sec
Reticulocyte count	0.5%–2.5% RBC	0.005–0.025
Vitamin B$_{12}$	205–876 pg/ml	150–674 pmol/L
Borderline	140–204 pg/ml	102.6–149 pmol/L

Miscellaneous Values

Carcinoembryonic antigen	0–2.5 ng/ml	0–2.5 µg/L

MINIMAL MI REQUIRED	NOTE	METHOD
5-B	Use heparin as anticoagulant	Beutler. In: Williams et al., eds. Hematology. New York: McGraw-Hill, 1972, p. 1375.
6-B	Use EDTA as anticoagulant	Gordon et al. Am J Dis Child 1955:90:669.
0.5-B	Use EDTA as anticoagulant; counts are performed on Clay Adams Ultraflow; when counts are low, results are confirmed by hand counting	(Hand count): Brecher et al. Am J Clin Pathol 1955:23:15
5-B	Use heparin as anticoagulant	Hargraves et al. Proc Staff Meet Mayo Clin 1949:24:234.
5-B	Use defibrinated blood	Barnes et al. J Invest Dermatol 1950:14:397.
4.5-P	Collect as in factor II determination	Benthaus. Thromb Diath Haemorrh 1959:3:311.
18-P	Collect as in factor II determination	Born. Nature 1962:194:927.
4.5-P	Collect as in factor II determination	Rabiner, Hrodek. J Clin Invest 1968:47:901.
0.1-B		Brecher. Am J Clin Pathol 1949:19:895.
12-S		Difco Manual, 9th ed. 1953, p. 221 (modified).
20-P	Must be sent on ice	Hansen et al. J Clin Res 1971:19:143

(continued)

DETERMINATION	REFERENCE RANGE	
	CONVENTIONAL	SI
Chylous fluid		
Digitoxin	17 ± 6 ng/ml	22 ± 7.8 nmol/L
Digoxin	1.2 ± 0.4 ng/ml	1.54 ± 0.5 nmol/L
	1.5 ± 0.4 ng/ml	1.92 ± 0.5 nmol/L
Duodenal drainage		
pH (urine)	5–7	5–7
Gastric analysis	Basal	
	Females: 2.0 ± 1.8 mEq/h	0.6 ± 0.5 μmol/sec
	Males: 3.0 ± 2.0 mEq/h	0.8 ± 0.6 μmol/sec
	Maximal (after histalog or gastrin)	
	Females: 16 ± 5 mEq/h	4.4 ± 1.4 μmol/sec
	Males: 23 ± 5 mEq/h	6.4 ± 1.4 μmol/sec
Gastrin-1	0–200 pg/ml	0–95 pmol/L

Immunologic Tests

Alpha-fetoprotein	Undetectable in normal adults	
α-1-antitrypsin	85–213 mg/100 ml	0.85–2.13 g/L
Rheumatoid factor	<60 IU/ml	
Antinuclear antibodies	Negative at a 1:8 dilution of serum	
Anti-DNA antibodies	Negative at a 1:10 dilution of serum	

MINIMAL MI REQUIRED	NOTE	METHOD
	Use fresh specimen	Todd et al. Clinical diagnosis, 12th ed. 1953, p. 624.
1-S	Medication with digitoxin or digitalis	Smith, Butler, Haber. N Engl J Med 1969:281: 1212.
1-S	Medication with digoxin 0.25 mg/day	Smith, Haber. J Clin Invest 1970:49:2377.
1-S	Medication with digoxin 0.5 mg/day	
	pH should be in proper range with minimal amount of gastric juice	
		Marks. Gastroenterology 1961:41:599.
4-P	Heparinized sample	Dent et al. Ann Surg 1972:176:360.
2-S		
10-B		Nephelometric assay
10 ml clotted blood	Fasting sample preferred	Nephelometric assay
2-S	Send to laboratory promptly	Immunofluorescence assay
2-S		*Crithidia lucilliae* assay

(continued)

DETERMINATION	REFERENCE RANGE	
	CONVENTIONAL	SI
Antibodies to Sm and RNP (ENA)	None detected	
Antibodies to SS-A (Ro) and SS-B (La)	None detected	
Autoantibodies to		
Thyroid colloid and microsomal antigens	Negative at a 1:10 dilution of serum	
Gastric parietal cells	Negative at a 1:20 dilution of serum	
Smooth muscle	Negative at a 1:20 dilution of serum	
Mitochondria	Negative at a 1:20 dilution of serum	
Interstitial cells of the testes	Negative at a 1:10 dilution of serum	
Skeletal muscle	Negative at a 1:60 dilution of serum	
Adrenal gland	Negative at a 1:10 dilution of serum	
Bence Jones protein	No Bence Jones protein detected in a 50-fold concentrate of urine	
Complement, total hemolytic	150–250 U/ml	
Cryoprecipitable proteins	None detected	0 arb. unit
C3	Range, 83–177 mg/100 ml	0.83–1.77 g/L

MINIMAL MI REQUIRED	NOTE	METHOD
10 ml clotted blood		Double diffusion
10 ml clotted blood		Double diffusion
2-S	Low titers in some elderly normal women	Doniach, Bottazzo, Drexhage. The autoimmune endocrinopathies. In: Lachmann, Peters, eds. Clinical aspects of immunology, vol. 2. Oxford: Blackwell Scientific, 1982, p. 903.
2-S		
2-S		
2-S		
2-S		
		Doniach et al. Protocol of autoimmunity laboratories. London: Middlesex Medical School.
50-U		
10-B	Must be sent on ice	Hook, Muschel. Proc Soc Exp Biol Med 1964:117:292.
10-S	Collect and transport at 37 °C	Barr et al. Ann Intern Med 1950:32:6 (modified).
2-S		Nephelometric assay

(continued)

DETERMINATION	REFERENCE RANGE	
	CONVENTIONAL	SI
C4	Range, 15–45 mg/100 ml	0.15–0.45 g/L
Factor B	12–30 mg/100 ml	
C1 esterase inhibitor	13.2–24 mg/100 ml	
Hemoglobin A_{1c}	3.8%–6.4%	0.038–0.064
Hypersensitivity pneumonitis screen	No antibodies to those antigens assayed	
Immuno-globulins		
IgG	639–1349 mg/100 ml	6.39–13.49 g/L
IgA	70–312 mg/100 ml	0.7–3.12 g/L
IgM	86–352 mg/100 ml	0.86–3.52 g/L
Viscosity	1.4–1.8 relative viscosity units	
Iontophoresis	Children: 0–40 mEq sodium/L	0–40 mM/L
	Adults: 0–60 mEq sodium/L	0–60 mM/L
Propranolol (includes bioactive 4-OH metabolite)	100–300 ng/ml	386–1158 mM/L
Stool fat	Less than 5 g in 24 h or less than 4% of measured fat intake in 3-day period	<5 g/day

MINIMAL MI REQUIRED	NOTE	METHOD
2-S		Nephelometric assay
5 ml clotted blood		Nephelometric assay
5 ml clotted blood		Nephelometric assay
5-P	Send EDTA tube on ice promptly to laboratory	Nathan et al. Clin Chem 1982:28:512.
5 ml clotted blood		Double diffusion
2-S		
2-S		
2-S		
10-B	Expressed as the relative viscosity of serum compared to water	Barth. Viscosimetry of serum in relation to the serum globulins. In: Sunderman, Sunderman, eds. Serum proteins and the dysproteinemias, 1964, p. 102.
	Value given in terms of sodium	Gibson, Cooke. Pediatrics 1959:23:545.
1-S	Obtain blood sample 4 h after last dose of beta-blocking agent	M.G.H. method of Rockson, Homcy, Haber: by radioimmunoassay
24- or 3-day specimen		Jover et al. J Lab Clin Med 1962:59:878.

(continued)

	REFERENCE RANGE	
DETERMINATION	CONVENTIONAL	SI
Stool nitrogen	Less than 2 g/day or 10% of urinary nitrogen	<2 g/day
Synovial fluid Glucose	Not less than 20 mg/100 ml lower than simultaneously drawn blood sugar	See Blood Glucose
D-Xylose absorption	5–8 g/5 h in urine; 40 mg per 100 ml in blood 2 h after ingestion of 25 g of D-xylose	33–53 mM/day 2.7 mM/L

MINIMAL MI REQUIRED	NOTE	METHOD
24-h or 3-day specimen		Peters, Van Slyke. Quantitative clinical chemistry, vol. 2 (Methods). 1932, p. 353.
1 ml of fresh fluid	Collect with oxalate-fluoride mixture	See Blood Glucose.
5-U 5-B	For directions see Benson et al. N Engl J Med 1957:256:335.	Roe, Rice. J Biol Chem 1948:173:507.

SI, Système international d'Unités; P, plasma, S, serum; B, blood; U, urine; L, liter; h, hour; sec, second.
Note: To update the normal reference values* of laboratory procedures recorded in the Case Records of the Massachusetts General Hospital and to give the methods used, the tabular summaries previously published have been revised. Both the conventional values and SI units are listed.
(Plumer A. Principles and practice of intravenous therapy. Boston: Little, Brown & Co, 1987.)

APPENDIX 10. Therapeutic Drug Levels

DRUG	ROUTE OF ADMINISTRATION	
	INTERMITTENT IV*	CONTINUOUS IV
Amikacin	P/T	—
Digoxin	T	—
Gentamicin	P/T	—
Heparin	T	†
Lidocaine	—	†
Phenobarbital	T	—
Phenytoin	T	—
Procainamide	T	†
Quinidine	T	—
Theophylline	P/T	†
Tobramycin	P/T	—

* When administering the drug intermittently, IV trough (T) level should be drawn 30 min before a scheduled dose. If T level is being drawn with a peak (P/T), both levels should be drawn after the dose, if possible. Intermittent IV peak (P) level is drawn 30 min after the completion of a 1-h infusion for amikacin, gentamicin, and tobramycin, and 90 min after an IM injection. Theophylline peaks are drawn 30 min after a 30-min infusion is completed.
† The level may be drawn at any time.
(Department of Pharmacy, St. Mary's Hospital, Richmond, VA.)

When are Serum Drug Levels Measured?

1. When drug toxicity is suspected.
2. When there is a question concerning compliance with a specific drug regime, such as the home IV antibiotic patient who must comply with a specific drug regime to achieve appropriate drug levels independent of professional nursing interventions.
3. When a disease process alters drug metabolism and elimination; for example, changes in hepatic function affect dosage requirements for theophylline and lidocaine, which are metabolized and eliminated by the liver.
4. When a disease process masks toxicity; the drug dosage may be inappropriately increased because the drug does not seem to be working.
5. When the possibility of drug interaction and subsequent change in serum level exists; for example, lidocaine hydrochloride interacts with cimetidine (Tagamet); the subsequent decreased metabolism of lidocaine raises its serum level. The serum lidocaine level should be monitored and the dosage adjusted as needed.

Concentration Time Curves

Volume The obvious body space into which a drug is distributed; volume represents the ratio of plasma concentration to total amount of drug in the body and is useful in calculating loading doses (mg/kg).

Plasma Clearance The rate (volume/time) at which plasma is purged of a drug.

Half-life The time required for a drug concentration to fall to one half its current value in the absence of drug input.

Drugs with Long Half-Lives

Take a blood sample immediately prior to giving another dose. This is the point at which the serum drug concentration reaches the trough level.

Drugs with Short Half-Lives

Take a blood sample for both peak and trough levels. These drugs reach peak serum levels 1–2 h after a dose.

Drugs Given by Continuous Infusion

Take a blood sample anytime after the drug reaches equilibrium (4 or 5 half-lives after infusion is initiated, unless a loading dose has been given). The sample should be drawn from the opposite extremity.

(continued)

Patients in Need of TDM
1. Those with renal dysfunction.
2. Those with third-spacing.
3. Those for whom therapeutic failure would prove catastrophic (ie, the septic neutropenic patient for whom aminoglycosides have been ordered).
4. Those who fail to respond to therapy despite appropriate dosing.

Nursing Responsibilities: TDM
1. Correct scheduling of the sampling time with respect to steady-state.
2. Accurate documentation of the sampling time.
3. Avoiding contamination by the presence of undistributed drug at the sampling site. (Obtain samples from sites other than that being used for infusion purposes.)
4. Maintain awareness of lab procedures; for example, many labs combine bound and unbound serum drug concentrations into one value. Toxicity as a result of protein binding may be masked by such reporting methods.
5. Preparation of the patient.
6. Use of good technique, consistent with institutional policy and aimed at patient safety and protection.

Case Presentation
Mr. J., a 78-year old man with a history of increasing shortness of breath, was admitted to the hospital with a preliminary diagnosis of chronic obstructive pulmonary disease, possibly exacerbated by an intercurrent respiratory infection and complicated by corpulmonale with mild right-sided congestive heart failure. He failed to respond to supportive therapy including theophylline and was placed on a therapeutic regimen of ampicillin initially and later chloramphenicol, oxacillin, gentamicin and hydrocortisone 300 mg every 8 h. On the 4th and 5th days of hospitalization, the theophylline concentrations in serum were 16.3 and 16.1 µg/ml, respectively.

On the 5th day of hospitalization, mechanical respiration was instituted because of continued respiratory decompensation. On the 7th day, pleural effusions were evident; on the 8th day, the patient became comatose despite normal electrolyte concentration and lack of any change in blood-gas values. Generalized edema was noted, and furosemide therapy was instituted. On the 9th day, atrial fibrillation developed, followed by ventricular fibrillation, both of which responded to appropriate therapy. Severe hemorrhage from the upper GI tract was noted. The theophylline concentration was 42.5 µg/ml even though there had been no change in dosage since the first day of hospitalization. Alkaline phosphatase activity and prothrombin time were now also abnormal. Theophylline therapy was discontinued.

Although the theophylline concentration began to fall, the patient continued to hemorrhage from the upper GI tract, and numerous blood transfusions were given. On the 17th hospital day, refractory hypotension developed and the patient died.

The progressively worsening heart failure, as indicated by increasing edema, increased alkaline phosphatase, abnormal prothrombin time, and the appearance of pleural effusions, along with chloramphenicol therapy (inhibitor of theophylline metabolism) probably explains the decrease in theophylline clearance and development of this toxicity.

This case illustrates the pitfalls of relying completely on standardized dose regimens when theophylline is administered.

(Therapeutic drug monitoring. Needham Heights, MA: Needham Clinical Laboratories, 1983:11)

APPENDIX 12. Medication Errors

Dispensing

1. Dispensing a wrong medication (drug, strength, quantity, route of administration or dosage form)
2. Causing the dispensing of an unordered medication or dispensing an unordered medication (adding a medication to the wrong patient's profile or placing unordered drugs in the cassette)
3. Dispensing a medication in an inappropriate container; for example, omission of an ultraviolet-light filter bag for certain IV fluids
4. Dispensing a medication with incomplete or improper labeling (strikeovers, misspellings, lack of accessory labels)
5. Dispensing a medication without sufficient education of the patient concerning use and effects
6. Dispensing a medication with an inappropriate or unordered dose or dosage schedule due to misinterpretation of physician's orders
7. Dispensing a medication that has no indication or is contraindicated for the patient's condition
8. Dispensing a medication without alerting the prescriber when the patient has a known or suspected sensitivity to the drug
9. Dispensing a medication that has the same pharmacologic intent as other drugs the patient is receiving, when such combination therapy is inappropriate
10. Dispensing, without alerting the prescriber, a medication that could possibly elicit a known, serious drug–drug interaction
11. Omission of a dose of medication or a lost medication order
12. Incorrect transcription
13. Miscellaneous nonadherence to pharmacy policy
14. Establishment of a therapeutic regimen not in compliance with the approved dosage regimen
15. Providing incorrect drug information

Prescribing

This list would detail information specific to the physician.

Administration

1. Omission of a dose of medication
2. Administration of a medication that has not been ordered by a licensed physician
3. Administration of medication by the wrong route or dosage form
4. Administration of an outdated medication
5. Omission of an ultraviolet-light filter bag for certain IV fluids

6. Incomplete labeling of medications and infusions in progress to which additives have been made by the nursing professional
7. Administration of a medication that has no indication or is contraindicated for the patient's condition
8. Administration of a medication that has the same pharmacologic intent as other drugs the patient is receiving
9. Administration of an IV medication at an incorrect and unsafe rate of administration
10. Dilution of medication with an incorrect and inappropriate diluent
11. Administration of a medication that could possibly elicit a known, serious drug–drug interaction
12. Administration of a medication at a time other than prescribed by the physician or not in compliance with the therapeutic regime
13. Failure to provide patient teaching concerning medication regime

(AJHP 1985;42:1724–1732. © 1985 American Society of Hospital Pharmacists, Inc. All rights reserved. Reprinted with permission.)

APPENDIX 13. Guidelines for Management of Hypersensitivity Reactions: Prevention, Recognition, and Management

I. Identifying Susceptible Patients

A. Obtain history of previous allergies, especially to drugs, on admission and prior to giving any intravenous drug.
   1. Determine type of allergy (eg, drug, food, hay fever).
   2. Note type and severity of previous symptoms.
   3. Questionable allergies should be evaluated by a physician.
B. With seriously ill or unresponsive patients, seek information from medical record, family members, medical identification tag or wallet ID card.

II. Instituting Preventive Measures

A. List specific drugs (and other substances) to which the patient is allergic on the front of the chart and in other pertinent parts of the medical record (eg, nursing history, problem list, medication record, Kardex).
B. Instruct patient regarding advisability of wearing a medical identification tag and assist in obtaining one as needed.
C. Be aware of related drugs that can produce cross-reactions: patients with penicillin allergies may also be allergic to ampicillin or semisynthetic penicillin (such as carbenicillin), or to the cephalosporins. Patients with known allergies to one aminoglycoside (eg, gentamicin, kanamycin, amikacin) may be allergic to others.
D. Be aware that individuals with multiple drug allergies are also prone to developing allergies to chemically unrelated drugs.
E. When an intravenous drug, especially penicillin, is ordered, determine whether the patient has received it previously. Prior exposure may have sensitized the person; subsequent doses can elicit an allergic response.
F. Avoid administering a drug to which the patient is known to be allergic, even if previous reactions were mild. In rare instances when such a drug must be given, follow the procedure below.

III. Monitoring for Signs of Allergic Reactions

A. For patients with *no* history of allergy:
   1. Remain with the patient for 5–10 min during infusion of the intial dose.
   2. Observe for and report: urticaria (hives), dyspnea, edema (especially on the face) or local reactions at the IV site.
   3. Without unduly alarming them, instruct appropriate patients to report any such symptoms. Patients who are unable to report symptoms should be checked periodically until dose has infused.

B. For patients with a positive history of allergies *or* when administering a drug that is likely to be allergenic (as indicated for specific drugs in this text):

1. Have emergency medications and supplies readily available (see treatment section).

2. Stay with patient throughout infusion of the first dose (or for 10–20 min if drug is in large volume infusion). Both for efficiency and to lessen patient apprehension, try to plan patient care that can be given while observing for allergic signs and symptoms.

3. After infusion of medication, check the patient every 30 minutes or so for the next few hours. Reactions occurring later are less likely to be severe. Check the temperature every 4 h for 24 h to detect occurrence of drug fever.

4. Instruct the patient to report any of the symptoms mentioned above, particularly breathing difficulties, swelling of the face or other parts of the body, or skin reactions.

5. At the first appearance of any allergic symptom, discontinue the drug and notify the physician immediately. Keep the intravenous line open in case any emergency medications are required. If allergic symptoms appear, consider any other drugs the patient is receiving concurrently, particularly parenteral ones that may be the source of the reaction.

6. If no allergic manifestations occur, observe the patient for 5–10 min during the administration of subsequent doses. Observe for late signs: fever, arthralgia, lymph node enlargement, skin eruptions (maculopapular type), and neuritis.

IV. Administering a Drug to Which a Patient is Known to Be Allergic

A. In rare instances, the benefits of giving a drug outweigh the risks of a potentially serious allergic reaction. For example, penicillins, including some penicillinase-resistant semisynthetic penicillins such as nafcillin, are the treatment of choice in specific kinds of bacterial endocarditis and septicemia. In rare instances, the patient may also be allergic to an unrelated second-line drug. In such a case, the first-line drug is given and steps are taken to minimize reactions.

B. The *physician* performs appropriate skin tests (first, a scratch test; if negative, then an intradermal test).

1. If results of both tests are negative, administer the drug, taking precautions outlined in III-B above.

2. If either test is positive, one of the following measures must be performed before the drug can be given.

(continued)

      (a) Rapid hyposensitization—*always done by the physician*—involves giving small, increasing doses of the drug every 2–6 h.

      (b) Drug suppression using either antihistamines or glucocorticoids. This requires a day of pretreatment followed by a test dose before the drug is started.

C. When the course of therapy is started, the first dose, and ideally the first several doses, should be administered by the physician. Emergency medications and equipment that must be kept close at hand throughout both the testing and drug therapy include:

      (a) Epinephrine, 1:1000 and 1:10,000 solutions

      (b) Antihistamines, such as diphenhydramine (Benadryl) for intravenous use

      (c) Glucocorticoids, hydrocortisone (Solu-Cortef) and methylprednisolone (Solu-Medrol)

      (d) Calcium preparations in case cardiac arrest should occur

      (e) Vasopressors (dopamine [Intropin], levarterenol [Levophed], isoproterenol [Isuprel])

      (f) Lidocaine

      (g) Airway and manual resuscitation bag (eg, Puritan, Hope, Ambu)

      (h) Endotracheal tube and laryngoscope

      (i) Tracheostomy tray, in case laryngeal edema or spasm prevents oral intubation

      (j) Intravenous fluids

V. Treatment of Allergic Reactions

A. *Anaphylactic shock.* Should anaphylaxis occur in spite of all possible precautions, it is essential that treatment be instituted immediately, because death can ensue in a matter of minutes. While specific regimens may vary slightly according to physician preference, essential elements of treatment generally include:

1. Aqueous epinephrine, 1:10,000, given intravenously by *slow* injection. The initial dose is 2–5 ml. For milder symptoms such as urticaria, 0.2–0.5 ml of 1:1000 strength can be initially given subcutaneously, repeated at 3-min intervals if required. A continuous infusion of epinephrine diluted with normal saline or 5% dextrose in water may be given.

2. Establish and/or maintain a patent airway. Endotracheal intubation or emergency tracheostomy may be required if airway obstruction, due to either laryngeal edema or bronchospasm, is present. In these instances, either antihistamines such as diphenhydramine (Benadryl) 50–80 mg IV or IM, or chlor-

pheniramine (Chlor-Trimeton), 10 mg IV; or aminophylline, 0.25–0.50 g IV (6 mg/kg over a 20-min period), may be given as adjunctive measures.

3. Establish a secure, preferably central, intravenous line if the one already present is at risk of dislodgement or infiltration.

4. Provide intravenous volume expansion with agents, such as dextran, saline, or albumin, and treat acidosis as needed.

5. If bronchospasm or hypotension persists, corticosteroids may be used.

6. Maintain close nursing observation of the patient for at least 24 h after the reaction or until stable. Monitoring of vital signs, particularly blood pressure, respiration, and pulse rate, is essential for the assessment of the patient's progress.

7. Following anaphylactic shock or any significant allergic reaction, it is vital that the patient, or the parent or responsible person when indicated, be informed of the allergy and its significance. With a school-aged child, the parents should be advised to inform the child's teacher or school nurse of the allergy so that the information can be entered into the health record. Another important aspect of the nurse's teaching responsibility includes explaining the value of wearing a medical identification tag and assisting the patient in obtaining one if indicated.

B. *Less severe allergic manifestations.* The primary measure is to discontinue the drug. In cases of mild reactions, this is often the only measure required; symptoms subside spontaneously. For more severe reactions, epinephrine may be given. Antihistamines may also be used, both to relieve symptoms and as a prophylaxis against serum sickness. If signs of exfoliative dermatitis appear, steroids are used. Drug fever and other isolated symptoms are often treated symptomatically. Nursing intervention in drug allergy includes:

1. Providing psychological support to help allay the patient's anxiety. Asthmatic or other symptoms which interfere with breathing, as well as extensive skin reactions, are particularly anxiety provoking.

2. Continuing close observation following discontinuation of the drug to be sure that the symptoms are not worsening.

3. Providing symptomatic relief for skin reactions, such as urticaria and rashes, with such measures as tepid baths, use of a bed cradle to prevent pressure and irritation from the bed linen and, unless the skin is broken, application of lotion to relieve itching.

(continued)

VI. Drug Extravasation

A. Prevention

1. When possible, select the largest vein available and use an appropriately sized needle or cannula for that vein.

2. If the drug is to be administered by infusion, avoid needle appliances such as scalp vein needles.

3. Ideally, the appliance should be inserted for infusion into the vein at a point away from elbow, wrist, and hand joints. Motion at these areas contributes to cannula displacement.

4. Avoid using scalp veins in babies.

5. Be certain that the cannula or needle is within the lumen of the vein before initiating an infusion or injecting the drug. There should be free return of venous blood, and a test injection of normal saline or another isotonic solution should not produce pain or swelling.

6. If an infusion is to be administered, the cannula must be secured with tape to prevent movement. If a vein that is near a joint must be used, use an armboard. Anchor tubing to prevent pull on the cannula. The taping technique should be designed to allow visibility of the skin surrounding the vein and insertion site.

7. When possible, instruct the patient on the importance of the drug, as well as on the hazards of extravasation and how he can participate in its prevention.

B. Recognition

1. Instruct the patient to report *undue* pain at the injection site. Some drugs normally cause burning along the vein tract; help him differentiate this from unusual pain.

2. Examine the tissues proximal to the injection or infusion site for blanching, swelling, or coolness. Do this every 30 min, or more frequently if an infusion pump is in use.

C. Management

1. If extravasation is suspected, stop the infusion or injection immediately. With infusion, if the drug is non-life-supporting, remove the cannula or needle. If the drug is life-supporting, quickly restart the infusion at another site.

2. Elevate the extremity.

3. Notify the physician immediately. Treatment must begin as soon as possible after detection of the problem.

4. Be prepared for the specific treatment for the drug in use. If a treatment is known for a drug, it will appear in the text of this book; otherwise, consult the pharmacist or drug-information department of your institution.

5. After treatment, continue to monitor the affected area for signs and symptoms of tissue damage:
   (a) Continuing pain or numbness
   (b) Redness
   (c) Swelling
   (d) Cyanosis or continuing blanching
   (e) Loss of pulses distal to the area
   (f) Bleb formation or tissue sloughing
6. Protect the area from further trauma and from infection.

(Sager, Bomar. Quick reference to intravenous medications. Philadelphia: JB Lippincott, 1983.)

APPENDIX 14. Guidelines for Handling Cytotoxic Agents

PREAMBLE

The mutagenic, teratogenic, carcinogenic, and local irritant properties of many cytotoxic agents are well established and pose a possible hazard to the health of occupationally exposed individuals. These potential hazards necessitate special attention to the procedures used in the handling, preparation, and administration of these drugs, and the proper disposal of residues and wastes. These recommendations are intended to provide information for the protection of personnel participating in the clinical process of chemotherapy. It is the responsibility of institutional and private health care providers to adopt and use appropriate procedures for protection and safety.

I. **Environmental Protection**
   A. Preparation of cytotoxic agents should be performed in a class II biologic safety cabinet located in an area with minimal traffic and air turbulence. Class II Type A cabinets are the minimal requirement. Class II cabinets which are exhausted to the outside are preferred.
   B. The biologic safety cabinet must be certified by qualified personnel at least annually or any time the cabinet is physically moved.

II. **Operator Protection**
   A. Disposable surgical latex gloves are recommended for all procedures involving cytotoxic agents.
   B. Gloves should routinely be changed about every 30 min when working steadily with cytotoxic agents. Gloves should be removed immediately after overt contamination.
   C. Protective barrier garments should be worn for all procedures involving the preparation and disposal of cytotoxic agents. These garments should have a closed front, long sleeves and closed cuff (either elastic or knit).
   D. Protective garments must not be worn outside the work area.

III. **Techniques and Precautions for Use in the Class II Biologic Safety Cabinet**
   A. Special techniques and precautions must be used because of the vertical (downward) laminar airflow.
   B. Clean surfaces of the cabinet using 70% alcohol and a disposable towel before and after preparation. Discard towel into a hazardous chemical waste container.
   C. Prepare the work surface of the biologic safety cabinet by covering

it with a plastic-backed absorbent pad. This pad should be changed when the cabinet is cleaned or after a spill.

D. The biologic safety cabinet should be operated with the blower on, 24 h/day, 7 days/wk. Where the biologic safety cabinet is used infrequently (eg, 1 or 2 times weekly) it may be turned off after thoroughly cleaning all interior surfaces. Turn on the blower 15 min before beginning work in the cabinet.

E. Drug preparations must be performed only with the view screen at the recommended access opening. Professionally accepted practices concerning the aseptic preparation of injectable products should be followed.

F. All materials needed to complete the procedure should be placed into the biologic safety cabinet before beginning work to avoid interruptions of cabinet airflow. Allow 2 or 3 min before beginning work for the unit to purge itself of airborne contaminants.

G. The proper procedures for use in the biologic safety cabinet differ from those used in the horizontal laminar hood because of the nature of the airflow pattern. Clean air descends through the work zone from the top of the cabinet toward the work surface. As it descends, the air is split, with some leaving through the rear perforation and some leaving through the front perforation.

H. The least efficient area of the cabinet in terms of product and personnel protection is within 3 inches of the sides near the front opening, and work should not be performed in these areas.

I. Entry into and exit from the cabinet should be in a direct manner perpendicular to the face of the cabinet. Rapid movements of the hands in the cabinet and laterally through the protective air barrier should be avoided.

IV. Compounding Procedures and Techniques

A. Hands must be washed thoroughly before gloving and after gloves are removed.

B. Care must be taken to avoid puncturing of gloves and possible self-inoculation.

C. Syringes and IV sets with Luer-Lok fittings should be used whenever possible to avoid spills due to disconnection.

D. To minimize aerosolization, vials containing cytotoxic agents should be vented with a hydrophobic filter to equalize internal pressure, or use negative pressure technique.

E. Before opening ampules, care should be taken to ensure that no liquid remains in the tip of the ampule. A sterile disposable sponge should be wrapped around the neck of the ampule to

(continued)

reduce aerosolization. Ampules should be broken in a direction away from the body.

F. For sealed vials, final drug measurement should be performed before removing the needle from the stopper of the vial and after the pressure has been equalized.

G. A closed collection vessel should be available in the biologic safety cabinet or the original vial may be used to hold discarded excess drug solutions.

H. Cytotoxic agents should be properly labeled to identify the need for caution in handling (eg, "Chemotherapy: Dispose of Properly").

I. The final prepared dosage form should be protected from leakage or breakage by being sealed in a transparent plastic container labeled, "Do Not Open if Contents Appear to be Broken."

V. Precautions for Administration

A. Disposable surgical latex gloves should be worn during administration of cytotoxic agents. Hands must be washed thoroughly before donning gloves and after gloves are removed.

B. Protective barrier garments may be worn. Such garments should have a closed front, long sleeves, and closed cuff (either elastic or knit).

C. Syringes and IV sets with Luer-Lok fittings should be used whenever possible.

D. Special care must be taken in priming IV sets. The distal tip or needle cover must be removed before priming. Priming can be performed into a sterile, alcohol-dampened gauze sponge. Other acceptable methods of priming such as closed receptacles (eg, evacuated containers) or back-filling of IV sets may be used. Do not prime sets or syringes into the sink or any open receptacle.

VI. Disposal Procedures

A. Place contaminated materials in a leakproof, punctureproof container appropriately marked as hazardous chemical waste. These containers should be suitable to collect bottles, vials, gloves, disposable gowns and other materials used in the preparation and administration of cytotoxic agents.

B. Contaminated needles, syringes, sets and tubing should be disposed of intact. To prevent aerosolization, needles and syringes should not be clipped.

C. Cytotoxic drug waste should be transported according to the institutional procedures for hazardous material.

D. There is insufficient information to recommend any preferred method for disposal of cytotoxic drug waste.

1. One acceptable method for disposal of hazardous waste is by

incineration in an Environmental Protection Agency (EPA) permitted hazardous waste incinerator.

2. Another acceptable method of disposal is by burial at an EPA permitted hazardous waste site.

3. A licensed hazardous waste disposal company may be consulted for information concerning available methods of disposal in the local area.

VII. Personnel Policy Recommendations

A. Personnel involved in any aspect of the handling of cytotoxic agents must receive an orientation to the agents, including their known risks, and special training in safe handling procedures.

B. Access to the compounding area must be limited to authorized personnel.

C. Personnel working with these agents should be supervised regularly to ensure compliance with procedures.

D. Acute exposures must be documented, and the employee referred for medical examination.

E. Personnel should refrain from applying cosmetics in the work area. Cosmetics may provide a source of prolonged exposure if contaminated.

F. Eating, drinking, chewing gum, smoking or storing food in areas where cytotoxic agents are handled should be prohibited. Each of these can be a source of ingestion if they are accidentally contaminated.

VIII. Monitoring Procedures

A. Policies and procedures to monitor the equipment and operating techniques of personnel handling cytotoxic agents should be implemented and performed on a regular basis with appropriate documentation. Specific methods of monitoring should be developed to meet the complexities of the function.

B. It is recommended that personnel involved in the preparation of cytotoxic agents be given periodic health examinations in accordance with institutional policy.

IX. Procedures for Acute Exposure or Spills

A. Acute Exposure

1. Overtly contaminated gloves or outer garments should be removed immediately.

2. Hands must be washed after removing gloves. Some cytotoxic agents have been documented to penetrate gloves.

3. In case of skin contact with a cytotoxic drug product, the

(continued)

affected area should be washed thoroughly with soap and water. Refer for medical attention as soon as possible.
4. For eye exposure, flush affected eye with copious amounts of water, and refer for medical attention immediately.
B. Spills
1. All personnel involved in the clean-up of a spill should wear protective barrier garments (eg, gloves, gowns). These garments and other material used in the process should be disposed of properly.
2. Double gloving is recommended for cleaning up spills.

POSITION STATEMENT

There are substantial data regarding the mutagenic, teratogenic and abortifacient properties of certain cytotoxic agents both in animals and humans who have received therapeutic doses of these agents. Additionally, the scientific literature suggests a possible association of occupational exposure to certain cytotoxic agents during the first trimester of pregnancy with fetal loss or malformation. These data suggest the need for caution when women who are pregnant, or attempting to conceive, handle cytotoxic agents. Incidentally, there is no evidence relating male exposure to cytotoxic agents with adverse fetal outcome.

No studies have addressed the possible risk associated with the occupational exposure to cytotoxic agents and the passage of these agents into breast milk. Nevertheless, it is prudent that women who are breast feeding should exercise caution in handling cytotoxic agents.

If all procedures for safe handling, such as those recommended by the Commission, are complied with, the potential for exposure is minimized.

Personnel should be provided with information to make an individual decision. This information should be provided in written form and it is advisable that a statement of understanding be signed.

It is essential to refer to individual state right-to-know laws to ensure compliance.

(National Study Commission on Cytotoxic Exposure, Boston, September 1987.)

APPENDIX 15. Vesicant Pharmacologic Agents and Antidotes

Vesicant*	Antidote
Calcium chloride	Hyaluronidase
Dacarbazine	Hyaluronidase or dexamethasone
Dactinomycin	Hyaluronidase or dexamethasone
Daunomycin	Hyaluronidase or dexamethasone
Dobutamine	Phentolamine
Dopamine	Phentolamine
Doxorubicin	Hyaluronidase or dexamethasone
Epinephrine	Phentolamine
Levarterenol	Phentomaline
Mechlorethamine	Sodium thiosulfate (use 2% solution for cleanup of spills)
Metaraminol	Phentolamine
Methoxamine	Phentolamine
Mitomycin	Dexamethasone
Nitroprusside	Sodium thiosulfate
Norepinephrine	Phentolamine
Phenylephrine	Phentolamine
Plicamycin	Dexamethasone
Tromethamine	Hyaluronidase or phentolamine
Vinblastine	Hyaluronidase
Vincristine	Hyaluronidase

Other Vesicant Pharmacologic Agents

Pyrazofurin	Idarubicin*†
Promethazine	MER-BCG*†
Mercaptopurine	Neocarzinustatin*†
Vindesine*†	AZQ*†
Estramustine	4-deoxydoxorubicin*†
BCG*†	

*Vesicant: An agent capable of causing or forming a blister or causing tissue destruction.
†Denotes investigational agent.

APPENDIX 16. Irritant Pharmacologic Agents and Antidotes

Irritant*

Carmustine
Etoposide
Teniposide

Antidote

Sodium bicarbonate
Hyaluronidase
Hyaluronidase

Other Irritant Pharmacologic Agents

Streptozocin
Mitoguazone
Bleomycin
Cyclophosphamide
Dantrolene
Diazepam
Diazoxide
Doxapram
Doxycycline
Mannitol
Propiomazine
Methocarbamol
Metronidazole
Mezlocillin
Sodium bicarbonate
Pentobarbital
Phenobarbital
Phenytoin
Promazine
Secobarbital
Trimethoprim-sulfamethoxazole
10% dextrose solution
Potassium chloride
Nafcillin
Radiocontrast media
Iron dextran
Phytonadione

Irritant: An agent capable of producing venous pain at the site or along the wall of the vein, with or without inflammatory reaction.

Canadian Drug Brand
and Proprietary Names

NONPROPRIETARY NAME	BRAND NAME (CANADIAN MANUFACTURER)
acetazolamide	Acetazolam (ICN), Apo-Acetazolamide (Apotex)
acyclovir	Zovirax (Burroughs Wellcome)
Albumin (human)	normal serum albumin (Winnipeg Plasma)
alteplase	Activase rt-PA (Genentech)
amikacin sulfate	Amikin (Bristol)
aminocaproic acid	Amicar (Lederle)
amphotericin B	Fungizone (Squibb)
ampicillin	Ampicin (Bristol), Ampilean (Organon)
bleomycin sulfate	Blenoxane (Bristol)
bretylium tosylate	Bretylate (Burroughs Wellcome)
calcium disodium edetate	Calcium Disodium Versenate (Riker/3M)
calcium folinate	Leucovorin Calcium (Lederle)
calcium gluconate	H-F Antidote Gel (Pharmascience)
carmustine	BiCNU (Bristol)
cefamandole nafate	Mandol (Lilly)
cefazolin sodium	Ancef (Smith Kline & French)
cefoperazone sodium	Cefobid (Pfizer)
cefotaxime sodium	Claforan (Roussel)
cefoxitin	Mefoxin (Merck Sharp & Dohme)
ceftriaxone	Rocephin (Roche)
cephapirin sodium	Cefadyl (Bristol)
cimetidine	Apo-Cimetidine (Apotex), Tagamet (Smith Kline & French)
cisplatin	Platinol (Bristol)
clindamycin	Dalacin C (Upjohn)
co-trimoxazole (sulfamethoxazole/ trimethoprim)	Apo-Sulfatrim (Apotex), Bactrim Roche (Roche)
cyclophosphamide	Cytoxan (Bristol), Procytox (Horner)
cyclosporine	Sandimmune (Sandoz)
cytarabine	Cytosar (Upjohn)
dacarbazine	DTIC (Miles)

(continued)

NONPROPRIETARY NAME	BRAND NAME (CANADIAN MANUFACTURER)
dactinomycin	Cosmegean (Merck Sharp & Dohme)
daunorubicin	Cerubidine (Rhone-Poulenc)
deferoxamine	Desferal (CIBA)
dextran	Hyskon (Pharmacia)
diazepam	Apo-Diazepam (Apotex)
diethylstilbestrol	Honvol (Horner)
digoxin	Lanoxin (Burroughs Wellcome)
diphenhydramine hcl	Allerdryl (ICN), Benadryl (Parke Davis)
dobutamine hcl	Dobutrex (Lilly)
dopamine hcl	Intropin (DuPont), Revimine (Rorer)
epinephrine hcl	Adrenalin (Parke Davis)
factor IX complex (human)	Coagulation Factor IX (Winnipeg Plasma)
furosemide	Lasix (Hoechst)
gentamicin sulfate	Cidomycin (Roussel), Garamycin (Schering)
heparin	Calciparine subcutaneous calcium (Anglo-French Laboratories), Hepalean (Organon), Heparin Leo (Leo)
insulin	Iletin Regular (Lilly), Insulin-Toronto (Connaught Novo)
lidocaine hcl	Xylocard (Astra)
lincomycin hcl monohydrate	Lincocin (Upjohn)
magnesium sulfate	Magnesium (Abbott; NovoPharm/LyphoMed)
mannitol	Osmitrol (Abbott)
methotrexate	methotrexate, amethopterin (Horner)
metoclopramide hcl	Emex (Beecham), Maxeran (Nordic)
metronidazole	Flagyl (Rhone-Poulenc), Neo-Metric (Neolab)
mitomycin	Mutamycin (Bristol)
morphine sulfate	Epimorph (Robins), Morphine H.P. (Sabex)
nafcillin sodium	Unipen (Wyeth)
penicillin G potassium	Ayercillin (Ayerst)
phenytoin	Dilantin (Parke Davis; NovoPharm/LyphoMed)

(continued)

NONPROPRIETARY NAME	BRAND NAME (CANADIAN MANUFACTURER)
piperacillin sodium	Pipracil (Lederle)
prochlorperazine	Stemetil (May & Baker)
Rho (D) immune globulin	Win Rho (Winnipeg Rh Institute)
terbutaline sulfate	Bricanyl (Astra)
tetracycline hcl	Achromycin (Lederle)
theophylline	Elixophyllin (Berlex Canada)
ticarcillin disodium	Ticar (Beecham)
vancomycin	Vancocin (Lilly)
vasopressin	Pitressin (Parke Davis)
verapamil hcl	Isoptin Parenteral (Knoll)
vidarabine	Vira-A (Parke Davis)
vinblastine sulfate	Velbe (Lilly)
vincristine sulfate	Oncovin (Lilly)
warfarin	Coumadin sodium (DuPont)

(Canadian Pharmaceutical Association. Compendium of pharmaceuticals and specialties. 24th ed. Ottawa, 1989)

SYSTEM OF INTERNATIONAL UNITS (SI)

The System of International Units (SI) is a fully international system of measurements useful to the nursing professional in calculations. It is the accepted international language for measurement in science, industry, and general use.

The basic unit is the measurement used in hospitals.

Meter: Unit of Length and Distance

kilometer	km	1000 m
meter	m	1 m
decimeter	dm	0.1 m
centimeter	cm	0.01 m
millimeter	mm	0.001 m
micrometer	μm	0.000001 m
nanometer	nm	0.000000001 m

Kilogram: Unit of Mass

kilogram	kg	1000 g
gram	g	
milligram	mg	0.001 g
microgram	μg	0.001 mg

Liter: Unit of Volume for Liquids and Gases

Pascal: Unit of Pressure

Joule: Unit of energy

1 diet calorie	4.2 kJ
1000 diet calories	4200 kJ

Mole: Unit of Substance

$$\text{Concentration in mM/L} = \frac{\text{Concentration in mg/100 ml} \times 10}{\text{molecular weight of substance}}$$

Degrees Celsius: Unit of Temperature

OTHER CALCULATIONS

Replacement of Present Losses

Fluid loss may be calculated by determining loss of body weight; 1 L body water equals 1 kg or 2.2 lb of body weight.

Maintenance Water

Maintenance water equals 1600 ml/m^2 of body surface area per day.

(Glenn J, McCaugherty D. SI units for nurses. Philadelphia: Lippincott Nursing Series, 1981; and Drug and Therapeutic Information Inc. Parenteral water and electrolyte solutions. Med Lett 1970;12[19]:77.)

Index

Official generic drug names are shown in boldface. *Trade names* are shown in italics, followed by the official generic name in parentheses. (CAN) after a trade name indicates the Canadian name.